Evidence-Based Approach to Urology

Evidence-Based Approach to Urology

Editor: Ezra Martin

AMERICAN
MEDICAL PUBLISHERS
www.americanmedicalpublishers.com

AMERICAN
MEDICAL PUBLISHERS
www.americanmedicalpublishers.com

Cataloging-in-Publication Data

Evidence-based approach to urology / edited by Ezra Martin.
p. cm.
Includes bibliographical references and index.
ISBN 979-8-88740-549-0
1. Urology. 2. Genitourinary organs--Diseases. 3. Urinary organs--Diseases.
4. Evidence-based medicine. I. Martin, Ezra.
RC871 .E85 2023
616.6--dc23

American Medical Publishers,
41 Flatbush Avenue,
1st Floor, New York,
NY 11217, USA

ISBN 979-8-88740-549-0 (Hardback)

Contents

Preface

Urology is a branch of medicine that focuses on medical conditions and diseases of the male and female urinary tract systems and reproductive organs. The different sub-specialties of urology include, but are not limited to female urology, andrology, neurourology, urologic oncology, reconstructive urology, and pediatric urology. Urology is involved in the medical and surgical treatment of various diseases and conditions such as bladder cancer, cystitis, vasectomy, kidney stone and erectile dysfunction. It also deals with prostate cancer and development of the urinary and reproductive organs. An evidence-based approach to urology offers practical recommendations for the care of patients. This book provides comprehensive insights into an evidence-based approach to urology. A number of latest researches have been included to keep the readers up-to-date with the global concepts in this area of study. The book aims to serve as a resource guide for students and experts alike and contribute to the growth of the discipline.

This book has been the outcome of endless efforts put in by authors and researchers on various issues and topics within the field. The book is a comprehensive collection of significant researches that are addressed in a variety of chapters. It will surely enhance the knowledge of the field among readers across the globe.

It gives us an immense pleasure to thank our researchers and authors for their efforts to submit their piece of writing before the deadlines. Finally in the end, I would like to thank my family and colleagues who have been a great source of inspiration and support.

Editor

1

Two-year outcomes of surgeon-tailored trans obturator tape for female stress urinary incontinence: A randomized, comparative, trial with traditional trans obturator tape

Salah E. Shebl*

Abstract

Background: Previously, we presented the short-term outcomes of surgeon-tailored mesh in patients with SUI undergoing TOT. In this report, we aim to highlight the two-year outcomes of surgeon tailored mesh in terms of subjective and objective cure rates, as well as late complications.

Methods: We performed a randomized, open-label comparative trial that recruited women with SUI who were scheduled to undergo TOT. Eligible patients were randomly allocated in a 1:1 ratio to receive traditional TOT mesh or surgeon-tailored polyethylene mesh. All patients were followed up for two years.

Results: At the end of the follow-up, there were 13 women in the traditional TOT mesh group and 14 patients in the surgeon-tailored polyethylene mesh group. Concerning the primary outcome of the present study, the cure rate was 100% in the surgeon-tailored polyethylene mesh (n = 14) and 92.9% in the traditional TOT mesh group ($p = 0.39$). One woman reported improved symptoms in the traditional TOT mesh group. There were no reported failures in both groups. Concerning safety, the incidence of de novo urgency was 0% in the surgeon-tailored polyethylene mesh group, compared to 7.1% in the traditional TOT mesh group ($p = 0.34$). None of the women in both groups reported mesh erosions, dyspareunia, or need for reoperation.

Conclusion: Surgeon-tailored mesh for patients undergoing TOT is a cost-effective technique, which has comparable long-term outcomes, in terms of cure rate and complications, to the traditional costly meshes. Larger multicentre studies should confirm our results.

Keywords: Stress urinary incontinence, Trans obturator tape, Long-term

Background

Stress urinary incontinence (SUI) is a prevalent disorder that is characterized by leakage of urine after physical stress [1]. Surgical procedures are widely performed for women with failed conservative management or women seeking definitive treatment [2]. Mid-urethral sling (MUS) is a highly effective, minimally-invasive, surgical approach for SUI that is based on the passing of a small band of a synthetic mesh into either the retropubic space (known as tension-free vaginal tape, TVT) or through the obturator foramen (known as trans-obturator tape, TOT or TVT-O, through the inside-out route) [3]. Previous reports showed that MUS achieves a cure rate of up to 94% [4], with a low risk of postoperative complications, such as visceral injuries and retention [5]. The current

*Correspondence: Salahshebl@yahoo.com; Salahshebl@azhar.edu.eg
Urology Department, Faculty of Medicine for Girls, Al-Azhar University, Cairo, Egypt

body of evidence demonstrated a well-established short- and long-term efficacy profile of MUS [6–8].

Nonetheless, TOT is a costly procedure, especially in developing countries, due to the need for prefabricated slings and specific needles or passers to reduce the risk of injuries to surrounding structures [9]. Thus, a number of surgeon-tailored meshes were proposed to reduce the cost of the procedure, with maintaining the postoperative and long-term outcomes [10]. Previously, we presented the short-term outcomes of surgeon-tailored mesh in patients with SUI undergoing TOT [11]. In this report, we aim to highlight the two-year outcomes of surgeon-tailored mesh in terms of subjective and objective cure rates, as well as late complications.

Materials and methods

The protocol of the current trial was approved by the local ethics committee of the Faculty of Medicine for Girls Al-Azhar University, Cairo, Egypt. All procedures run in compliance with the standards of the Declaration of Helsinki [12]. We prepared the following manuscript in concordance with CONSORT guidelines [13].

Study design and patients

We performed a randomized, open-label comparative trial that recruited women with SUI who were scheduled to undergo TOT at Al Zahraa University Hospital through the period from the end of December 2016 to the end of April 2021. Women were considered eligible if they fulfilled the following criteria: female patients aged more than 18 years old, patients with an established diagnosis of genuine SUI, and patients who did not exhibit a significant response to conservative management. We included women regardless of their parity status. On the other hand, we excluded patients with mixed incontinence, urge incontinence, acute infection, malignancies, overactive bladder, bleeding disorders, internal sphincteric deficiency, concomitant prolapse, post-void residual urine more than 150 cc, and/or bladder capacity less than 250 cc. Pregnant and lactating women were excluded as well.

Eligible patients were randomly allocated in a 1:1 ratio to receive traditional TOT mesh or surgeon-tailored polyethylene mesh by a computer software program (www.Randmizer.org), and allocation sequences were done by opaque closed envelopes.

Study's procedures and follow-up

All eligible women were subjected to standardized preoperative history taking and local gynecological examination. Patients underwent routine abdominopelvic ultrasonography (US) and cystometry by Andromeda Urodynamic apparatus.

The full surgical procedure was described previously [11]. After placing the patients in the lithotomy position, the surgeon introduced a 16 French catheter into the bladder and inflated the balloon. Then, the vaginal wall was incised in the midline for a one-cm distance, approximately one cm from the urethral meatus. This was followed by the incision of mucosa and submucosa, and dissection of periurethral fascia bilaterally towards the inferior pubic ramus. A skin incision was then performed medial to the genito-femoral fold at the base of the adductor longus tendon, approximately at the level of the clitoris. A needle with fixed tape was introduced from the obturator to the vaginal incisions. Patients in the surgeon-tailored polyethylene mesh group received 30×1 cm polypropylene strips, which were prepared by splitting the 30×30 prolene mesh and re-sterilized by plasma machine. All patients were asked to cough to assess continence after the bladder was filled with 250 ml saline. The skin and vaginal incisions were closed by 3-0 vicryl in sub-cuticular and interrupted fashions, respectively. All patients were followed up for two years.

Study's outcomes

The primary outcome of the present study was the two-year objective success rate. The objective success year was categorized into the following three categories: cure, which donates that the women have no stress-induced urine leak on cough test and that the women exhibited satisfactory control of their urine; improved, which donates that the women had urine leak on severe exertion only and they express subjective improvement in their symptoms; and failure, which donates that the women still exhibit the same level of preoperative urine leak on cough test and they are not satisfied with their condition. The secondary outcomes of this study included the incidence of late postoperative complications, such as reoperation, mesh erosion, de novo urgency, and dyspareunia.

Statistical analysis

Retrieved data were summarized and processed with IBM SPSS statistical software (version 25). Frequencies were used to describe gynecological history, Ultrasound findings, postoperative complications, and success rates. On the other hand, age, ALPP, duration surgery, and hospital stay were summarized, according to normality, into mean ($\pm$standard deviation [SD]) or median (range). The hypothesize of significant differences between the type of mesh and primary or secondary outcomes was challenged using the independent t-test or Chi-square test for continuous and categorical data, respectively. P value < 0.05 was regarded as statistically significant.

Results

Initially a total of 63 women were screened for eligibility; of them, 35 women were deemed eligible and 30 of them agreed to sign the informed consent. The 30 women were randomly allocated to the traditional TOT mesh (n = 15 women) or surgeon-tailored polyethylene mesh (n = 15 women). At the end of follow-up, there were 13 women in the traditional TOT mesh group and 14 patients in the surgeon-tailored polyethylene mesh group (Fig. 1).

The mean age between the traditional TOT mesh and the surgeon-tailored polyethylene mesh groups was comparable (46.79 ± 7.567 vs. 40.67 ± 7.93 years old; $p = 0.85$). There were no significant differences between both groups in terms of parity ($p = 0.36$), number of previous vaginal deliveries ($p = 0.13$), number of previous Cesarean section ($p = 0.18$), use of pad ($p = 0.63$), and residual urine by US ($p = 0.39$). The mean operative time was slightly lower in the surgeon-tailored mesh group (15.67 ± 2.06 vs. 20.86 ± 3.35 min in the traditional TOT mesh group), without statistically significant difference ($p = 0.075$). Likewise, the mean ALPP was comparable between both groups (25.72 ± 6.87 vs. 33.72 ± 9.73,

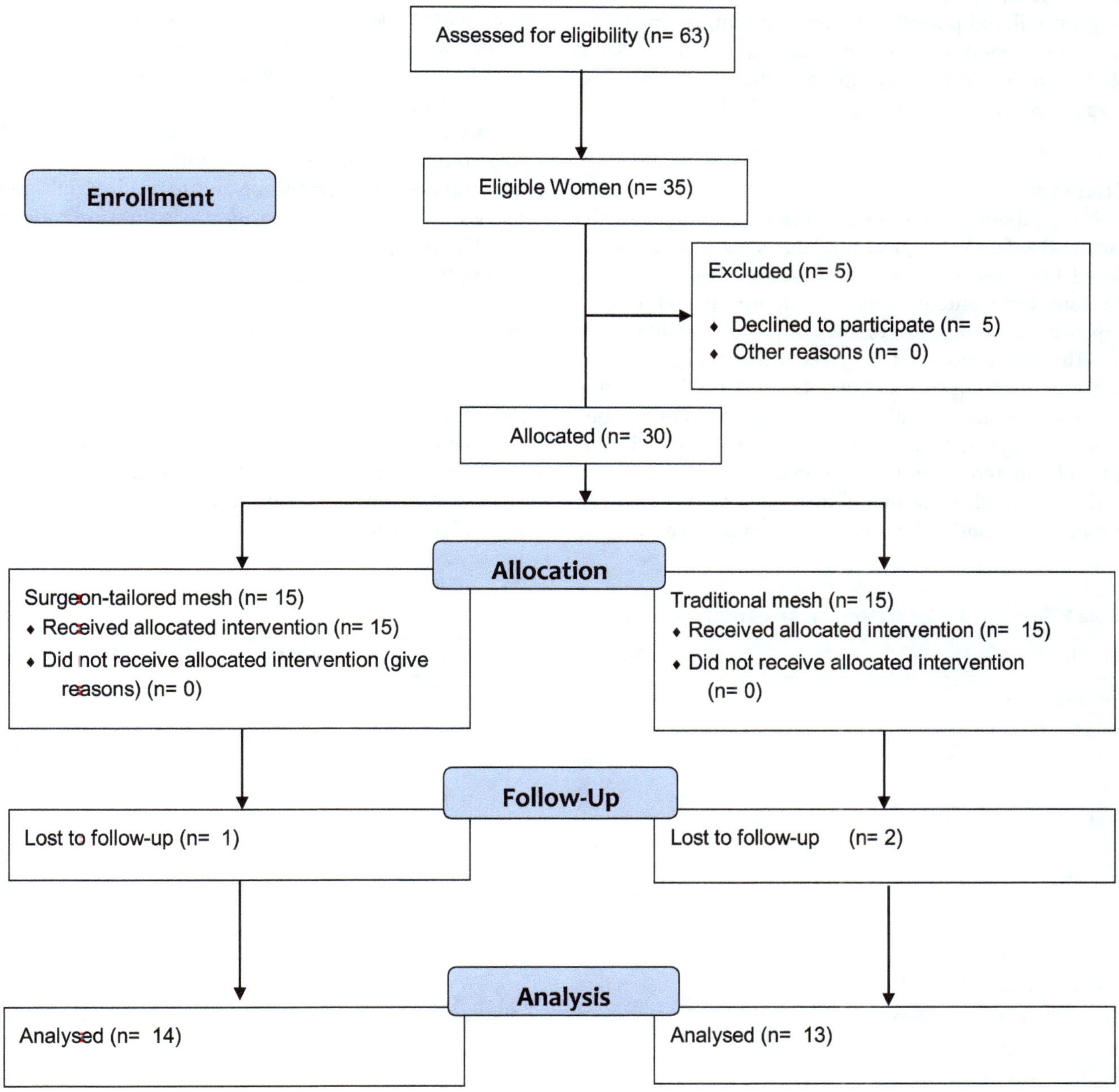

Fig. 1 Checklist of the study

respectively; $p=0.51$). The incidence of intraoperative vaginal wall injury was 0% in the surgeon-tailored polyethylene mesh group, compared to 7.7% in the traditional TOT mesh group ($p=0.34$). The incidence of UTI or vaginal infection (23.1% versus 0% in the traditional TOT mesh and the surgeon-tailored polyethylene mesh groups, respectively), with $p=0.088$ (Table 1).

Concerning the primary outcome of the present study, the cure rate was 100% in the surgeon-tailored polyethylene mesh (n = 14) and 92.3% in the traditional TOT mesh group ($p=0.39$). One woman reported improved symptoms in the traditional TOT mesh group. There were no reported failures in both groups (Fig. 2). With regard to safety, the incidence of de novo urgency was 0% in the surgeon-tailored polyethylene mesh group, compared to 7.7% in the traditional TOT mesh group ($p=0.34$). None of the women in both groups reported mesh erosions, dyspareunia, or need for reoperation (Table 2).

Discussion

Although there is a plethora of evidence about the efficacy and safety of surgical modalities for SUI, the published literature still lacks high-quality evidence about the long-term outcomes of new approaches aiming to improve the financial outcomes of these modalities [14, 15]. Thus, we conducted the present trial to highlight the two-year outcomes of surgeon tailored mesh in terms of subjective and objective cure rates and late complications. Our results showed the lack of statistically significant difference between surgeon-tailored mesh and traditional mesh in terms of cure rate (100% vs. 85.7%, respectively). Both techniques had comparable de novo urgency, mesh erosion, and dyspareunia rates at the end of the second year of follow-up.

TOT is a widely utilized, minimally-invasive technique that has proven its usefulness in patients with SUI; the technique is associated with optimal cure rates and diminished risks of major postoperative complications, such as injuries to surrounding structures and retention [3, 5]. Previous reports showed that the TOT exhibited acceptable levels of cure rate and safety profile on long-term follow-up among women with SUI [8, 16]. TOT was proven to be associated with lower direct cost than laparoscopic Burch colposuspension [17]. However, it is well-recognized that the TOT procedure is associated with a considerable financial burden on the patients and healthcare systems due to the high cost of its equipment, including meshes and passengers. Mesh erosion can put a further cost burden on the patients [18]. Thus, the need for alternative, less costly alternatives were deemed critical, particularly in developing countries [19]. Previous reports showed that the use of tailored polypropylene mesh resulted in satisfactory results and a less costly procedure for patients with SUI. Our previous report confirmed such findings showing that the surgeon-tailored mesh was associated with a high cure rate similar to traditional mesh [11]. Nonetheless, the current body of evidence shows scarcity of the long-term outcomes of this modified cheap approach. The present report found that the surgeon-tailored was associated with high cure rates at the end of the second year of follow-up, which donates its satisfactory long-term outcomes. In concordance with our findings, ElSheemy et al. [9], showed that the use of tailored polypropylene mesh in women undergoing TVT

Table 1 Perioperative Characteristics of the Follow-up Cohort (n = 27)

Variables	Traditional mesh (n = 13)	Surgeon-tailored mesh (n = 14)	*P* value
Age in years, mean ± SD	46.79 ± 7.567	40.67 ± 7.93	0.85
Parity, no. (%)			
P2	2 (15.4%)	5 (28.6%)	0.36
P3	7 (53.8%)	4 (28.4%)	
P4	2 (15.4%)	0	
> P4	2 (15.4%)	5 (28.6%)	
MOD, no. (%)			0.13
NVD	7 (53.8%)	5 (28.6%)	
CS	6 (46.2%)	9 (71.4%)	
Use of pad, no. (%)	2 (15.4%)	1 (7.1%)	0.63
Residual urine by US, no. (%)	2 (15.4%)	0	0.39
Operative time in minutes, mean ± SD	15.67 ± 2.06	20.86 ± 3.35	0.075
Intraoperative vaginal wall injury, No. (%)	1 (7.7%)	0	0.34
ALPP, mean ± SD	25.72 ± 6.87	33.72 ± 9.73	0.51
UTI or vaginal infection, No. (%)	3 (23.1%)	0	0.088

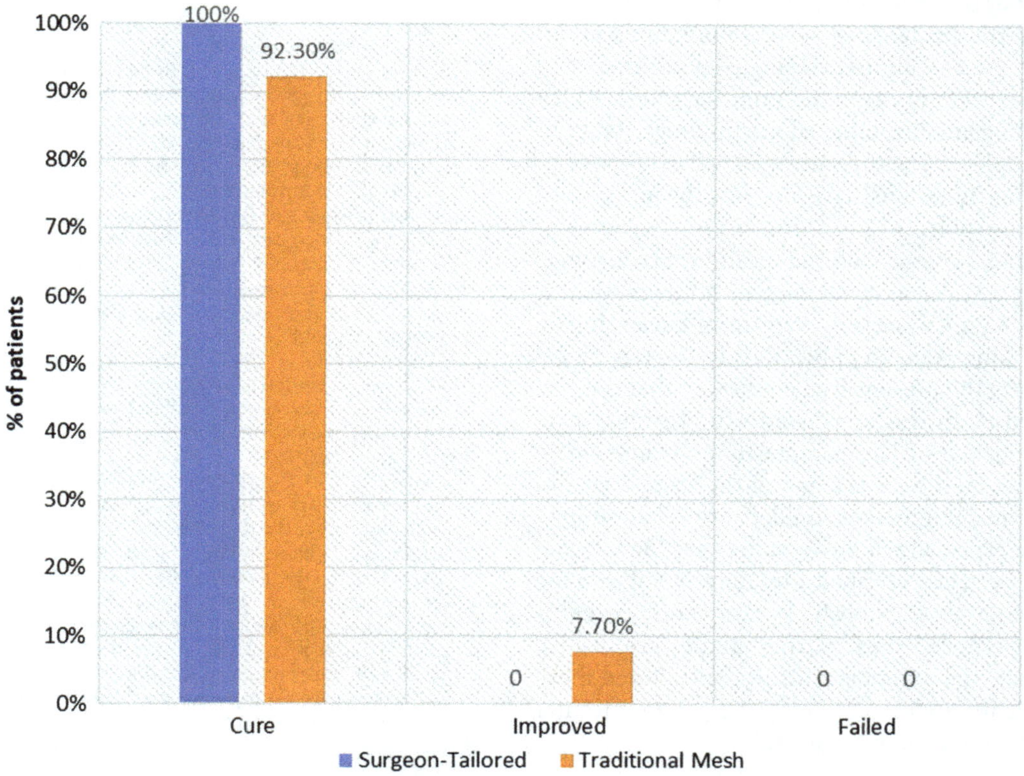

Fig. 2 Outcome of the procedure

Table 2 Safety outcomes of the follow-up cohort (n = 27)

Variables	Traditional mesh (n = 13)	Surgeon-tailored mesh (n = 14)	*P* value
De novo urgency, no. (%)	1 (7.7%)	0	0.34
Mesh erosions, no. (%)	0	0	–
Dyspareunia, no. (%)	0	0	–
Need for reoperation, no. (%)	0	0	–

was associated with a cure rate of 91%. Another long-term comparative study by the same group showed that the tailored polypropylene mesh was associated with a comparable cure rate to the traditional mesh in women undergoing TVT [10]. In a Chinese report, Chen et al. [18], reported that the tailored polypropylene mesh led to a cure rate of 96% at the end of the first year of follow-up. Our findings are in line with short and medium-term results reported by Imamura et al. [15], in which the TOT achieved higher cure rates than other procedures.

The surgical management of SUI can be associated with a high rate of treatment failure and reoperation. It was previously noted that up to 4% of patients undergoing surgery need reoperation due to recurrent SUI. Nonetheless, the rate of reoperation is not consistent across various surgical approaches for SUI [20]. TOT is thought to increase the risk of reoperation due to synthetic mesh, which may be exposed in the long term and need removal. The synthetic mesh may also lead to chronic pain and voiding dysfunction requiring reoperation [3]. Several risk factors were implicated in the need for reoperation among women undergoing TOT, such as obesity, diabetes, revision surgery, and mixed UI [21]. More recently, Illiano et al. [22], noted that technical errors play a significant role in TOT failure and reoperation, which can be reduced by translabial ultrasound. However, it should be noted that long-term studies demonstrated a low rate of TOT failure and need for reoperation, with a follow-up period of nearly 13 years [23]. Other systematic reviews demonstrated similar findings [8, 16]. In the present study, we demonstrated that the use of surgeon-tailored mesh was associated with a similar risk of failure and reoperation compared to traditional mesh. Our findings are similar to the reports by ElSheemy et al. [9, 10] and Chen et al. [18].

To our knowledge, only a few reports have attempted to explore the outcomes of surgeon-tailored mesh for SUI patients undergoing TOT; nonetheless, we acknowledge the existence of several limitations in our trial. Our study was limited to single-center only, and all procedures were done by the same surgeons, which can affect the generalizability of our findings. In addition, the sample size was relatively small. The postoperative voiding functions have not also been assessed using validated tools.

In conclusion, surgeon-tailored mesh for SUI patients undergoing TOT is a cost-effective strategy that is associated with a comparable long-term cure rate and incidence of long-term complications to the traditional costly meshes. The present trial confirmed that the surgeon-tailored mesh was associated with a similar cure rate and incidence of late complications compared to the traditional meshes at the end of the second year of follow-up. Thus, surgeons should consider these low-cost meshes, especially in low-resource settings. Nonetheless, the current published literature is still limited by the low number of published cases and low quality of published reports; thus, further studies are needed to characterize the outcomes of surgeon-tailored mesh for SUI patients undergoing TOT. Larger multicenter studies should confirm our results.

Abbreviations

TOT: Trans obturator tape; SUI: Stress urinary incontinence; MUS: Mid-urethral sling; PVS: Pubo-vaginal sling; TVT: Tension-free vaginal tape; ALPP: Abdominal leak point pressure; US: Ultrasonography.

Acknowledgements

The author thanks Dr. Sayeda E, Aly and Dr. Ahmed A. El Gammal (urology department faculty of medicine for girls Al-Azhar University) for their participation in short-term outcomes of surgeon tailored mesh in patients with SUI undergoing TOT.

Authors' contributions

SES was responsible for data collection, study design, and final revision and proofreading of the final draft, data analysis, presentation, the writing process, and agreed that the final version of the manuscript was ready for publication. The author read and approved the final manuscript.

Competing interests

The authors declare that they have no conflict of interest.

References

1. Komesu YM, Schrader RM, Ketai LH, Rogers RG, Dunivan GC. Epidemiology of mixed, stress, and urgency urinary incontinence in middle-aged/older women: the importance of incontinence history. Int Urogynecol J. 2016;27(5):763–72.
2. Pandey D, Maturi C, Dhakar BPS, Jain G, Kyalakond K. Interventions and quality of life in stress urinary incontinence. Gynecol Minim Invasive Ther. 2019;8(3):106–12.
3. Karim NB, Lo TS, Nawawi EA, Wu PY. Review on midurethral sling procedures for stress urinary incontinence. Gynecol Minim Invasive Ther. 2015;4:33–6.
4. Ford AA, Rogerson L, Cody JD, Aluko P, Ogah JA. Mid-urethral sling operations for stress urinary incontinence in women. Cochrane Database Syst Rev. 2017;7(7):CD006375.
5. Ogah J, Cody JD, Rogerson L. Minimally invasive synthetic suburethral sling operations for stress urinary incontinence in women. Cochrane database Syst Rev. 2009;4:CD006375.
6. Jain P, Jirschele K, Botros SM, Latthe PM. Effectiveness of midurethral slings in mixed urinary incontinence: a systematic review and meta-analysis. Int Urogynecol J. 2011;22:923–32.
7. Jiao B, Lai S, Xu X, Zhang M, Diao T, Zhang G. A systematic review and meta-analysis of single-incision mini-slings (MiniArc) versus transobturator mid-urethral slings in surgical management of female stress urinary incontinence. Medicine. 2018;97:e0283.
8. Leone Roberti Maggiore U, Finazzi Agrò E, Soligo M, Li Marzi V, Digesu A, Serati M. Long-term outcomes of TOT and TVT procedures for the treatment of female stress urinary incontinence: a systematic review and meta-analysis. Int Urogynecol J. 2017;28:1119–30.
9. ElSheemy MS, Elsergany R, ElShenoufy A. Low-cost transobturator vaginal tape inside-out procedure for the treatment of female stress urinary incontinence using ordinary polypropylene mesh. Int Urogynecol J Pelvic Floor Dysfunct. 2015;26(4):577–84.
10. ElSheemy MS, Fathy H, Hussein HA, Elsergany R, Hussein EA. Surgeon-tailored polypropylene mesh as a tension-free vaginal tape-obturator versus original TVT-O for the treatment of female stress urinary incontinence: a long-term comparative study. Int Urogynecol J. 2015;26(10):1533–40. https://doi.org/10.1007/s00192-015-2725-6.
11. Sayeda E, Ahmed A, Shebl M, Salah E. Assessment of correction of female stress urinary incontinence with trans obturator tape; traditional versus tailored. Med J Cairo Univ. 2021;89(6):845–50.
12. JAVA. Declaration of Helsinki world medical association declaration of Helsinki. Bull World Health Organ. 2013;79(4):373–4.
13. Moher D, Hopewell S, Schulz KF, Montori V, Gøtzsche PC, Devereaux PJ, et al. CONSORT 2010 explanation and elaboration: updated guidelines for reporting parallel group randomised trials. Int J Surg. 2012;10:28–55.
14. Wu Y, Welk B. Revisiting current treatment options for stress urinary incontinence and pelvic organ prolapse: a contemporary literature review. Res Rep Urol. 2019;11:179–88.
15. Imamura M, Hudson J, Wallace SA, Maclennan G, Shimonovich M, Omar MI, et al. Surgical interventions for women with stress urinary incontinence: Systematic review and network meta-analysis of randomised controlled trials. BMJ. 2019;365:l1842.
16. Tommaselli GA, Di Carlo C, Formisano C, Fabozzi A, Nappi C. Medium-term and long-term outcomes following placement of midurethral slings for stress urinary incontinence: a systematic review and metaanalysis. Int Urogynecol J Pelvic Floor Dysfunct. 2015;26:1253–68.
17. Lo K, Marcoux V, Grossman S, Kung R, Lee P. Cost comparison of the laparoscopic burch colposuspension, laparoscopic two-team sling procedure, and the transobturator tape procedure for the treatment of stress urinary incontinence. J Obstet Gynaecol Can. 2013;35(3):252–7.
18. Chen X, Jiang M, Tong X, Li H, Qiu J, Shao L, et al. A modified inexpensive transobturator vaginal tape inside-out procedure versus tension-free vaginal tape for the treatment of SUI: a prospective comparative study. Arch Gynecol Obstet. 2011;284(6):1461–6. https://doi.org/10.1007/s00404-011-1871-4.
19. Chen X, Li H, Fan B, Yang X, Tong X. An inexpensive modified transobturator vaginal tape inside-out procedure for the surgical treatment of female stress urinary incontinence. Int Urogynecol J Pelvic Floor Dysfunct. 2009;20(11):1365–8. https://doi.org/10.1007/s00192-009-0961-3.
20. Wu M-P, Long C-Y, Liang C-C, Weng S-F, Tong Y-C. Trends in reoperation for female stress urinary incontinence: a nationwide study. Neurourol Urodyn. 2015;34(7):693–8.
21. Stav K, Dwyer PL, Rosamilia A, Schierlitz L, Lim YN, Lee J. Risk factors of treatment failure of midurethral sling procedures for women with urinary stress incontinence. Int Urogynecol J. 2010;21(2):149–55.
22. Illiano E, Trama F, Li Marzi V, Mancini V, Carrieri G, Ruvolo CC, et al. Translabial ultrasound: a non-invasive technique for assessing "technical errors" after TOT failure. Int Urogynecol J. 2021. https://doi.org/10.1007/s00192-021-04897-6.
23. Tulokas S, Rahkola-Soisalo P, Gissler M, Mikkola TS, Mentula MJ. Long-term re-procedure rate after mid-urethral slings for stress urinary incontinence. Int Urogynecol J. 2020;31(4):727–35.

2

Complete remission of Cdx-2 positive primary testicular carcinoid tumor: 10-years follow-up and literature review

Eugen Widmeier[1], Hannah Füllgraf[2] and Cornelius F. Waller[3*]

Abstract

Background: The neuroendocrine cells can cause a variety of malignancies throughout the human body known as the neuroendocrine tumors (NETs) or carcinoid tumors. The primary testicular carcinoid tumor (PTCT) accounts for less than 1% of the testicular neoplasms and for only 0.2% of all carcinoid tumors representing already a very rare neoplastic entity. Here, we present a patient with a history of an exceptionally rare primary testicular carcinoid tumor, staining positive for Cdx-2 along with a literature review.

Case presentation: A 44-year old patient without significant past medical history was diagnosed in September 2009 with primary testicular carcinoid tumor, which was surprisingly staining positively for Cdx-2, too. At the time of the initial diagnosis the tumor was already showing histopathological infiltration of veins. DOTA-TATE-PET/CT imaging and endoscopy studies did not show any signs of distant metastases and in particular no gastrointestinal manifestation following no further medical indication for systemic chemotherapy. The continuous and close follow-up of the patient has reached a total of over 10 years at the time of publication remaining in complete remission.

Conclusion: The diagnosis of primary testicular carcinoid is based on histopathology. The detailed histopathologic assessment of biomarkers based on immunohistochemistry is very important for the classification and the prognosis of the primary testicular carcinoid tumor. Primary testicular carcinoid tumor with Cdx-2 positive stain outlines an exceptionally rare neoplastic entity without a consensus about general follow-up guidelines, requiring close clinical and imaging aftercare and consideration in Cdx-2 positive metastatic tumor of unknown origin.

Keywords: Neuroendocrine tumor, Primary testicular carcinoid tumor, Histopathology, Biomarkers, Cdx-2 positivity, Metastatic tumor of unknown origin, Case report

Background

The neuroendocrine cells can cause a variety of malignancies throughout the human body known as the neuroendocrine tumors (NETs). These types of tumors, likewise called carcinoid tumors, are able to produce hormone-like molecules, which can mimic characteristic hormonal syndromes [1]. Carcinoid tumors occur predominantly in the gastrointestinal tract (67.5%) and in the bronchopulmonary system (25.3%) [2]. The primary testicular carcinoid tumor (PTCT) accounts for less than 1% of the testicular neoplasms [3] and for only 0.2% of all carcinoid tumors representing a very rare neoplastic entity [4, 5]. The distinction of the origin in primary or metastatic circumstance is of the outmost importance for the prognosis of the testicular carcinoid tumor and the treatment [6]. Here, we present a case history of a primary testicular carcinoid tumor with exceptionally rare Cdx-2 positive stain and complete remission along

*Correspondence: cornelius.waller@uniklinik-freiburg.de
[3] Department of Medicine I, Medical Center – University of Freiburg, Faculty of Medicine, University of Freiburg, Hugstetter Strasse 55, 79106 Freiburg, Germany
Full list of author information is available at the end of the article

with 10 years recurrence-free follow-up and a literature review.

Case presentation

We report a 44-year old patient, who saw his urologist in September 2009 due to a painless and for approximately 6 month continuously growing left testicular swelling. The patient did not report any further clinical signs or symptoms of general disease especially no history of sudden hot flushes. The past medical history reveals solely strumectomy due to Grave's disease and atopic diathesis. On clinical exam no additional noticeable problems aside the one-sided testicular mass, especially no inguinal lymphadenopathy, were detected. The complete blood count and metabolic panel studies were all in normal range. Due to suspected testicular malignancy on clinical exam the patient underwent a near-time radical inguinal left-sided orchiectomy. The histological analysis of the testicular tissue revealed the diagnosis of a primary testicular carcinoid tumor, which was positive for chromogranin A, CD56, Ep4 and Cdx-2. The nuclear MIB-1 expression was detected in patches of the tumor cells

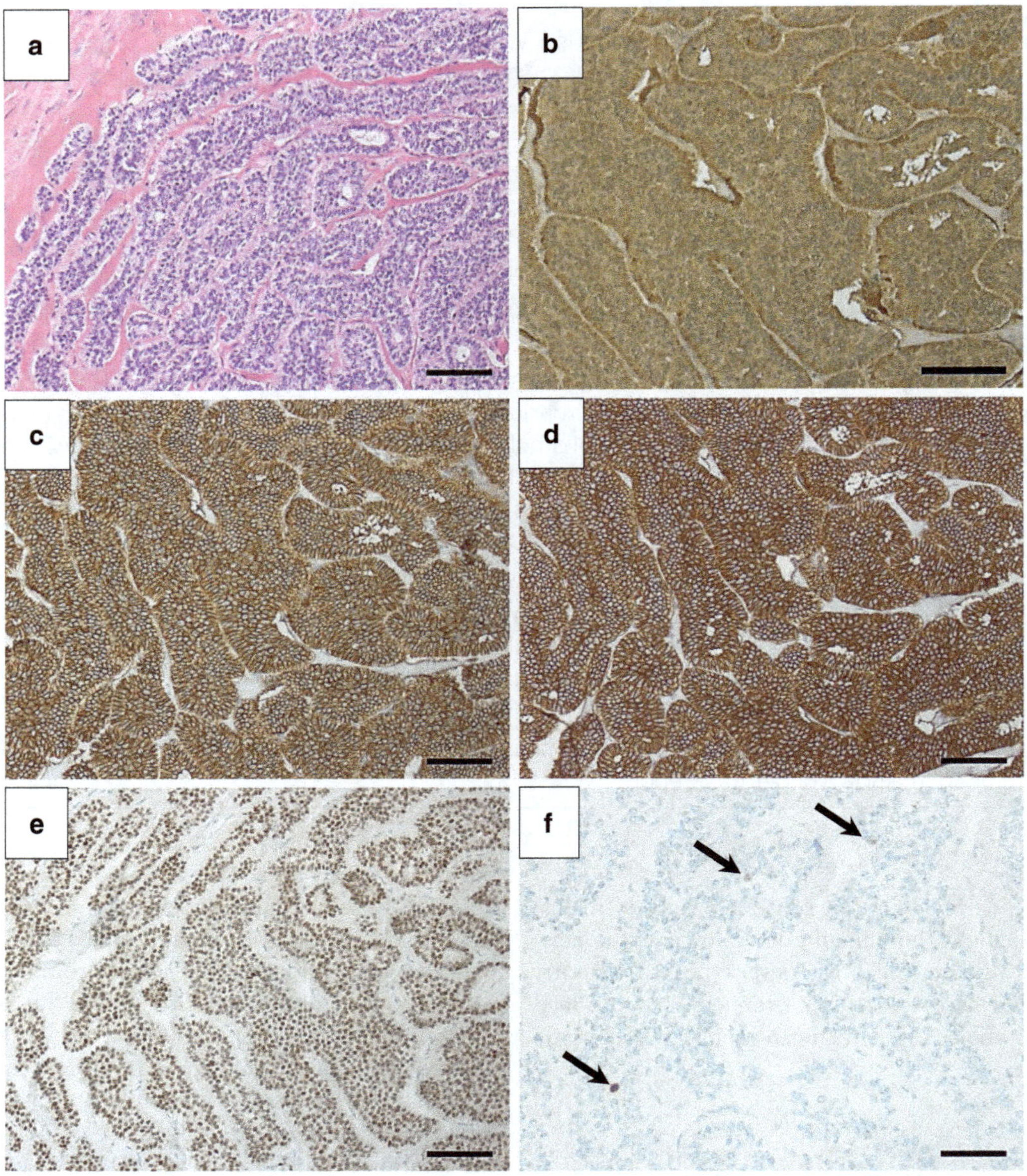

Fig. 1 Histological and immunohistochemical analysis of primary testicular carcinoid tumor tissue. Histological analysis (H&E staining) shows nested cuboidal cells with prominent round nuclei and reduced amount of cytoplasm, arranged in a ribbon-like structure and surrounded by moderate fibrotic stroma (**a**), with a positive immunohistochemical staining for Chromogranin A (**b**), CD 56 (**c**), Ep-4 (**d**), Cdx-2 (**e**) and Mib-1(**f**) pointed out by arrows. Scale bars 100 μm

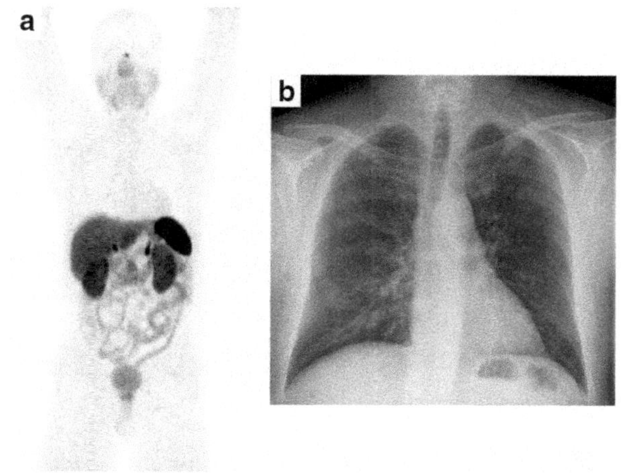

Fig. 2 Imaging studies in the context of aftercare. Imaging studies show no signs of primary testicular carcinoid tumor recurrence 3 years DOTA-TATE-PET/CT (**a**) and 10 years Chest X-ray (**b**) after initial diagnosis

with an MIB-1 index of approximately 2% (Fig. 1). At the time of the initial diagnosis the tumor was already showing histopathological infiltration of veins (cN0, cM0, R0 and V1). However the 24-h urine study showed a normal level of 5-Hydroxyindolacetic acid. Based on these findings the patient subsequently underwent DOTA-TATE-PET/CT imaging and endoscopy studies showing no signs of distant metastases and in particular no gastrointestinal manifestation following no further medical indication for systemic chemotherapy. Furthermore the patient was undergoing continuous clinical, abdominal sonography and imaging postsurgical care (Fig. 2). The follow-up of the patient has reached a total of over 10 years at the time of publication remaining in complete remission

Discussion

Historically, the nomenclature of "carcinoid" was describing the tumor entity of neuroendocrine cells with low malignancy in the gastrointestinal tract (GI) [7]. However the histopathogenesis of the primary testicular carcinoid remains under debate suggesting respective hypothesis: originating from the same precursor cell as the Leydig cells do or resulting from chromosomal irregularity [8, 9]. The diagnosis of primary testicular carcinoid is based on histopathology. The detailed histopathologic assessment is very important for the classification and the prognosis of the primary testicular carcinoid tumor [3]. Mitotic activity and vascular or tunica albuginea invasion were found not to increase the malignancy of the carcinoid tumors. However the occurrence of a low-degree of tumor differentiation, symptoms of a carcinoid syndrome as well as a tumor size correlate with increased metastatic potential [10, 11]. A precise detection of biomarkers assessed by immunohistochemistry (IHC) enables the subtyping and accurate classification of PTCT [12]. In general it is considered and it was described by Abbosh et al. that caudal type homeobox 2 (Cdx-2), a marker for neuroendocrine tumor cells originating from GI tract, is negative in PTCT [9, 13]. Lee et al. and Bing et al. described malignant germ cell tumors of the testes stained positive for Cdx-2 suggesting precaution in making a diagnosis in metastatic tumor with unknown origin and thereby considering an occult testicular malignancy rather than of GI origin [14, 15]. Albeit Atalay et al. demonstrated a strong significant Cdx-2 staining, as it is observed in tumor cells with GI origin, merely in testicular teratoma [16]. To the best of our knowledge, there is in the literature only one reported case of Cdx-2 positve PTCT [17]. In our case, the exceptionally rare Cdx-2 stain positivity was found as well, albeit no GI origin of carcinoid tumor cells was detected. This data suggests that the analytic specificity of Cdx-2 marker needs to be assessed critically and distinct in each case. The standard treatment of PTCT remains the radical inguinal orchiectomy [6]. The recurrence of PTCT may occur up to 17 years after the initial diagnosis and treatment requiring close clinical and imaging aftercare [18]. Since the data is based on single cases there is no consensus about general follow-up guidelines [6, 19]. In summary PTCT has a good prognosis with the 5-year overall survival rate of 78.7% and the 5-year specific survival rate of 84.3% and should be alternatively considered in Cdx-2 positive metastatic tumor of unknown origin [19].

Conclusion

Primary testicular carcinoid tumor with Cdx-2 positive stain outlines an exceptionally rare neoplastic entity. The standard treatment of PTCT remains the radical inguinal orchiectomy. PTCT have a good prognosis albeit some prognostic factors increase metastatic potential. The recurrence can appear almost 2 decades after initial diagnosis requiring close clinical and imaging aftercare.

Abbreviations

CD56: Cluster of differentiation 56; Cdx-2: Caudal type homeobox 2; DOTA-TATE-PET/CT: Tetraazacyclododecanetetraacetic acid–DPhe1-Tyr3-octreotate positron emission tomography/computed tomography; Ep4: Prostaglandin E receptor 4; GI: Gastrointestinal tract; IHC: Immunohistochemistry; MIB-1: Marker of proliferation Ki-67; NET: Neuroendocrine tumor; PTCT: Primary testicular carcinoid tumor.

Acknowledgements
We are grateful to the patient for his contribution.

Authors' contributions
E.W. and C.F.W. were involved in patient's medical care. A.F performed and analyzed pathological studies. E.W. and C.F.W. gathered detailed clinical information and analyzed data. E.W. and C.F.W. wrote the paper. E.W. and C.F.W. Conceived of and directed the project. The manuscript was critically reviewed by all authors. All authors read and approved the final manuscript.

Competing interests
The authors declare that they have no competing interests.

Author details
[1] Department of Medicine IV, Medical Center – University of Freiburg, Faculty of Medicine, University of Freiburg, Freiburg, Germany. [2] Institute of Surgical Pathology, Faculty of Medicine, University of Freiburg, Freiburg, Germany.
[3] Department of Medicine I, Medical Center – University of Freiburg, Faculty of Medicine, University of Freiburg, Hugstetter Strasse 55, 79106 Freiburg, Germany.

References
1. Yao JC, et al. One hundred years after "carcinoid": epidemiology of and prognostic factors for neuroendocrine tumors in 35,825 cases in the United States. J ClinOncol. 2008;26:3063–72.
2. Modlin IM, Lye KD, Kidd M. A 5-decade analysis of 13,715 carcinoid tumors. Cancer. 2003;97:934–59.
3. Wang WP, et al. Primary carcinoid tumors of the testis: a clinicopathologic study of 29 cases. Am J SurgPathol. 2010;34:519–24.
4. Kato N, et al. Primary carcinoid tumor of the testis: Immunohistochemical, ultrastructural and FISH analysis with review of the literature. Pathollnt. 2003;53:680–5.
5. Berdjis CC, Mostofi FK. Carcinoid tumors of the testis. J Urol. 1977;118:777–82.
6. Stroosma OB, Delaere KP. Carcinoid tumours of the testis. BJU Int. 2008;101:1101–5.
7. D'Arrigo L, et al. Primary carcinoid tumour of the testis: a case-report. Arch ItalUrolAndrol. 2014;86:231–2.
8. Mai KT, Park PC, Yazdi HM, Carlier M. Leydig cell origin of testicular carcinoid tumour: immunohistochemical and electron microscopic evidence. Histopathology. 2006;49:548–9.
9. Abbosh PH, et al. Germ cell origin of testicular carcinoid tumors. Clin Cancer Res. 2008;14:1393–6.
10 Zavala-Pompa A, et al. Primary carcinoid tumor of testis: immunohistochemical, ultrastructural, and DNA flow cytometric study of three cases with a review of the literature. Cancer. 1993;72:1726–32.
11. Penke M. Primary neuroendocrine tumor of the testis and osseous, cardiac, and lymph node metastases in a young patient. Case Rep Oncol. 2014;7:815–8.
12. Duan K, Mete O. Algorithmic approach to neuroendocrine tumors in targeted biopsies: practical applications of immunohistochemical markers. Cancer Cytopathol. 2016;124:871–84.
13. Lin F, Liu H. Immunohistochemistry in undifferentiated neoplasm/tumor of uncertain origin. Arch Pathol Lab Med. 2014;138:1583–610.
14. Lee MJ, Vogt AP, Hsiao W, Osunkoya AO. CDX-2 expression in malignant germ cell tumors of the testes, intratubular germ cell neoplasia, and normal seminiferous tubules. Tumour Biol. 2012;33:2185–8.
15. Bing Z, Pasha T, Tomaszewski JE, Zhang P. CDX2 expression in yolk sac component of testicular germ cell tumors. Int J SurgPathol. 2009;17:373–7.
16 Oz Atalay F, AytacVuruskan B, Vuruskan H. CDX2 immunostaining in primary and metastatic germ cell tumours of the testis. J Int Med Res. 2016;44:1323–30.
17. AbouZahr R, et al. Primary carcinoid tumor of the testis: a case report and review of the literature. Case Rep Urol. 2018;2018:3614387.
18. Hayashi T, et al. Primary carcinoid of the testis associated with carcinoid syndrome. Int J Urol. 2001;8:522–4.
19. Amine MM, et al. Neuroendocrine testicular tumors: a systematic review and meta-analysis. CurrUrol. 2017;10:15–25.

3

Prevalence and associated factors of urinary incontinence in women living in China

Kaikai Xue[1,2], Mary H. Palmer[3] and Fang Zhou[1*]

Abstract

Background: This review of studies on urinary incontinence (UI) was focused primarily on UI prevalence rates and associated factors across the adult lifecourse of Chinese women. UI is a urologic symptom that can have a significant impact on women's physical and mental health and quality of life. In addition, women with UI may experience socioeconomic burdens due to UI's effect on their ability to work and function in society. Although researchers from many countries have reported prevalence rates and associated factors for UI, little is known about the prevalence of UI in China's large female population. Language may act as a barrier to the inclusion of published studies in English-language journals. To overcome this barrier and to add to the global knowledge base about UI in women, the authors reviewed and discussed findings from epidemiological studies published in China and in Chinese language.

Methods: The authors retrieved research studies from the Wanfang database using the following search terms: "Subject: (Female) × Subject: (Urinary incontinence) × Subject: (Prevalence) × Date: 2013 to 2019". Searches employed the China National Knowledge Infrastructure Database, VIP Database for Chinese Technical Periodicals and China Biology Medicine Database. The authors also used PubMed to search English-language studies published in Chinese journals on UI in Chinese women.

Results: This literature review includes 48 articles published between January 2013 and December 2019. The overall UI prevalence rates reported in adult Chinese women ranged from 8.7 to 69.8%, representing 43–349 million women, respectively. For women aged 17–40 years, 41–59 years, and 60 years and older, prevalence rates ranged from 2.6–30.0, 8.7–47.7, to 16.9–61.6%, respectively. Significant associated factors for overall UI included age, body mass index, constipation, parity, and menopause. Despite the 17–40 age range being peak reproductive years, the literature revealed little focus on UI prevalence rates. For women aged 41–59 years, the main associated factors included those related to pregnancy and gynecologic diseases. For women 60 years and older, chronic diseases represented most of the associated factors.

Conclusions: About 43–349 million Chinese women may experience UI. Many of the identified associated factors could be mitigated to reduce UI incidence and prevalence rates. Little is known about the prevalence rates and associated factors for UI among young (aged 17–40) Chinese women. Future research should investigate UI in young women to improve bladder health across their lifecourse.

Keywords: Women, Urinary incontinence, Bladder, Prevalence, China

Background

Urinary incontinence (UI), which is defined as the complaint of the involuntary loss of urine [1], is one of the most frequently reported lower urinary tract symptoms

*Correspondence: meadow_zh@hotmail.com
[1] School of Nursing, Xuzhou Medical University, Xuzhou, China
Full list of author information is available at the end of the article

in women [2]. The three main types of UI are stress urinary incontinence (SUI), urgency urinary incontinence (UUI), and mixed urinary incontinence (MUI) [1]. The definition of each UI type is as follows: SUI is "the complaint of involuntary loss of urine on effort or physical exertion (e.g., sporting activities) or on sneezing or coughing"; UUI is the "observation of involuntary leakage from the urethra synchronous with the sensation of a sudden, compelling desire to void that is difficult to defer"; and MUI is the "complaint of involuntary loss of urine associated with urgency and also with effort or physical exertion or on sneezing or coughing" [1].

Prevalence rates of UI for women reported globally can differ as a result of variations in methods used in studies or reports, women's underreporting of their symptoms, and providers underdiagnosing the condition [3]. As an example, the UI prevalence rate for women between 45 and 60 years old living in Brazil was 23.6% [4], whereas the prevalence rates for adult women (over 18 years old) in Germany, Denmark, and Norway were 48.3%, 46.4% [5], and 18.7% [6], respectively. The number of women with UI in the United States has been estimated to be about 28.4 million [7]. Previous research suggests that 31.9% (approximately 160 million) women in China are affected by UI [8], indicating an urgent need for health and social resources to manage and treat UI.

Many factors are associated with UI [8], including unmodifiable factors (e.g., age, gender, menopause, history of vaginal delivery) and potentially modifiable factors (e.g., smoking, alcohol intake, toileting behaviors [9], constipation, and obesity). Besides UI's impact on women's physical and mental health, UI affects women's quality of life by limiting social activities [10] and interactions, interfering with the ability to work [11], and increasing the financial burden on women and society [12–14]. Therefore, UI should be viewed as both a women's health issue and a public health issue [15].

Studies of UI prevalence rates and associated factors often appear in English-language journals, but research findings published in non-English-language journals or English-language journals not published outside of China are seldom disseminated widely. The resultant knowledge gap could negatively affect potential research and clinical advances with regard to Chinese women's bladder health. This gap could also delay the development of culturally appropriate interventions to prevent and treat UI across women's lifecourse. Thus, the need to close the knowledge gap is important, especially considering China's large female population. For example, 650 million women were living in China in 2010, with more than 500 million women over 20 years old [16].

The aims of this study were to: (1) summarize findings from studies in non-English-language journals and English-language journals published in China that investigate UI prevalence in Chinese women, (2) categorize the findings by life stage (i.e., age range categories), and (3) facilitate dissemination of this existing information to researchers and clinicians to aid in their planning to prevent, manage, and treat female UI.

Methods

Literature search

The authors searched the relevant literature using five databases: the Wanfang full-text database (a Chinese professional academic database covering journals, meeting minutes, papers, academic achievements and academic conference papers), China National Knowledge Infrastructure (CNKI) Database (the largest continuously updated China journal full-text database in the world. It contains more than 9100 important journals in China, mainly including academic, technical, policy guidance, higher science popularization and education, and some basic education, popular science and technology, popular culture and literature and art works, covering natural science, engineering technology, agriculture, philosophy, medicine, humanities and Social Sciences and other fields, there are more than 32.52 million full-text documents), VIP Database (it analyzes the contents and citations of more than 14,000 kinds of science and technology periodicals and 57 million full-text periodicals published in China), and China Biology Medicine database (it involves basic medicine, clinical medicine, preventive medicine, pharmacy, traditional Chinese medicine, traditional Chinese medicine and other biomedical fields. It is an important retrieval tool for medical literature in China at present) for Chinese Technical Periodicals, and PubMed for English-language articles. The Wanfang full-text database search expression was Subject (Female/Women) × Subject (Urinary incontinence) × Subject (Prevalence) × Date: 2013–2019 or Subject: (Lower urinary tract symptoms) × Subject (Prevalence) × Date: 2013 to2019. The authors used the same search strategy for the other four databases: China National Knowledge Infrastructure, VIP, China Biology Medicine, and PubMed. After the electronic retrieval of relevant articles, the authors obtained further studies from the references cited in those articles. The search was conducted in two phases: initially the review included studies published between January 2013 and December 2017, and was subsequently updated to include literature published between January 2018 and December 2019.

Eligibility criteria

The inclusion criteria for this review were: (1) studies must be a cross-sectional research design; (2) study participants were adult women (≥ 17 years old) living in China; (3) studies discussed prevalence rates and/or associated factors of UI; and (4) sample sizes were greater than or equal to 100 women. The exclusion criteria were (1) narrative or systematic reviews, meta-analyses, or clinical guidelines; (2) case–control studies of UI treatment or care; and (3) studies focused on UI mechanisms. (4) Study participants were currently pregnant or up to 3 months postpartum.

Study selection

Two native Chinese-speaking reviewers (proficient in English) independently screened the article titles and abstracts. Duplicate articles were excluded. Full texts were obtained for the selected studies to assess their eligibility and their reference lists were scanned for further relevant articles. Any disagreement that arose between the reviewers regarding the inclusion or exclusion of articles was resolved through discussion. See Fig. 1.

Data extraction and analysis

The study team developed a standardized abstraction table. Data extraction was performed by two reviewers. One author independently read the included studies and extracted data from them, but consulted with the other authors to resolve ambiguities. The studies were described and then summarized using a narrative descriptive approach. Data in the abstraction table were double checked by reviewers.

The age ranges of the participants differed among the studies selected for review. Thus, we adopted the following age range categories to examine the studies more closely in terms of participant age: 17–40 years old for young women, 41–59 years old for middle-aged women, and 60 years old and over for older women. Two reviewers independently extracted data onto a data extraction summary sheet regarding prevalence rates and associated factors for UI in young, middle-aged, and older Chinese women. Factors that were significantly associated with urinary incontinence ($p < 0.05$) were included in the review.

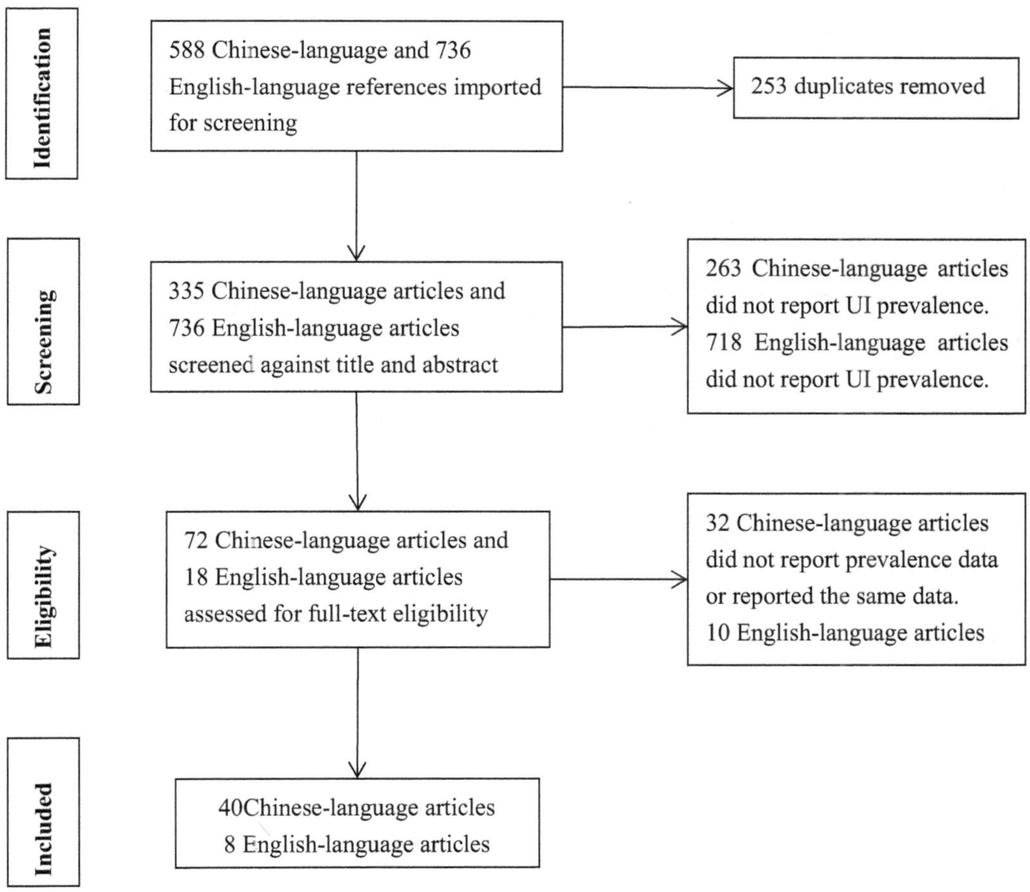

Fig. 1 PRISMA flow diagram for the review process

Results

The articles initially retrieved included 335 Chinese-language and 736 English-language articles, after removing 253 duplicates. Of those articles, 72 Chinese-language articles and 18 English-language articles were retained after screening titles and abstracts. We then reviewed the full texts of each article and identified 40 Chinese-language and 8 English-language articles for final analyses (Fig. 1). Among the Chinese-language articles, there were four Master's thesis [17–20].

Studies selected for review were conducted in 22 different provinces and regions in China including: Shanghai [21], Beijing [22], Chongqing [23], Hebei [24], Shanxi [25], Gansu [26], Xinjiang [27, 28], Guangzhou [29], and Taiwan [30, 31] etc. Figure 2 presents a map of China that reported prevalence rates of UI in various areas throughout the country.

Based on the eligibility criteria, all the included articles were cross-sectional research design. The sample sizes range from 146 to 18,992. Almost all of the studies reported that trained interviewers surveyed face to face with standardized questionnaire and some of the researchers also conducted gynecological examination for participants [32–34]. All the studies focused on the associated factors of any UI or SUI. Two article focused on the associated factors of the other type (UUI) [19, 22]. No articles that focused on the associated factors of MUI were located.

The prevalence rates and associated factors for female UI in China are presented in the "Appendix". The reported prevalence rates of overall UI (overall UI includes all types of UI) in Chinese adult women ranged from 8.7 [34] to 69.8% [35]. Where prevalence of specific UI types were reported, the following ranges were: SUI prevalence rates ranged from 6.7 [34] to 44.0% [35], UUI

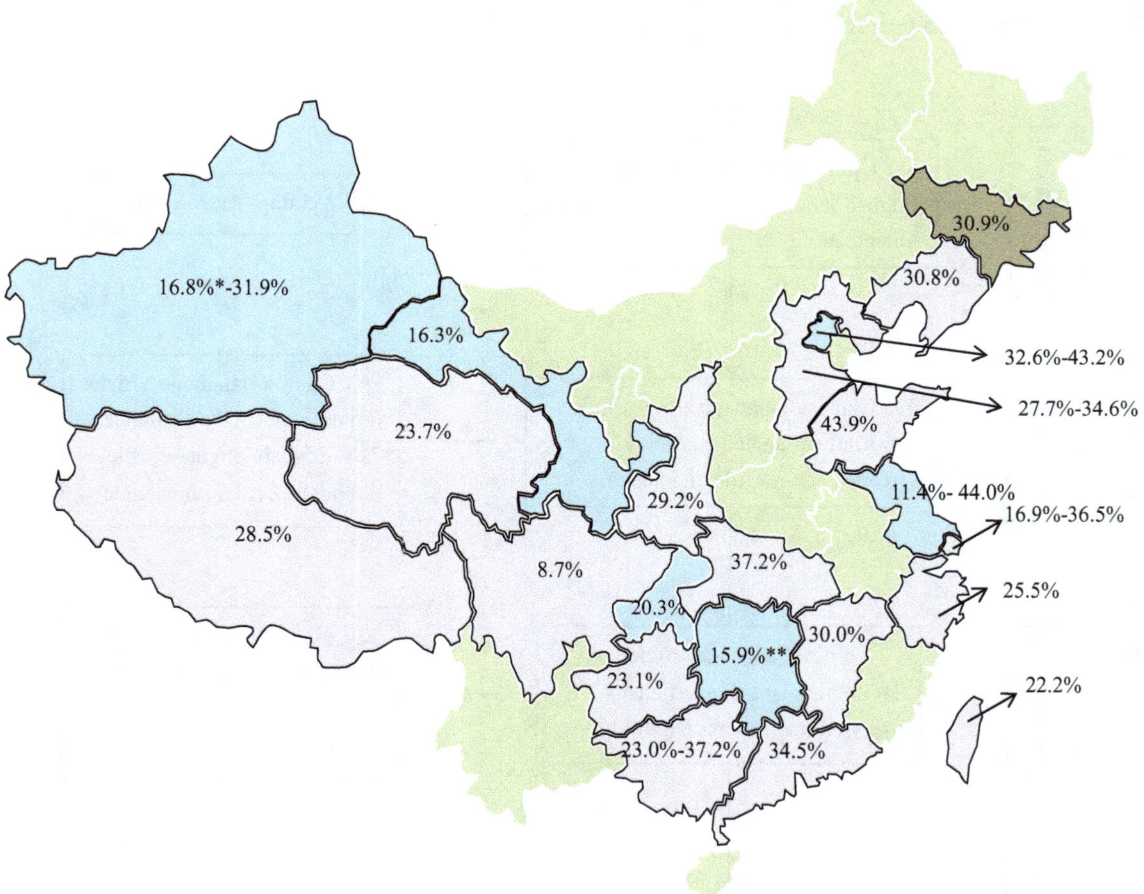

Fig. 2 Prevalence rates of female urinary incontinence by location in China (This figure is created by authors with Word of Microsoft Office Home and Student 2019 (https://www.microsoftstore.com.cn/office/office-home-student-2019). It does not represent all the territory of China (China Sea Islands etc.).). [ ] UI (UI: Urinary incontinence, type not specified) of adult women (≥ 18 or 20 years old). [ ] SUI (SUI: Stress urinary incontinence) of adult women (≥ 18 years old). [ ] UI of older women (≥ 60 or older). [ ] No prevalence of UI reported. Two studies including women with 17 years old: *[20]. **[40]

prevalence rates ranged from 1.2 [17] to 21.0% [22], and MUI prevalence rates ranged from 1.5 [17] to 15.7% [36]).

Definitions for UI, SUI, UUI, and MUI differed across some of the studies. Most of the authors used the International Continence Society (ICS) definition of UI: "complaint of involuntary loss of urine" [1]. Five studies [37–41] did not include a definition for UI. Other definitions used varied slightly from the ICS definition, including: (1) UUI was defined as, "the occurrence of urinary frequency, urgency, increased frequency of nocturnal discharge and decreased urine output; or cannot control urine leaking out, waited too late to urinate leading to leakage of urine" [42, 43]; and (2) UUI was defined as, "urinating without any warning or a weak or faint amount of early warning, sudden urge sensation resulting in uncontrolled urine outflow" [22]. SUI was defined as "urine leaks out when exercising" [22]. The "Appendix" includes the UI definitions used in the reviewed studies.

Only one article reported UI prevalence rates and associated factors specifically for young women (18–26 years old) [44]. It found that age (21–26 years old comparing with 18–20 years old) (OR = 0.87, 95% CI = 0.77–0.98), constipation (OR = 2.40, 95% CI = 1.49–3.84), alcohol consumption (OR = 1.76, 95% CI = 1.11–2.79), often/always delayed urination (OR = 1.74, 95% CI = 1.31–2.31), and/or often/always strained to urinate (OR = 1.43, 95% CI = 1.11–1.85) were associated with UI. The prevalence of UI in this study was 23.6% [44]. Based on the data extracted from studies that included adult women, UI prevalence rates for community-living young women (18 to40 years old) ranged from 2.6 [45] to 30.0% [46], and the prevalence rates of SUI, UUI, and MUI were reported as 4.7 [21]–24.5% [47], 0 [48]–8.1% [42], and 0.7 [49]–10.7% [50], respectively. Eight articles [29, 30, 34, 51–55] were focused on middle-aged, perimenopausal, and menopausal women, and seven articles [41, 43, 56–60] were focused on older women. The prevalence rates of UI for middle-aged women ranged from 8.7 [34] to 47.7% [36], and the prevalence rates of UI for older women ranged from 16.9 [57] to 61.6% [60]. Table 1 provides a summary of the UI prevalence rates and associated factors of different age group of women. Table 2 reports the number of articles that investigated underlying factors and number of articles in which these factors were found to be significantly associated.

Discussion

The studies selected for this review revealed a wide range of prevalence rates for overall UI and the specific types of UI, which may be due, in part, to the country's size. China is a large country with 9.6 million square kilometers and it includes numerous cultures in urban and rural locations. Genetic factors, diet, lifestyle, local environment, climate, economic development level, occupation types, and toileting behaviors may differ across these regions. These factors could act as determinants of UI, and thus affect variation in UI prevalence rates. Other important reasons for the variations in UI prevalence rates and UI types are the different research definitions and statistical and sampling methods used in the selected studies. For example, researchers used different methods when creating samples (i.e., based on general outpatient [40] or gynecological clinics [38] or physical examination [61] or nursing institutions [60]). The study participants had different occupations (i.e., medical personnel [62], nurses [22] and railway workers [63]), and different

Table 1 Prevalence Rates and Factors Associated with Urinary Incontinence in Chinese Women

Population	Age	Prevalence	Associated factors
Young women	17[#] to 40 years	UI 2.6–30.0% SUI 4.7–24.5% UUI 0–8.1% MUI 0.7–10.7%	Age, constipation, alcohol consumption, delayed urination, strained to urinate
Middle-aged women	41–59 years	UI 8.7–47.7% SUI 6.7–40.5% UUI 2.1–62.9% MUI 1.2–20.4%	Age, overweight, BMI, level of education, monthly income, constipation, menstrual disorders, menstrual disorders, parity, perineal laceration, postpartum urinary incontinence, pelvic operation history, POP, menopause, atrophic vaginitis, history of hormone replacement therapy, urinary tract infection, mental disease, hyperlipidemia, chronic bronchitis or asthma, respiratory system diseases, fecal incontinence
Older women	≥ 60 years	UI 16.9–61.6% SUI 10.0–62.4% UUI 3.3–21.1% MUI 3.3–26.6%	Age, more than 80 years old, BMI, low level of education, spouse, mental labor, alcohol consumption, delayed voiding, medical payment method, constipation, parity, pregnancy > 4 times, leakage of urine, gynecological diseases, urinary tract infection, malnutrition, autonomic activity limitation, activities of daily living, chronic pain, sleep disorders, chronic respiratory, urinary, cardiovascular disease, diabetes, drugs, indwelling catheterization

UI urinary incontinence, *SUI* stress urinary incontinence, *UUI* urgency urinary incontinence, *MUI* mixed urinary incontinence, *BMI* Body Mass Index, *POP* pelvic organ prolapse

Table 2 Number of articles investigated underlying factors and number of articles in which the factors significantly associated with urinary incontinence (N=48)

Factors[a]	Number of articles[b]	Significantly associated[c]
Age	37	29
BMI/weight	28	22
Constipation	27	19
Parity	23	15
Vaginal delivery	23	10
Hypertension	22	8
Menopause	21	8
Educational	19	8
POP	15	8
Pelvic surgery/hysterectomy	20	7
Alcohol consumption	17	7
Chronic pelvic pain	8	7
Urinary tract infections	8	7
Diabetes	23	6
Cough	8	6
Smoking	18	5
Occupation	13	5

POP pelvic organ prolapse

[a] Factors: the top seventeen associated factors according to the investigated frequencies

[b] Number of articles: the number of articles that investigated underlying factors

[c] Significantly associated: number of articles in which these factors were found to be significantly associated with urinary incontinence

living conditions (i.e., rural [64] and urban [45]). Also, in some studies, clinicians conducted physical examinations and documented medical histories, which may have yielded different results from women's self-reported questionnaires.

Researchers identified several factors associated with overall UI in Chinese women. Some of these factors are modifiable, such as weight, BMI, education, smoking and drinking alcohol. Some factors can be remedied or controlled (i.e., constipation, hypertension, chronic cough, diabetes, respiratory diseases, and vaginitis). Lastly, although some of the identified factors are unmodifiable (i.e., age, vaginal delivery, cesarean section delivery, and menopause), interventions can nonetheless be designed and tested to promote bladder health and help delay the onset or slow worsening of UI.

Age is often associated with UI risk factors such as education level, number of pregnancies and deliveries, menopause, and chronic conditions such as hypertension, diabetes, and respiratory diseases. Thus, studying clusters of factors that increase UI risk across the lifecourse is important. Moreover, using a lifecourse perspective is advocated in bladder health research [65].

Chinese scholars have largely confined their research on prevalence of UI in adult women ($\geq$17 years old), but in their findings of subgroup analyses for discrete age groups were not reported. Despite this limitation, when using the prevalence rate range of 2.6 [45]–30% [46] for young women aged 17–40 years old, the number of Chinese women in this age group who are affected by UI is estimated to be between 6.6 million and 75.8 million. This finding alone indicates that screening young women for risk factors, especially modifiable ones, and taking actions to minimize or eliminate the effects of these factors could potentially prevent or delay incident cases of UI throughout the lifecourse and especially later in life.

In a prospective cluster-randomized controlled trial of UI among young women (18–40 years), SUI prevalence was 14.3% [66]; 49.5% of these women had SUI during pregnancy, 43.6% had postpartum SUI, and 6.9% had SUI before pregnancy. Because muscle, connective, and nervous system pelvic structures are subjected to anatomical, morphological, functional, and hormonal changes during pregnancy, clinicians should initiate primary prevention interventions [67]. The pelvic floor also undergoes an enormous amount of stretching to allow the passage of a newborn during vaginal delivery [68]. Evident or hidden injuries to the pelvic floor may manifest as urinary and fecal incontinence, prolapse symptoms, or sexual dysfunction, all of which have a considerable impact on quality of life. Because pregnancy and childbirth can put young women at risk of developing UI [69], research and clinical attention should be focused on understanding the underlying mechanisms of UI as well as developing effective strategies (perform pelvic floor muscle training, maintain normal weight, avoid constipation [70]) to preserve bladder health for young Chinese nulligravid women.

In our research, there was only one study focused on the young women (18–26 years old) and it found that age (21–26 years old comparing with 18–20 years old), constipation, alcohol consumption, often/always delayed urination, and/or often/always strained to urinate were associated with UI. The prevalence of UI in this study was 23.6% [44]. Evidence from studies of young women who live outside of China also provides compelling evidence that UI in young women should be investigated further and intentionally. For example, the prevalence rate of UI for Swedish women (N=653) between the ages of 18 and 30 years was 12% [71]. In nulligravid Australian women aged 16–30 years (average age 22.5 $\pm$ 3.2 years), the prevalence of overall UI was 12.6% [72], and women who were sexually active and those who were not using oral contraceptives had the highest rates of UI [72]. Mishra et al.'s study found that the UI prevalence rate for Australian women aged 22–27 years was 6.8% at baseline and increased to 16.5% nine years later [73]. These researchers also reported that women with depressive symptoms or a history of depression were more likely than those without depressive symptoms to report subsequent UI symptoms [73]. For nulligravid women living in Italy between 15 and 25 years old, age, BMI, depression/anxiety/panic attacks, eating disorders, and constipation were risk factors for UI [74]. Participating in organized sports that involves high-volume exercise for competition also increased the risk of developing UI (OR = 2.53, 95% CI = 1.3–2.7) [75]. Other studies conducted outside of China showed that UI is an issue for many nulliparous female athletes [76].

Cultural differences may be evident with regard to UI risk and associated factors in China and abroad. A relatively new factor under investigation is toileting behaviors, i.e., actions women take immediately prior to and during urination [77–80]. Toileting behaviors play a role in developing or worsening urinary symptoms, but more research is required, especially studies that focus on young women in China [44]. It is often during youth and young adulthood when women develop habitual behaviors and form beliefs and attitudes about bladder health for themselves and their children. This period in women's lifecourse may be pivotal in influencing prevalence rates because evidence is mounting that research to prevent or reduce UI in this age stage is important [65].

This review also found that UI prevalence rates for middle-aged Chinese women ranged from 8.7 [34] to 47.7% [36], which represents 15.5–85.0 million middle-aged women with UI. The UI prevalence rate for women between 45 and 60 years old living in Brazil was 23.6% [4]. The associated factors relate mainly to obstetrics-related ones, such as parity, perineal laceration, and postpartum UI, and gynecological factors, such as menstrual disorder, menopause, pelvic organ prolapse, pelvic operation history, and hormone replacement therapy (see Table 1). UI prevalence rate was found to be significantly higher in a postmenopausal group than a premenopausal age group [81], which may be related to the change of hormone levels in postmenopausal women [82]. Research conducted in China found that the protective effect of cesarean section delivery compared with vaginal delivery was more obvious at five years postpartum than at one year postpartum [83]. Vaginal delivery appears to aggravate pelvic floor structure injuries. Compared to this study, studies conducted in other countries had similar findings. In Norway, a survey of middle-aged women (average age 47 years) who had delivered either vaginally or by Caesarian sections 15–23 years previously had 46.9% UI prevalence. In addition, caesarian section delivery was a protective factor as UI prevalence was lower than in this group of women as compared to women who delivered vaginally.[84]. Further research is needed to determine the mechanism(s) of injury during childbirth and identify associated factors and interventions that prevent or lessen adverse effects of childbirth on bladder health.

Although UI is common across the lifecourse, its prevalence peaks in the older age group of women [3]. China's older female UI prevalence rate ranged from 16.9 [57] to 61.6% [60], which translates to more than 12.8–46.7 million older Chinese women living with UI. Scholars outside of China have found similar UI prevalence rates for older women. A survey of 622 older women living in Brazil (average age 64 years) revealed that the UI prevalence rate was 52.3% [85] and for women over 65 years old living in Turkey the UI prevalence was 51.6% [86]. In China, risk factors associated with UI include being 80 years old and over, BMI, malnutrition, low educational level, sleep disorders [58], unspecified number and types of medications, history of pregnancy, urine leakage during pregnancy, chronic respiratory disease, cardiovascular disease, gynecological diseases, diabetes, urinary tract diseases [31], chronic pain, constipation, and restricted activity [41] (see Table1). Compared to middle-aged women, older women have a higher prevalence of chronic diseases (i.e., respiratory disease, hypertension, diabetes, etc.), limited physical activity, malnutrition, and other factors that could be contributing risk factors for UI. A longitudinal study of older women (baseline ages of 51–74 years) conducted in the United States years who did not have UI found the incidence of UI was 37.2% ten years later [87]. This study also found that UI prevalence in later in life had strong associations with obesity, functional ability, and medical comorbidities, but not with parity [87].

Although we used rigorous methods to conduct this epidemiological review, some limitations are noted. First, although we searched one English database (i.e., PubMed), and the PRISMA review process was followed, we may have inadvertently overlooked eligible articles. Second, research into UI prevalence rates has not been conducted in all 34 provinces in China (e.g., 22 of the 34 provinces are represented in the included studies), which could result in an incomplete picture of the distribution of UI across the Chinese female adult population. The quality of the included studies was not formally assessed in order to include a broad representation of the literature. It is recommended that future studies include this important element. This paper, however, provides important information and raises awareness about prevalence of UI in women living in China.

Conclusions

Most of the information in this review has been previously unavailable to researchers in countries outside of China. Thus, in addition to adding to the specific knowledge about UI in Chinese women, this review adds to the global knowledge base about female UI. Findings from the reviewed studies revealed that UI prevalence rates for Chinese women range from 8.7 to 69.8%. Most of the studies focused on middle-aged and older women. Little information about UI prevalence for women in their teens and twenties was found. Given the prevalence of UI and size of China's female population, research is needed to better understand the risk, and protective, factors for UI across the lifecourse of women. This information should stimulate interest in further multi-country comparisons and the development and testing of evidence-based interventions to prevent UI.

Abbreviations

BMI: Body Mass Index; ICS: International Continence Society; MUI: Mixed urinary incontinence; POP: Pelvic organ prolapse; SUI: Stress urinary incontinence; UI: Urinary incontinence; UUI: Urgency urinary incontinence.

Authors' contributions

KKX analyzed and interpreted the literature data regarding UI and was a major contributor in writing the manuscript. FZ and MHP made substantial contributions to the conception and design strategy and revised the article for important intellectual content. All authors read and approved the final manuscript.

Competing interests

The authors declare that they have no competing interests.

Author details

[1] School of Nursing, Xuzhou Medical University, Xuzhou, China. [2] School of Nursing and Midwifery, Jiangsu College of Nursing, Huai'an, China. [3] School of Nursing, University of North Carolina at Chapel Hill, CB 7460, Chapel Hill, USA.

Appendix

See Table 3.

Table 3 Prevalence and associated factors of urinary incontinence for three age groups

First author	Date range of study	Location (provinces)	Age (characteristic)	Instrument (methods)[a]	Prevalence (n/N (%))	Authors' definitions of UI and UI types	Associated factors [odds ratio (OR), 95% confidence interval (95% CI)]
Zhang and Lei [8]	February 2006–July 2006	Northwest, Northeast, North, Southwest, East, and South-central China	> 20 years	ICIQ-FLUTS[b] (face to face interviews by trained interviewers using a standardized questionnaire)	UI 6052/18992 (31.9) SUI 3592/18992 (18.9) UUI 488/18992 (2.6) MUI 1788/18992 (9.4)	ICS[c] definitions	UI: Age 30–39 years (1.55, 1.34–1.80), 40–49 years (2.66, 2.29–3.10), 50–59 years (2.80, 2.32–3.38), 60–69 years (2.46, 1.98–3.06), 70–79 years (3.02, 2.39–3.81), 80–89 years (3.32, 2.52–4.31), ≥ 90 years (5.87, 3.58–9.65), BMI ≥ 28 kg/m^2 (1.77, 1.52–2.06), menopause (1.41, 1.24–1.61), residence (urban: 0.90, 0.84–0.97), constipation (1.87, 1.70–2.06), pelvic organ prolapse (POP) (1.96, 1.47–2.60), hypertension (1.29, 1.16–1.44), alcoholism (1.51, 1.35–1.68), vaginal delivery (1.63, 1.49–1.79)
Sun and Wenyu [17]	2012–2013	Qinghai	20–80 years	(Face to face) Bristol Standardized Questionnaire-FLUTS)	UI 253/1066 (23.7) SUI 222/1066 (20.8) UUI 13/1066 (1.2) MUI 16/1066 (1.5)	ICS definitions	UI: Age (1.08, 1.05–1.12), natural vaginal delivery (0.002, 0.00–0.01), obstetric forceps vagina delivery (8.17, 1.49–44.77), parity (668.8, 146.09–3061.86), chronic cough (7.62, 1.84–31.57), constipation (2.72, 1.29–5.73)

Table 3 (continued)

First author	Date range of study	Location (provinces)	Age (characteristic)	Instrument (methods)[a]	Prevalence (n/N (%))	Authors' definitions of UI and UI types	Associated factors [odds ratio (OR), 95% confidence interval (95% CI)]
Liu and Tingting [18]	March 2013–October 2013	Guangxi	20–90 years	(Face to face) Nanning UI Epidemiological questionnaire	UI 663/2883 (23.0) SUI 376/2883 (13.0)	ICS definitions	SUI: Age (1.53, 1.13–2.00), chronic pelvic pain (0.73, 0.58–0.93), chronic respiratory disease (5.24, 1.17–21.27), BMI (1.53, 1.37–1.75), recurrent urinary tract infection (1.97, 1.08–3.65)
Li and Jingxuan [19]	October 2012–June 2013	Shandong	18–90 years (married)	(Face to face) Bristol Standardized Questionnaire-Female LUTS	UI 1142/2600 (43.9) SUI 571/2600 (22.0) UUI 199/2600 (7.7) MUI 372/2600 (14.3)	ICS definitions	SUI: parity = 1 (1.24, 1.17–1.76), parity = 2 (2.96, 1.17–2.61), parity (3.25, 1.23–1.96), menopause (2.45, 1.01–2.35), constipation (1.39, 1.26–3.32), history of pelvic surgery (1.20, 1.00–1.73), BMI ≥ 28.0 kg/m^2 (2.07, 1.52–3.54) UUI: Parity = 1 (1.10, 1.17–1.76), parity = 2 (2.01, 1.17–2.61), parity ≥ U (2.93, 1.23–3.32), constipation (1.52, 1.26–3.32), BM I(2.93 kg/m^2 (2.07, 1.52–3.54); MUI: Age 50–59 (3.15, 1.20–3.07), age 60–69 (1.55, 1.01–2.46), age 70–79 (1.25, 1.14–1.88), age ≥ 80 years (1.11, 1.10–1.96), constipation (2.01, 1.26–3.32), menopause (1.11, 1.01–1.96)

Table 3 (continued)

First author	Date range of study	Location (provinces)	Age (characteristic)	Instrument (methods)[a]	Prevalence (n/N (%))	Authors' definitions of UI and UI types	Associated factors [odds ratio (OR), 95% confidence interval (95% CI)]
Arzigul [20]	June 2010–November 2010	Xinjiang	Y: 17–78 years	(Face to face) Questionnaires (general condition, UI prevalence situation, childbirth and chronic diseases)	SUI 338/2009 (16.8)	ICS definitions	SUI: Prolonged delivery (4.72), Difficult birth (1.85), perineum tear (1.73), chronic pelvic pain (1.50), pelvic surgery (6.68), chronic cough (2.60). (No 95% CI is reported)
Liu and Bo [21]	March 2010–September 2012	Shanghai	≥ 20 years	Bristol Standardized Questionnaire-FLUTS (face to face interviews by researchers with standardized questionnaire)	UI 1266/5433 (23.3) SUI 761/5433 (14.0) UUI 164/5433 (3.0) MUI 341/5433 (6.3)	ICS definitions	UI: Age (2.38, 2.16–2.63), education (2.80, 2.32–3.53), residence rural (1.95,1.64–2.31), manual labor (6.90,5.66–8.47), exercise frequency < 8 times/months (0.56, 0.47–0.68), hyperlipidemia (1.99, 1.56–2.53), no nervous system disease (0.31, 0.18–0.55), diabetes (1.69,1.20–2.38), nocturia (8.20, 6.72–10.01), constipation (7.53, 6.01–9.43), eating less greasy food (0.80, 0.73–0.88), respiratory diseases (2.67, 2.19–3.27), POP (7.37, 3.68–14.76), chronic pelvic pain (2.94, 2.20–3.91), urinary tract infection (7.75, 5.06–11.89)

Table 3 (continued)

First author	Date range of study	Location (provinces)	Age (characteristic)	Instrument (methods)[a]	Prevalence (n/N (%))	Authors' definitions of UI and UI types	Associated factors [odds ratio (OR), 95% confidence interval (95% CI)]
He and Chongjun [22]		Beijing	19–58 years (nurses)	Beijing nurse Questionnaire LUTS	SUI 349/1070 (32.6)	SUI*	SUI: Occupational stress of nurses: unclear about task expectations, business stress. (No ORs and 95% CI is reported)
					UUI 225/1070 (21.0)	UUI*	UUI: Occupational stress of nurses: unclear about task expectations, task conflicts, work environment, tension of interpersonal relationship. (No ORs and 95% CI is reported)
Xie and Jiangling [23]	June 2011–December 2012	Chongqing	20–78 years	(Face to face) Self-designed questionnaire (refer to Bristol Standardized Questionnaire-FLUTS)	SUI 135/666 (20.3)	ICS definitions	BMI, pelvic surgery history, hypertension, diabetes, chronic cough, constipation and other chronic diseases, perimenopausal period, multiple pregnancy abortions, parity, lateral episiotomy, perineal laceration. (No ORs and 95% CI is reported)

Table 3 (continued)

First author	Date range of study	Location (provinces)	Age (characteristic)	Instrument (methods)[a]	Prevalence (n/N (%))	Authors' definitions of UI and UI types	Associated factors [odds ratio (OR), 95% confidence interval (95% CI)]
Jiang and Yan [24]	January 2016–May 2016	Hebei	18–91 years	(Face to face) self-designed questionnaire (refer to ICIQ-LUTS)	UI 667/2408 (27.7) SUI 557/2408 (23.1) UUI 38/2408 (1.6) MUI 72/2408 (3.0)	ICS definitions	UI: Age 40–49 years (5.76, 1.68–19.69), 50–59 years (8.76, 2.58–29.74), 60–69 years (8.85, 2.61–29.99), 70–79 years (6.43, 1.86–22.25), ≥ 80 years (4.55, 1.24–16.71), daily drinking water ≥ 1500 ml (0.75, 0.62–0.91), urinary system diseases (1.96, 1.32–2.91), respiratory diseases (1.62, 1.19–2.21), vaginitis (2.32, 1.32–4.10), abortion 1–2 times (1.51, 1.21–1.87), abortion ≥ 3 times (2.59, 1.41–4.75), hypertension (1.90, 1.52–2.38), chronic low back pain (1.52, 1.24–1.86), cesarean delivery (0.365, 0.20–0.69), postpartum infection (2.00, 1.10–3.65), dysmenorrhea (1.28, 1.04–1.57)
Song and Yingchun [25]	July 2012–November 2012	Shanxi	20–87 years	(Face to face) ICIQ-LUTS	UI 882/3017 (29.2) SUI 547/3017 (18.1) UUI 138/3017 (4.6) MUI 184/3017 (6.1)	ICS definitions	UI: Age (1.70, 1.35–2.14), BMI (2.19, 1.68–2.84), organ prolapse (3.14, 2.49–3.95), cesarean delivery (2.38, 1.26–4.48), manual labor (2.67, 1.95–3.65), chronic cough (3.01, 1.47–6.61), constipation (2.23, 1.22–4.07), smoking (2.00, 1.37–2.91)

Table 3 (continued)

First author	Date range of study	Location (provinces)	Age (characteristic)	Instrument (methods)[a]	Prevalence (n/N (%))	Authors' definitions of UI and UI types	Associated factors [odds ratio (OR), 95% confidence interval (95% CI)]
Wang and Lihong [26]	March 2012–September 2012	GANSU	30–70 years	General survey	SUI 975/6000 (16.3)	ICS definitions	SUI: Age, parity, mode of delivery, place of residence, weight. (No ORs and 95% CI is reported)
Wan and Xiaohui [27]	April 2011to August 2011	Xinjiang	20–85 years (have sex or married)	(Face to face) ICIQ-LUTS	SUI 960/3403 (28.2) UUI 71/3403 (2.1) MUI 392/3403 (11.5)	ICS definitions	SUI: BMI (1.67, 1.08–2.58), parity (5.09, 3.89–6.67), weight of infant (5.62, 3.33–9.48), mode of delivery (2.25, 1.63–3.09), perineum lateral incision (4.45, 3.11–6.36), menopause (5.15, 3.61–7.33), chronic pelvic pain (3.87, 1.05–14.25), POP (3.50, 2.51–4.89)
Liu and Zhaochun [28]	July 2015–September 2015	Xinjiang	30–70 years (Gynecology and obstetrics outpatient)	(Face to face) ICIQ-UI	SUI 53/166 (31.9)	ICS definitions	SUI: Menopause, parity, delivery, puerperal incontinence. (No ORs and 95% CI is reported)
Wu and Yonghong [29]	February 2013–June 2013	Guangdong	40–55 years (Peri-menopausal period)	(Face to face) ICIQ-UI	SUI 211/1200 (17.6)	ICS definitions	Reported that UI was not associated with age

Table 3 (continued)

First author	Date range of study	Location (provinces)	Age (characteristic)	Instrument (methods)[a]	Prevalence (n/N (%))	Authors' definitions of UI and UI types	Associated factors [odds ratio (OR), 95% confidence interval (95% CI)]
Horng and Shiow-Shiun [30]	2005	Taiwan	35–64 years	The short form 36 (SF-36) health survey (interview survey)	UI 1036/4661 (22.2)	ICS definitions	UI: Age 44–54 (1.53, 1.27–1.83), age 55–64 (1.88, 1.49–2.37), parity 1 time (1.87, 1.17–2.99), parity 2 time (2.58, 1.73–3.85), parity ≥ 3 times (2.83, 1.90–4.23), BMI 24–26.9 kg/m^2 (1.48, 1.25–1.76), BMI.47.0 kg/m^2 (2.33, 1.71–3.61), history of hormone replacement therapy (1.53, 1.17–1.99), psychiatric disease (1.45, 1.07–2.07), hyperlipidemia (1.35, 1.11–1.65), respiratory disease (1.62, 1.07–2.46)
Chen and Cong [32]	January 2014–May 2014	Zhejiang	≥ 20 years	Face to face questionnaire administration, Gynecological examination	SUI 244/986 (24.7) UUI 47/986 (4.8) MUI 53/986 (5.4)	ICS definitions	SUI: Age > 40 years (1.4, 1.0–2.0), vaginal delivery (2.6, 1.6–4.2), hypertension (1.7, 1.1–2.5), chronic coughing (3.6, 2.1–6.2), BMI ≥ 25 kg/m^2 (1.7, 1.1–2.4), educational level ≤ middle school (1.4, 1.4–1.9)
Hu and Mengyan [33]	May 2010–July 2010	Zhejiang	20–82 years (gynecological outpatient and married)	face to face interview, Gynecologic examination	SUI 194/500 (38.8)	SUI**	SUI: Age, BMI, vaginal delivery, hypertension, diabetes, recurrent urinary tract infection, constipation, chronic diseases, anterior and posterior vaginal wall touch, uterine prolapse. (No ORs and 95% CI is reported)

Table 3 (continued)

First author	Date range of study	Location (provinces)	Age (characteristic)	Instrument (methods)[a]	Prevalence (n/N (%))	Authors' definitions of UI and UI types	Associated factors [odds ratio (OR), 95% confidence interval (95% CI)]
Han and Daihua [34]	January 2015–September 2016	Sichuan	35–64 years	(Face to face) ICIQ-UI, Gynecological examination	UI 455/5217 (8.7) SUI 348/5217 (6.7) UUI 45/5217 (0.9) MUI 62/5217 (1.2)	ICS definitions	UI: Age (0.82, 0.70–0.95), education level (1.49, 1.23–1.90), chronic bronchitis or asthma (1.55, 1.02–2.35), parity (0.79, 0.66–0.95), postpartum incontinence (8.87, 6.57–11.99), BMI (0.96, 0.93–0.99), POP (1.64, 1.09–2.49)
Sun and Yanling [35]	September 2018–December 2018	Jiangsu	≥ 18 years (urban and rural)	(Face to face) ICIQ-LUTS	Urban UI 245/443(55.3) SUI 128/443 (28.9) UUI 79/443 (17.8) MUI 38/443 (8.6) Rural UI 268/384 (69.8) SUI 169/384 (44.0) UUI 51/384 (13.3) MUI 48/384 (12.5)	ICS definitions	Urban UI: Age (1.35, 1.04–1.43), occupation (1.82, 1.16–2.89), alcohol consumption (7.37, 1.06–28.76), smoking (1.23, 1.15–2.67), sitting > 2 h/day (5.43, 1.10–21.82) Rural UI: Age (1.06, 1.02–1.09), occupation (2.86, 1.25–6.56), alcohol consumption (7.85, 1.57–29.24), smoking (1.09, 1.01–2.52), sitting > 2 h/day (6.31, 1.59–26.86), load frequently > 3 kg (3.65, 1.38–16.79)

Table 3 (continued)

First author	Date range of study	Location (provinces)	Age (characteristic)	Instrument (methods)[a]	Prevalence (n/N (%))	Authors' definitions of UI and UI types	Associated factors [odds ratio (OR), 95% confidence interval (95% CI)]
Deng and Li [36]	July 2012–December 2012	Guangxi	22–78 years	(Face to face) ICIQ-LUTS	UI 91/1052 (37.2) SUI 202/1052 (19.2) UUI 24/1052 (2.3) MUI 165/1052 (15.7)	ICS definitions	UI: Age 40–49 years (1.96, 1.02–3.78), natural vaginal delivery (8.66, 4.78–15.68), perineum lateral incision (2.89, 1.64–5.27), cesarean delivery (2.31, 1.29–4.17), hypertension (1.98, 0.91–3.37), menopause (2.11, 1.10–3.56), pelvic surgery (2.38, 1.04–5.47), chronic cough (2.65, 1.43–4.92), constipation (2.11, 1.39–3.22)
Wen and Fang [37]	October 2014–November 2014	Guizhou	18–70 years (married)	(Face to face) ICIQ-UI-short form	UI 68/294 (23.1)	Not reported	UI: Age (1.04, 1.01–1.07), ethnicity (2.53, 1.31–4.89), place of delivery (3.15, 1.42–6.99), mode of delivery (2.34, 1.09–5.05)
Zhang and Lijuan [38]	September 2011–June 2013	Jiangsu	20–72 years (gynecological outpatient)	Questionnaire investigation, routine physical examination	SUI 302/2655 (11.4)	Not reported	SUI: Parity (1.52, 1.13–2.36), age (1.29, 1.03–1.63), constipation (1.79, 1.30–6.84), vaginal delivery (2.95, 1.10–7.56), Prolonged delivery (3.54, 1.43–9.37), hysterectomy (3.75, 3.19–9.58), perineum laceration (1.35, 1.09–1.35)
Li and Jianjun [39]	March 2011–June 2011	Hunan	17–75 years (gynecological outpatient)	ICIQ-LUTS (long form)	SUI 122/769 (15.9) UUI 35/769 (4.6) MUI 23/769 (3.0)	Not reported	Not reported

Table 3 (continued)

First author	Date range of study	Location (provinces)	Age (characteristic)	Instrument (methods)[a]	Prevalence (n/N (%))	Authors' definitions of UI and UI types	Associated factors [odds ratio (OR), 95% confidence interval (95% CI)]
Li and Fang [40]	October 2012	Shanxi	≥ 20 years (gynecological outpatient)	(Face to face) Questionnaire administration	UI 210/421 (49.9)	Not reported	UI: Age, BMI, education, daily water intake, more pregnancy, Parity, vaginal delivery, and intensity of labor. (No ORs and 95% CI is reported)
Wang and Xin [41]	January 2012–October 2012	Jilin	60–87 years (urban)	ICIQ-UI	UI 305/986 (30.9) SUI 98/986 (10.0) UUI 69/986 (7.0) MUI 138/986 (14.0)	Not reported	UI: Respiratory diseases (1.50, 1.10–2.50), urinary diseases (2.60, 1.30–4.20), cardiovascular diseases (2.20, 1.20–4.20), gynecologic diseases (3.30, 1.90–5.40), parity > 4 times (1.80, 1.20–2.10), restriction of autonomic activity (2.40, 1.50–4.10)
Shi and Lihua [42]	April 2014–April 2015	Jiangxi	20–80 years	Bristol Standardized Questionnaire-FLUTS, pad testing	UI 150/500 (30.0) SUI 93/500 (18.6) UUI 37/500 (7.4) MUI 20/500 (4.0)	SUI:ICS UUI** MUI:SUI and UUI exist at the same time	Not reported
Xin and Chunyan [43]	April 2013–September 2014	Xinjiang	≥ 65 years	(Face to face) Questionnaire administration (refer to ICIQ-UI)	UI 682/1148 (59.4) SUI 335/1148 (29.2) UUI 83/1148 (7.2) MUI 264/1148 (23.0)	SUI:ICS definitions UUI** MUI*	Not reported
Zhou and Fang [44]	October 2017–December 2017	Jiangsu	18–26 years (college students)	(Face to face) ICIQ-FLUTS	UI 219/929 (23.6)	ICS definitions	Age: 21–26 years old comparing with 18–20 years old (0.87, 0.77–0.98), constipation (2.40, 1.49–3.84), alcohol consumption (1.76, 1.11–2.79), often/always delayed urination (1.74, 1.31–2.31), often/always strained to urinate (1.43, 1.11–1.85)

Table 3 (continued)

First author	Date range of study	Location (provinces)	Age (characteristic)	Instrument (methods)[a]	Prevalence (n/N (%))	Authors' definitions of UI and UI types	Associated factors [odds ratio (OR), 95% confidence interval (95% CI)]
Chu and Lei [45]	January 2012–September 2012	Shanghai	20–83 years	(Face to face interviews) Bristol Standardized Questionnaire-FLUTS	UI 2103/7314 (28.8) SUI 1719/7314 (23.5) UUI 154/7314 (2.1) MUI 183/7314 (2.5)	ICS definitions	UI: Postmenopausal (1.10, 1.04–1.17), pelvic surgery (1.38, 1.29–1.49), more than twice vaginal delivery history (1.49, 1.25–1.44), more than 20 weeks of pregnancy history (1.34, 1.25–1.44), the first vaginal delivery at < 20 years old (1.58, 1.46–1.71), obstetric forceps vagina delivery (2.75, 2.54–2.97), diabetes (1.16, 1.06–1.28), education (0.95, 0.90–0.99), hypertension (1.33, 1.23–1.43), BMI ≥ 30 kg/m^2 (2.37, 2.22–2.54)
Gao and Jixue [46]	May 2010–April 2013	Shanxi	21–72 years	(Face to face) Questionnaire administration, provocative test	UI 210/589 (35.7) SUI 128/589 (21.7)	ICS definitions	SUI: Age, BMI, alcohol consumption, educational level. (No ORs and 95% CI is reported)

Table 3 (continued)

First author	Date range of study	Location (provinces)	Age (characteristic)	Instrument (methods)[a]	Prevalence (n/N (%))	Authors' definitions of UI and UI types	Associated factors [odds ratio (OR), 95% confidence interval (95% CI)]
Luo and Xiaomei [47]	March 2015–September 2015	Xizang	≥ 20 years	(Face to face) Self-designed questionnaire (health characteristics and UI occurrence)	SUI 342/1200 (28.5)	ICS definitions	SUI: Urinary tract infection (1.67, 1.42–1.98), menopause (1.22, 1.16–1.29), uterine prolapse (1.49, 1.34–1.66), Anterior vaginal prolapse (1.68, 1.63–1.73), Posterior vaginal prolapse (1.08, 1.07–1.10), BMI (1.13, 1.11–1.16), perineal laceration, postpartum labor, chronic bronchitis (1.26, 1.23–1.29), cardiovascular disease (1.16, 1.15–1.18), constipation (1.13, 1.12–1.15), occupation (1.39, 1.36–1.42), education level low (1.10, 1.09–1.11), smoking (1.13, 1.11–1.56)
Xu and Ling [48]	June 2011	Shanghai	≥ 30 years	Face to face interviews Bristol Standardized Questionnaire-FLUTS	UI 218/597 (36.5) SUI 104/597 (17.4) UUI 32/597 (5.4) MUI 82/597 (13.7)	ICS definitions	Not reported
Wang and Yuliang [49]	October 2012–Jane 2013	Northwest, northeast, north, central, and south China	≥ 18 years	ICIQ-FLUTS (face to face interviews with questionnaires)	SUI 265/1472 (17.4) UUI 56/1472 (3.8) MUI 47/1472 (3.2)	ICS definitions	All LUTS: Age, alcohol consumption, smoking, parity (No ORs and 95% CI is reported)
Huang and Dong [50]	2011	Guangdong	≥ 20 years	Face to face questionnaire administration (health characteristics and UI occurrence)	UI 2373/6870 (34.5) SUI 1150/6870 (16.7) UUI 309/6870 (4.5) MUI 914/6870 (13.3)	ICS definitions	UI: Age (1.94, 1.51–3.99), mode of delivery (2.01, 1.08–5.02), process of childbirth (2.22, 0.52–9.89), constipation (2.78, 1.77–5.52), urinary tract infection (1.31, 1.01–3.66), and oral contraceptive drugs (1.59, 1.18–3.82)

Table 3 (continued)

First author	Date range of study	Location (provinces)	Age (characteristic)	Instrument (methods)[a]	Prevalence (n/N (%))	Authors' definitions of UI and UI types	Associated factors [odds ratio (OR), 95% confidence interval (95% CI)]
Li and Hong [51]	May 2014–March 2015	HUBEI	45–55 years (Peri-menopausal period)	(Face to face) ICIQ-UI	SUI 526/2057 (25.6)	ICS definitions	SUI: Age (1.63, 1.41–1.83), parity (2.35, 1.89–2.86), POP (2.10, 1.65–4.02), pelvic surgery (2.06, 1.90–3.32), urinary tract infection (2.40, 1.76–3.05)
Lu and Shi [52]	April 2014–October 2014	Hubei	40–65 years	(Face to face) ICIQ-UI short form	UI 397/1067 (37.2) SUI 344/1067 (32.2) UUI 230/1067 (21.6) MUI 177/1067 (16.6)	ICS definitions	UI: Menstrual disorder (1.54, 1.06–2.24), menopause (1.41, 1.03–1.93), BMI 18.5–25.0 kg/m^2 (2.98, 1.17–7.60), BMI > 25 kg/m^2 (3.37, 1.24–9.12), atrophic vaginitis (1.49, 1.08–2.04), constipation (1.82, 1.32–2.51), POP (5.07, 3.37–7.63), chronic pelvic pain (1.82, 1.32–2.51), fecal incontinence (2.89, 2.31–3.34)
Li and Tao [53]	April 2014–Oct ober 2014	HUBEI	40–65 years (peri-menopausal)	(Face to face) ICIQ-UI-short form	SUI 504/1519 (33.2) UUI 366/1519 (24.1) MUI 264/1519 (17.4)	ICS definitions	SUI: Age: 60–65 years old (3.40, 1.92–6.04), Cesarean Sect. (0.62, 0.40–0.92), atrophic vaginitis (1.36, 1.03–1.80), constipation (1.44, 1.07–1.93), chronic pelvic pain (2.17, 1.90–4.03), POP (2.81, 1.36–5.79), fecal incontinence (3.32, 2.03–5.43), monthly income: 2000–3999 comparing with ≤ 1999 (0.063, 0.40–0.92)

Table 3 (continued)

First author	Date range of study	Location (provinces)	Age (characteristic)	Instrument (methods)[a]	Prevalence (n/N (%))	Authors' definitions of UI and UI types	Associated factors [odds ratio (OR), 95% confidence interval (95% CI)]
Lu and Shi [54]	April 2014–December 2014	HUBEI	40–65 years (peri-menopausal)	(Face to face) ICIQ-UI-short form	UI 585/1519 (38.5) SUI 482/1519 (31.9) UUI 366/1519 (24.1) MUI 264/1519 (17.4)	ICS definitions	UI: Age: over 50 years old (2.0, 1.21–3.29), overweight (BMI: 25–30 kg/m^2) (2.85, 1.33–6.07), irregular menstruation (1.45, 1.03–2.06), gyneco-logical diseases (1.31, 1.01–1.70), chronic pelvic pain (2.32, 1.48–3.64), POP (2.33, 1.61–3.37), constipa-tion (1.42, 1.07–1.88), fecal incontinence (3.29, 2.33–4.65)
Wang and Bingyi [55]	No time is reported	Beijing	35–64 years	(Face to face) ICIQ-UI-short form	UI 59/126 (46.8)	ICS definitions	Age (No ORs and 95% CI is reported)
Chang and kengming [56]		Taiwan	$\geq$60 years	Face to face interview	UI 485/1517 (32.0)	ICS definitions	UI: Age (1.04, 1.02–1.07), diabetes mellitus (1.65, 1.11–2.47), previous urinary disease (3.46, 2.26–5.30), BMI (1.06, 1.01–1.11)
Li and Ruixia [57]	Apr 2013–Jun 2013	Shanghai	60–70 yeas	(Face to face) ICIQ-UI	UI 332/1962 (16.9) SUI 237/1962 (12.1)	ICS definitions	UI: BMI, pregnancy, pregnancy leak-age, gynecological diseases, constipation, urinary tract infection, chronic respiratory disease. (No ORs and 95% CI is reported)

Table 3 (continued)

First author	Date range of study	Location (provinces)	Age (characteristic)	Instrument (methods)[a]	Prevalence (n/N (%))	Authors' definitions of UI and UI types	Associated factors [odds ratio (OR), 95% confidence interval (95% CI)]
Gao and Maolong [58]	January 2013–May 2013	Beijing	≥ 60 years	(Face to face) Author-designed Questionnaire (Social and health characteristics)	UI 164/694 (23.6)	Patient reported	UI: Age 80–84 years (1.72, 0.96–3.08), age ≥ 85 years (2.49, 1.22–5.06), malnutrition (1.69, 1.08–2.65), chronic pain (1.47, 1.01–2.14), cognitive disorder (1.56, 1.08–2.24), sleep disorders (1.76, 1.22–2.53), drugs 1–4 types (2.23, 1.04–4.76), drug ≥ 5 types (5.07, 2.30–11.19)
Li and Yan [59]	2017	Sichuan	60–97 years (pension institutions)	(Face to face) ICIQ-UI-short form,	UI 102/205 (49.8) SUI 35/205 (17.1) UUI 21/205 (10.2) MUI 41/205 (20.0)	ICS definitions	UI: BMI < 24 kg/m^2 (0.38, 0.18–0.78), spouse (2.54, 1.20–5.38), Mental labour (0.25, 0.12–0.53), no alcohol consumption (0.40, 0.16–0.96), no delayed voiding (0.12, 0.05–0.30), number of chronic disease < 2 types (0.39, 0.18–0.83), parity ≥ 4 (2.82, 1.18–6.75), age of the first parity < 21 years (2.76, 1.03–7.43)
Chen and Mina [60]	No time is reported	Zhejianng	60–100 years (medical and nursing institutions)	(Face to face) ICIQ-UI-short form,	UI 217/352 (61.6)	ICS definitions	Education (0.59, 0.41–0.86), income (0.58, 0.37–0.92), medical payment method (1.64, 1.09–2.49), have no other disease (0.27, 0.13–0.58), activities of daily living (1.37, 1.12–1.67), indwelling catheterization (13.31, 2.35–75.22)

Table 3 (continued)

First author	Date range of study	Location (provinces)	Age (characteristic)	Instrument (methods)[a]	Prevalence (n/N (%))	Authors' definitions of UI and UI types	Associated factors [odds ratio (OR), 95% confidence interval (95% CI)]
Zhu and Zhichao [61]	January 2014–December 2014	Zhejiang	20–81 years	ICIQ-UI	UI 301/1178 (25.5)	UI*	UI: Age (1.02, 1.00–1.05), natural vaginal delivery (2.53, 1.10–5.84), difficult vaginal delivery (4.54, 1.63–12.64), Cesarean delivery (3.07, 1.10–1.45), parity (1.10, 1.00–1.21), BMI 20–25 kg/m^2 (1.43, 1.14–1.80), BMI > 25 kg/m^2 (1.40, 1.17–1.89), hypertcn sion (1.32, 1.01–1.74), diabetes (1.49, 1.17–1.89), other diseases (1.21, 1.02–1.45)
Che and Xinyan [62]	July 2018	Beijing	Mean: 39.4 ± 9.9 years (medical staff)	(Face to face) ICIQ-UI-short form,	SUI 63/146(43.2)	ICS definitions	Constipation (4.95, 1.81–13.53), Natural delivery (3.50, 1.49–8.21)
Liu and Yanjuan [63]	Nov 2010–Nov 2011	Hebei	≥ 20 years (railway workers)	(Face to face) ICIQ-UI	UI 474/1368 (34.6) SUI 296/1368 (21.6) UUI 52/1368 (3.8) MUI 126/1368 (9.2)	ICS definitions	Not reported
Li and Hui [64]	2014	Liaoning	≥ 18 years	(Face to face) ICIQ-LUTS	UI 1063/3456 (30.8) SUI 750/3456 (21.7) UUI 97/3456 (2.8) MUI 176/3456 (5.1)	ICS definitions	Not reported

E English-language articles searched from PubMed. *POP* pelvic organ prolapse

[a] All the questionnaires used in the studies were pencil and paper questionnaires

[b] ICIQ-FLUTS: Chinese version of the International Consultation on Incontinence Questionnaire-Female Lower Urinary Tract Symptoms

[c] ICS: International Continence Society

*UI**: [88]

SUI*: Urine leakage during exercise

SUI**: In the past year, loss of urine more than twice when abdominal pressure is increased (including stress, laughing, coughing, etc.)

UUI*: Urinating without any warning or a small amount of early warning, sudden stimulation results in uncontrolled urine outflow

UUI**: Occurrence of urinary frequency, urgency, increased frequency of nocturnal discharge and decreased urine output, or cannot control, too late, leading to urine leakage

MUI*: SUI and UUI exist at the same time

References

1. Haylen BT, de Ridder D, Freeman RM, Swift SE, Berghmans B, Lee J, et al. An International Urogynecological Association (IUGA)/International Continence Society (ICS) joint report on the terminology for female pelvic floor dysfunction. Neurourol Urodyn. 2010;29(1):4–20.
2. Aoki Y, Brown HW, Brubaker L, Cornu JN, Daly JO, Cartwright R. Urinary incontinence in women. Nat Rev Disease Primers. 2017;3:17042.
3. Searcy JAR. Geriatric urinary incontinence. Nurs Clin North Am. 2017;52(3):447–55.
4. Juliato CR, Baccaro LF, Pedro AO, Gabiatti JR, Lui-Filho JF, Costa-Paiva L. Factors associated with urinary incontinence in middle-aged women: a population-based household survey. Int Urogynecol J. 2017;28(3):423–9. nnn
5. Schreiber Pedersen L, Lose G, Hoybye MT, Elsner S, Waldmann A, Rudnicki M. Prevalence of urinary incontinence among women and analysis of potential risk factors in Germany and Denmark. Acta Obstet Gynecol Scand. 2017;96(8):939–48.n
6. Marit HE, Steinar H, Guri R, Yngvild SH. Prevalence, incidence and remission of urinary incontinence in women: longitudinal data from the Norwegian HUNT study (EPINCONT). BMC Urol. 2013;13:27.nnn
7. Wu JM, Hundley AF, Fulton RG. Forecasting the prevalence of pelvic floor disorders in US women 2010–2050. Obst Gynecol. 2009;114(6):1278–83. nn
8. Zhang L, Zhu L, Xu T, Lang J, Li Z, Gong J, et al. A population-based survey of the prevalence, potential risk factors, and symptom-specific bother of lower urinary tract symptoms in adult Chinese Women. Eur Urol. 2015;68(1):97–112.n
9. Zhou F, Newman DK, Palmer MH. Urinary urgency in working women: What factors are associated with urinary urgency progression? J Women's Health. 2018;27(5):575–83.nn
10. Coyne KS, Kvasz M, Ireland AM, Milsom I, Kopp ZS, Chapple CR. Urinary incontinence and its relationship to mental health and health-related quality of life in men and women in Sweden, the United Kingdom, and the United States. Eur Urol. 2012;61(1):88–95.n
11. Hung KJ, Awtrey CS, Tsai AC. Urinary incontinence, depression, and economic outcomes in a cohort of women between the ages of 54 and 65 years. Obstet Gynecol. 2014;123(4):822–7.nn
12. Wilson L, Brown JS, Shin GP, Luc KO, Subak LL. Annual direct cost of urinary incontinence. Obstet Gynecol. 2001;98(3):398–406.nn
13. Chang KM, Hsieh CH, Chiang HS, Lee TS. Trends in inpatient female urinary incontinence surgery and costs in Taiwan, 1997–2011. Taiwan J Obstet Gynecol. 2017;56(1):32–6.nn
14. Milsom I, Coyne KS, Nicholson S, Kvasz M, Chen CI, Wein AJ. Global prevalence and economic burden of urgency urinary incontinence: a systematic review. Eur Urol. 2014;65(1):79–95.n
15. Palmer MH, Wu JM, Marquez CS, Rupp B, Conover MM, Newman DK. "A secret club": focus groups about women's toileting behaviors. BMC Womens Health. 2019;19(1):44.nn
16. The State Council of Office of Population Censuses and Surveys. Data of the 2010 Census in China. China Statistics Press. 2012, 3.
17. Sun WY. The analysis of high risk factors on the adult female urinary incontinence of Qinghai. Beijing: Qinghai University; 2014.nnn
18. Liu TT. Nanning city related risk factors of female stress urinary incontinence and biomimetric electrical stimulation treatment. Beijing: Guangxi University of Chinese Medicine; 2014.nn
19. Li JX. Epidemiologic investigation of married woman with urinary incontinence in rural areas in Laiwu city. Beijing: Taishan Medical University; 2014.n
20. Arzigul A. Epidemiology and risk factors of female stress urinary incontinence in some counties and townships of Xinjiang of Hotan. Beijing: Xinjiang Medical University; 2013.n
21. Liu B, Wang L, Huang SS. Prevalence and risk factors of urinary incontinence among Chinese women in Shanghai. Int J Clin Exp Med. 2014;7(4):686–96.nn
22. He CJ, Zhang CF, Hai T, Yu LP, Wang Q, Gu BW, et al. Prevalence of overactive bladder and other lower urinary tract symptoms in female nurses in Beijing and its association with occupational stress. Chin J Urol. 2013;34(8):565–71.n
23. Xie JL, She X, Yang YW, Chen D. A survey on the incidence and risk factors of adult female stress urinary incontinence in Southeast Chongqing. J Mod Urol. 2013;18(6):590–3.n
24. Jiang Y, Yan L, Du FD, Zhen PT, Zhang L, Jiang L, et al. Prevalence and associated factors of female urinary incontinence in Hebei province. Chin J Obstet Gynecol. 2016;51(12):914–20.n
25. Song YC, Zhang PL, Xie L, Wang SQ, Zhao XL, Fan LJ, et al. Study on the epidemiology of urinary incontinence and the impact on the quality of life of adult female in Xi'an. Shanxi Med J. 2014;43(2):225–8.
26. Wang LH. Analysis of 1830 cases with female pelvic floor dysfunction in Suzhou district of Jiuquan City Gansu Province. Chin J Family Plan Gynecotokol. 2014;6(6):69–71.nn
27. Wan XH, Ding Y, Gulina A, Zainuer A, Lin L, Manrepa T. Epidemiologic study on the risk factors of the adult female urinary incontinence in Uygur of Kashi in Xinjiang. Chin J Obstet Gynecol. 2013;48(12):916–9.nn
28. Liu ZC, Wei XH, Liu XL, Luo MM, Hao Y. Investigation on female stress urinary incontinence in reclamation area. China Modern Doctor. 2015;53(36):120–3.n
29. Wu YH, Hu HW, Han CY. Survey on the current status of stress urinary incontinence among women during their menopausal transition in communities of Nanshan District. Shenzhen Chin Gener Pract. 2014;17(12):1400–3.nn
30. Horng S-S, Huang N, Wu S-I, Fang Y-T, Chou Y-J, Chou P. The epidemiology of urinary incontinence and it's influence on quality of life in Taiwanese middle-aged women. Neurourol Urodyn. 2013;32(4):371–6.nn
31. Chang KM, Hsieh CH, Chiang HS, Lee TS. Risk factors for urinary incontinence among women aged 60 or over with hypertension in Taiwan. Taiwan J Obst Gynecol. 2014a;53(2):183–6.
32. Chen C, Lu Y, Peng JW, Hu YJ, Lin XH, Wu XQ. Epidemiologic investigation on pelvic floor dysfunction among female in Wenzhou. J Wenzhou Med Univ. 2016;46(3):194–8.
33. Hu MY. Investigation and analysis of related factors of stress urinary incontinence of married women in Jiaojiang. Chin J Rural Med. 2013;20(9):69–70.
34. Han DH, Yuan JY, Bin XY, Yan LP. Prevalence and influence factors of urinary incontinence in 35–64 year old women in Chengdu Shuangliu District. J Pub Health Prev Med. 2017;28(2):139–42.n
35. Sun Y, Xue K, Su M, Xu H, Zhou F. Investigation and analysis of urinary incontinence in urban and rural adult women in Xuzhou City, Jiangsu Province. J Nurs Train. 2019;34(20):1881–3.nn
36. Deng L, Wei YP, Zhang LY, Liu J, Liu LL, Huang Y, et al. Epidemiological survey of adult female urinary incontinence in Nanning. J Guangxi Med Univ. 2013;30(6):963–6.nn
37. Wen F, Yang YJ, Zi D, Luo C, Chen GQ, Wu JJ. The status and comparison of 294 women with pelvic floor dysfunction dieseases among Miao, Buyi and Han nationalities. J Guizhou Med Univ. 2017;42(1):86–90.n
38. Zhang LJ, Chen YF, Qin WH, Huang HP. Epidemiological investigation on pelvic floor dysfunction in Wuxi. China Matern Child Health Care. 2015;30(16):2613–5.n
39. Li JJ, Guo HC, Wang XL, Wang BN, Wei J. Investigation and analysis of urinary tract symptoms among Changsha hospital gynecological clinic women. Guangdong Med J. 2013;34(22):3486–8.n
40. Li F, Liu J, Lie TT. An investigation of risk factors for adult female stress urinary incontinence in outpatient clinic. Shanxi Med J. 2014;43(6):756–7. nn
41. Wang X, Li ZG, Wang W, Hou J, Li JQ. Prevalence, quality of life and risk factors of urinary incontinence of elderly women in Jilin City. Chin J Gerontol. 2013;33(21):5422–3.nn
42. Shi LH, Wang WH, Li P, Tang HY, Zhang FY, Cao H, et al. A survey of the prevalence of stress urinary incontinence of women in Pingxiang. Contemp Med. 2016;22(33):34–5.n
43. Xin CY, Ge YH, Zhang CP. Incidence of urinary incontinence and quality of life of women aged 65 years and older in four communities in Urumqi. Chin J Gerontol. 2014;34(14):3979–81.nn
44. Zhou F, Xue K, Liu Y, Zhuo L, Tu S, Palmer MH. Toileting behaviors and factors associated with urinary incontinence in college-aged female students in China. Int Urogynecol J. 2019;31:961–71.n

45. Chu L, Wang JJ, Fan BZ, Sun J, Cao GY, Xu MJ, et al. The prevalence and risk factors of urinary incontinence among women in Shanghai. Prog Obstet Gynecol. 2015;24(6):421–4.nn
46. Gao JX, He XL, Li Y, Bai AS, Guo W, Ma YD, et al. Epidemiological analysis of female stress urinary incontinence in Yan'an City. J Kunming Med Univ. 2015;36(4):31–3.nn
47. Luo XM, Zhuoma, Liu CH, Ren NJ, Li D, Chen W. Epidemio ogical investigation of female stress urinary incontinence in Shannan City. J Clin Res. 2017;34(1):94–7.n
48. Xu L, Yang Y. Status quo of adult female urinary incontinence and quality of life in Shanghai. J Shanghai Jiaotong Univ (Med Sci). 2013;33(5):552–60. nn
49. Wang Y, Hu H, Xu K, Wang X, Na Y, Kang X. Prevalence, risk factors and the bother of lower urinary tract symptoms in China: a population-based survey. Int Urogynecol J. 2015;26(6):911–9.n
50. Huang D, Yang MY, Lin XM, Zhang L. Epidemiological studies of adult female urinary incontinence in Zhanjiang. China Matern Child Health Care. 2013;28(36):6019–22.
51. Li H, Liu XL, Cheng L. Epidemiological investigation and analysis of factors affecting stress urinary incontinence in climacteric women. China Matern Child Health Care. 2015;30(29):2613–5.
52. Lu S, Zhang H-L, Zhang Y-J, Shao Q-C. Prevalence and risk factors of urinary incontinence among perimenopausal women in Wuhan. J Huazhong Univ Sci Technol (Med Sci). 2016;36(5):723–6.
53. Li T, Zhang YJ, Zhang HL, Ding XH, Yu ZJ, Lu S. Prevalence and risk factors of stress urinary incontinence among perimenopausal women and its influence on daily life in women with sexual desire problem. Curr Med Sci. 2019;39(4):615–21.
54. Lu S, Zhang Y, Ding X, Zhang H. Investigation on the influencing factors of urinary incontinence among perimenopausal women in some areas of Hubei Province. Mater Child Health Care China. 2017;32(16):3896–900.n
55. Wang B, Zhang A. The incidence of urinary incontinence among women aged 35 to 64 in Changping district of Beijing and its impact on quality of life. Womens Health Res. 2019;19:15–46.nn
56. Chang KM, Hsieh CH, Chiang HS, Lee TS. Risk factors for urinary incontinence among women aged 60 or over with hypertension in Taiwan. Taiwan J Obstet Gynecol. 2014b;53(2):183–6.nn
57. Li RX, Ma M, Xiao XR, Xu Y, Li B. Analysis of prevalence and life quality and associared factors of stress urinary incontinence of the women aged 60–70 years in Shanghai. Geriatr Health Care. 2015;21(3):149–52.nn
58. Gao ML, Wang J, Wang JT, Song YT. Study on the prevalence of urinary incontinence among elderly people of residential community in Beijing city and the risk factors. Pract Geriatr. 2014;28(3):230–2.nn
59. Li Y, Zhang X, Liang X, Wang H, Zheng Y. Analysis and intervention of risk factors of urinary incontinence in elderly care institutions. Chin J Gerontol. 2019;39(2):461–4.n
60. Chen M, Chen X, Ding W, Zhang T, Feng W, Wang Q, et al. Survey of prevalence and influencing factors of elderly patients with urinary incontinence in medical and nursing institutions. Nurs Res. 2018;32(23):3791–5. nn
61. Zhu ZC, Zhu JM, Shao SH, Jiang RJ. Epidemiological investigation of female urinary incontinence in Yuhang City. Chin J Hum Sex. 2016;25(5):74–7.
62. Che X, Wu S, Chen Y, Huang Y, Yang Y. A survey of risk factors and quality of life in female medical staff with urinary incontinence. J Peking Univ (Health Sci). 2019;51(4):706–10.
63. Liu YJ, Qiao J, Yan H, et al. Prevalence of urinary incontinence and stress urinary incontinence on quality of life among female workers in Baoding railway Hebei Province. Occup Health. 2013;29(3):287–90.nn
64. Li H, Bai F, Zhang J, Bai H, Sun B. Epidemiological investigation of urinary incontinence in rural women in Liaoning. Chin For Health Digest. 2014;6:288–9.n
65. Harlow BL, Bavendam TG, Palmer MH, Brubaker L, Burgio KL, Lukacz ES, et al. The Prevention of Lower Urinary Tract Symptoms (PLUS) research consortium: a transdisciplinary approach toward promoting bladder health and preventing lower urinary tract symptoms in women across the life course. J Womens Health. 2018;27(3):283–9.nnn
66. Zhang N, He Y, Wang J, Zhang Y, Ding J, Hua KQ. Effects of a new community-based reproductive health intervention on knowledge of and attitudes and behaviors toward stress urinary incontinence among young women in Shanghai: a cluster-randomized controlled trial. Int Urogynecol J. 2016;27(4):545–53.n
67. Pelaez M, Gonzalez-Cerron S, Montejo R, Barakat R. Pelvic floor muscle training included in a pregnancy exercise program is effective in primary prevention of urinary incontinence: a randomized controlled trial. Neurourol Urodyn. 2014;33(1):67–71.
68. Paul Abrams, Wagg A. Incontinence. 6th ed. 2017.
69. Zhu L, Li L, Lang J-H, Xu T. Prevalence and risk factors for peri- and postpartum urinary incontinence in primiparous women in China: a prospective longitudinal study. Int Urogynecol J. 2012;23(5):563–72.
70. Palmer MH, Cockerell R, Griebling TL, Rantell A, van Houten P, Newman DK. Review of the 6th International Consultation on Incontinence: Primary prevention of urinary incontinence. Neurourol Urodyn. 2019.
71. Hagglund D, Olsson H, Leppert J. Urinary incontinence: an unexpected large problem among young females. Results from a population-based study. Fam Pract. 1999;16(5):506–9.
72. O'Halloran T, Bell RJ, Robinson PJ, Davis SR. Urinary incontinence in young nulligravid women: a cross-sectional analysis. Ann Intern Med. 2012;157(2):87–93.
73. Mishra GD, Barker MS, Herber-Gast GC, Hillard T. Depression and the incidence of urinary incontinence symptoms among young women: results from a prospective cohort study. Maturitas. 2015;81(4):456–61.
74. Bardino M, Di Martino M, Ricci E, Parazzini F. Frequency and determinants of urinary incontinence in adolescent and young nulliparous women. J Pediatr Adolesc Gynecol. 2015;28(6):462–70.
75. Da Roza T, Brandao S, Mascarenhas T, Jorge RN, Duarte JA. Urinary incontinence and levels of regular physical exercise in young women. Int J Sports Med. 2015;36(9):776–80.
76. Casey EK, Temme K. Pelvic floor muscle function and urinary incontinence in the female athlete. Phys Sportsmed. 2017;2017:1–9.
77. Palmer MH, Willis-Gray MG, Zhou F, Newman DK, Wu JM. Self-reported toileting behaviors in employed women: Are they associated with lower urinary tract symptoms? Neurourol Urodyn. 2017. https://doi.org/10.1002/nau.23337.
78. Wan X, Wu C, Xu D, Huang L, Wang K. Toileting behaviours and lower urinary tract symptoms among female nurses: a cross-sectional questionnaire survey. Int J Nurs Stud. 2017;65:1–7.
79. Palmer MH, Newman DK. Women's toileting behaviours: an online survey of female advanced practice providers. Int J Clin Pract. 2015;69(4):429–35.
80. Liu Y. Prevalence of lower urinary tract symptoms in female nurses and its relationship with toileting behavior. Beijing: Shandong University; 2013.
81. Zhu L, Lang J, Wang H, Han S, Huang J. The prevalence of and potential risk factors for female urinary incontinence in Beijing. China Menopause. 2008;15(3):566–9.
82. Walters MD. Urinary incontinence in women comes and goes, and reasons remain elusive. BJOG. 2015;122(6):824.
83. Zhang L. A population-based epidemiology survey of the lower urinary tract symptoms in adult Chinese women—cross-sectional study. London: Peking Union Medical College; 2015.
84. Volløyhaug I, Mørkved S, Salvesen Ø, Salvesen K. Pelvic organ prolapse and incontinence 15–23 years after first delivery: a cross-sectional study. BJOG. 2015;122(7):964–71.
85. Reigota RB, Pedro AO, de Souza Santos Machado V, Costa-Paiva L, Pinto-Neto AM. Prevalence of urinary incontinence and its association with multimorbidity in women aged 50 years or older: a population-based study. Neurourol Urodyn. 2016;35(1):62–8.
86. Kasikci M, Kilic D, Avsar G, Sirin M. Prevalence of urinary incontinence in older Turkish women, risk factors, and effect on activities of daily living. Arch Gerontol Geriatr. 2015;61(2):217–23.
87. Erekson EA, Cong X, Townsend MK, Ciarleglio MM. Ten-year prevalence and incidence of urinary incontinence in older women: a longitudinal analysis of the health and retirement study. J Am Geriatr Soc. 2016;64(6):1274–80.nn
88. Jian F, Liyan Z. Urinary incontinence classification criteria and stress urinary incontinence diagnosis. J Pract Obst Gynecol. 2003;19(2):71–3.

4

High dose versus low dose standardized cranberry proanthocyanidin extract for the prevention of recurrent urinary tract infection in healthy women

Asma Babar[1,2], Lynne Moore[2], Vicky Leblanc[3], Stéphanie Dudonné[3], Yves Desjardins[3], Simone Lemieux[3], Valérie Bochard[4], Denis Guyonnet[5] and Sylvie Dodin[1,2,6*]

Abstract

Purpose: Our objective was to assess the efficacy of a high dose cranberry proanthocyanidin extract for the prevention of recurrent urinary tract infection.

Material and methods: We recruited 145 healthy, adult women with a history of recurrent urinary tract infection, defined as ≥ 2 in the past 6 months or ≥ 3 in the past 12 months in this randomized, controlled, double-blind clinical trial. Participants were randomized to receive a high dose of standardized, commercially available cranberry proanthocyanidins (2 × 18.5 mg daily, n = 72) or a control low dose (2 × 1 mg daily, n = 73) for a 24-week period. During follow-up, symptomatic women provided urine samples for detection of pyuria and/or bacteriuria and received an appropriate antibiotic prescription. The primary outcome for the trial was the mean number of new symptomatic urinary tract infections during a 24-week intervention period. Secondary outcomes included symptomatic urinary tract infection with pyuria or bacteriuria.

Results: In response to the intervention, a non-significant 24% decrease in the number of symptomatic urinary tract infections was observed between groups (Incidence rate ratio 0.76, 95%CI 0.51–1.11). Post-hoc analyses indicated that among 97 women who experienced less than 5 infections in the year preceding enrolment, the high dose was associated with a significant decrease in the number of symptomatic urinary tract infections reported compared to the low dose (age-adjusted incidence rate ratio 0.57, 95%CI 0.33–0.99). No major side effects were reported.

Conclusion: High dose twice daily proanthocyanidin extract was not associated with a reduction in the number of symptomatic urinary tract infections when compared to a low dose proanthocyanidin extract. Our post-hoc results reveal that this high dose of proanthocyanidins may have a preventive impact on symptomatic urinary tract infection recurrence in women who experienced less than 5 infections per year.

Keywords: Women, Urinary tract infections, Proanthocyanidins, Cranberry, Prevention

*Correspondence: sylvie.dodin@fmed.ulaval.ca
[1] CHU de Québec-Laval University Research Center, Québec City, Canada
Full list of author information is available at the end of the article

Introduction

Urinary tract infection (UTI) is one of the main reasons for emergency medical consultation. One in three women over the age of 18 will experience a UTI, and many of them will have repeated infections [1]. Increasing resistance of pathogens to prescribed antibiotics, both in treatment and prophylaxis, as well as the side effects of antibiotics, reinforce the demand for alternatives that are effective and well tolerated [2].

Cranberry products are the most promising natural health alternatives for the prevention of UTIs [3]. Cranberry has been shown to inhibit the adhesion of uropathogenic *Escherichia coli* to uroepithelial cells [4]. In vitro, cranberry proanthocyanidins (PACs) with type A-linkages, have been identified as responsible for this anti-adhesion effect [5]. Clinical trials have been conducted to test the efficacy of cranberry products, mainly in the form of juices, but their results remain discordant [3]. This discrepancy is mainly explained by a lack of compliance, lack of statistical power and variable PAC concentrations in the tested products. Indeed, PAC concentrations are not disclosed in the majority of clinical trials. According to ex vivo clinical studies (dose–effect studies evaluating the optimal dose for urine anti-adhesion effect), the quantification of PACs requires standardized, reproducible methods and should be at least 36 mg/day [5, 6]. We hypothesize that the efficacy of cranberry products on the prevention of recurrent UTIs in women could be improved with the use of an optimal PACs dose (standardized at 2 × 18.5 mg/day).

Materials and methods

The Cranberry Extract for Prevention of Recurrent UTI Trial (PACCANN) was a randomized, double blind, controlled, clinical trial performed at the Institute of Nutrition and Functional Foods (INAF). The study was conducted according to the guidelines of the Helsinki Declaration (2013 revision). The protocol, consent form and all procedures were approved by the institutional ethics committee of Laval University. Written informed consent was obtained from all study participants. The protocol was registered on ClinicalTrials.gov on October 9, 2015 (NCT02572895) and has been published in BMC Urology [7].

Study population

We enrolled sexually active non-pregnant women aged 18 years and over presenting with recurrent UTI as diagnosed by a physician (defined as ≥ 2 UTIs in the past 6 months or ≥ 3 UTIs in the past 12 months). Women were recruited in the Laval University community in Quebec City, Canada, through e-mail list serves and local clinician referrals as well as posters in medical clinics, social media, paid advertising and word of mouth. Eligibility of potential participants was verified by the study coordinator according to inclusion and exclusion criteria (Table 1). The risks and benefits of the study have been thoroughly discussed and the consent form was signed at the first of three visits at INAF.

Study product

The high dose intervention consisted of twice daily intake of commercially available 120 mg Urophenol™, a purified cranberry extract from whole fruit (*Vaccinium macrocarpon* Aiton) standardized at min 15% PACs. The control dose was standardized at 1% PACs which is comparable to the majority of cranberry products approved by Health Canada [8]. Cranberry PACs were manufactured by Nutra Canada (now part of Diana Food Canada) and similar in size, smell and taste. Capsules were distributed in opaque packaging in order to conceal slight colour variations from the research team. Total PAC content of each treatment was validated at INAF's analytical laboratory using the 4-dimethylaminocinnamaldehyde (BL-DMAC) method [9] ("Appendix 1"). PACs were also characterized by normal-phase analytical HPLC coupled with fluorescence detection, as previously described [10].

Randomization

Concealed randomization was generated using computer assisted randomization by blocks of 10. Eligible women were assigned 1:1 to either high PAC (2 × 18.5 mg capsules per day) or low PAC (2 × 1 mg capsules per day) content cranberry capsules for 24 weeks. All clinical investigation, laboratory analysis, data collection and assessment were blinded to the randomization allocation.

Table 1 Admissibility criteria

Inclusion criteria
Sexually active healthy women
Aged 18 years and older
Recent history of recurrent urinary tract infections[a]
≥ 2 UTIs in the past 6 months and/or
≥ 3 UTIs in the past 12 months
No consumption of cranberry product, polyphenol or antioxidant supplements in the last 2 weeks
Exclusion criteria
Pregnancy
History of anatomical urogenital anomalies, urogenital tract surgery
History of acute or chronic renal failure, nephrolithiasis
History of intestinal diseases causing malabsorption
Anticoagulant medication in the last month
Known allergy or intolerance to cranberry

[a] UTIs diagnosed by a clinician and treated with antibiotic therapy

Clinical follow-up

Each visit (0, 12 and 24 weeks) included a short questionnaire documenting socio-demographic characteristics (T=0 only), medication and natural health product intake, quality of life (SF-12) [11], risk factors for UTIs, and a validated food frequency questionnaire [12] modified for our study to specifically include sixty-one foods containing PACs. Participants were instructed to obtain a midstream urine sample on which dipstick urinalysis and pregnancy tests were performed.

During their participation, women were asked to contact the study coordinator if they presented symptoms of UTI to schedule a visit at INAF in order to confirm the clinical diagnosis, provide a urine sample and receive an appropriate antibiotic prescription. A dipstick urinalysis using Chemstrip 9 (Roche Diagnostics USA) was used to confirm pyuria and urine samples were outsourced to the Laval University Hospital Center microbiology laboratory for culture. In line with the pragmatic aspect of this trial, women who were unable to present themselves to the research facility during a symptomatic episode were provided with an empiric antibiotic by prescription of the clinician.

Women that discontinued the intervention were asked to present themselves at the 12 and 24-week visit to complete intention to treat analysis. All participants were asked not to consume other products containing cranberry derivatives for the duration of the study.

Outcomes

The primary outcome was the number of symptomatic UTIs during the 24-week follow-up period. Symptomatic UTI was defined as acute urinary symptoms such as urine frequency, urgency, dysuria, pelvic pain, and hematuria in the absence of alternate diagnoses as assessed by study staff. The choice of symptomatic UTI was based on local [13] and international guidelines [14] as well as on realistic clinical settings in North America where empirical therapy is prescribed on the basis of clinical symptoms [14]. This outcome increased our capture of UTI episodes and trial conduct as we anticipated that certain women would be unable to present themselves to the research facilities to provide a urine sample.

Secondary outcomes were symptomatic UTI with pyuria and symptomatic UTI with bacteriuria. Women who presented both symptoms and a positive leukocyte esterase dipstick result, were diagnosed as having symptomatic UTI with pyuria. Episodes were categorized as symptomatic UTI with bacteriuria in the presence of $\geq 10^3$ CFU/ml of uropathogenic bacteria. Women with antibiotic treatment for symptomatic UTI during the study period continued to take the cranberry capsules and remained in the study for 24 weeks.

Compliance and side effects

Participants completed a daily journal to record compliance and were asked to bring capsule bottles to each visit in order to count remaining capsules. A bi-weekly email reminder was sent to encourage participation. Side effects were evaluated at each visit and participants were asked to document symptoms in their daily journal.

Sample size and statistical analysis

We estimated that 35% of patients in the control group would present at least one UTI during the 24-week follow-up period [3]. We needed to recruit 126 women to detect a clinically significant difference of 25% between the 2 groups (10% of women assigned to the experimental group would experience at least 1 UTI with a power of 80%). We estimated that 15% of randomized participants would be lost to follow-up [15], therefore 148 women needed to be recruited in order for at least 126 participants to complete the 24-week intervention.

The Poisson regression model was used to compare the incidence of symptomatic UTI during the 24-week follow-up. A Kaplan Meier estimate with a log-rank test was used to compare time to first UTI between the two treatment arms. Intention to treat analyses were performed in all randomly assigned subjects with the observation time censored at the date that the participant abandoned or the date of last contact (either a scheduled study visit or visit for UTI treatment). All statistical analyses were performed using SAS University Edition software (SAS Institute Inc., Cary, NC, USA).

Post-hoc and sensitivity analysis

In the case of imbalanced groups, we generated relative rate estimates adjusted for potential confounding variables. Univariate regression analyses were performed for relevant variables collected at the baseline visit and data collected from post-hoc questions. Missing data was excluded from analyses for post-hoc questions. Variables with a p value < 0.20 in univariate analysis were included in the multivariate regression model. Interactions with the treatment groups were tested in multivariate regression model using a backward elimination method. Interactions with a p value < 0.05 are presented in the results by subgroup of the effect-modifying factor.

The incidence of UTI with pyuria or bacteriuria was estimated using a statistical imputation method for missing urine samples with two extreme assumptions: symptomatic UTI episodes without urine samples were classified as (1) no symptomatic UTI with pyuria or bacteriuria; and (2) symptomatic UTI with pyuria or bacteriuria.

Results

Between August 2015 and December 2016, 267 potential participants were assessed for eligibility, of which 122 were excluded mainly because they did not meet criteria for recurrent UTI (Fig. 1). From August 2015 to April 2017, 145 women were recruited and randomly assigned to consume the high dose or low dose PAC capsules for a 24-week period. Reasons for discontinuing the intervention and abandoning study are shown in Appendices 2 and 3. The groups were well balanced in terms of

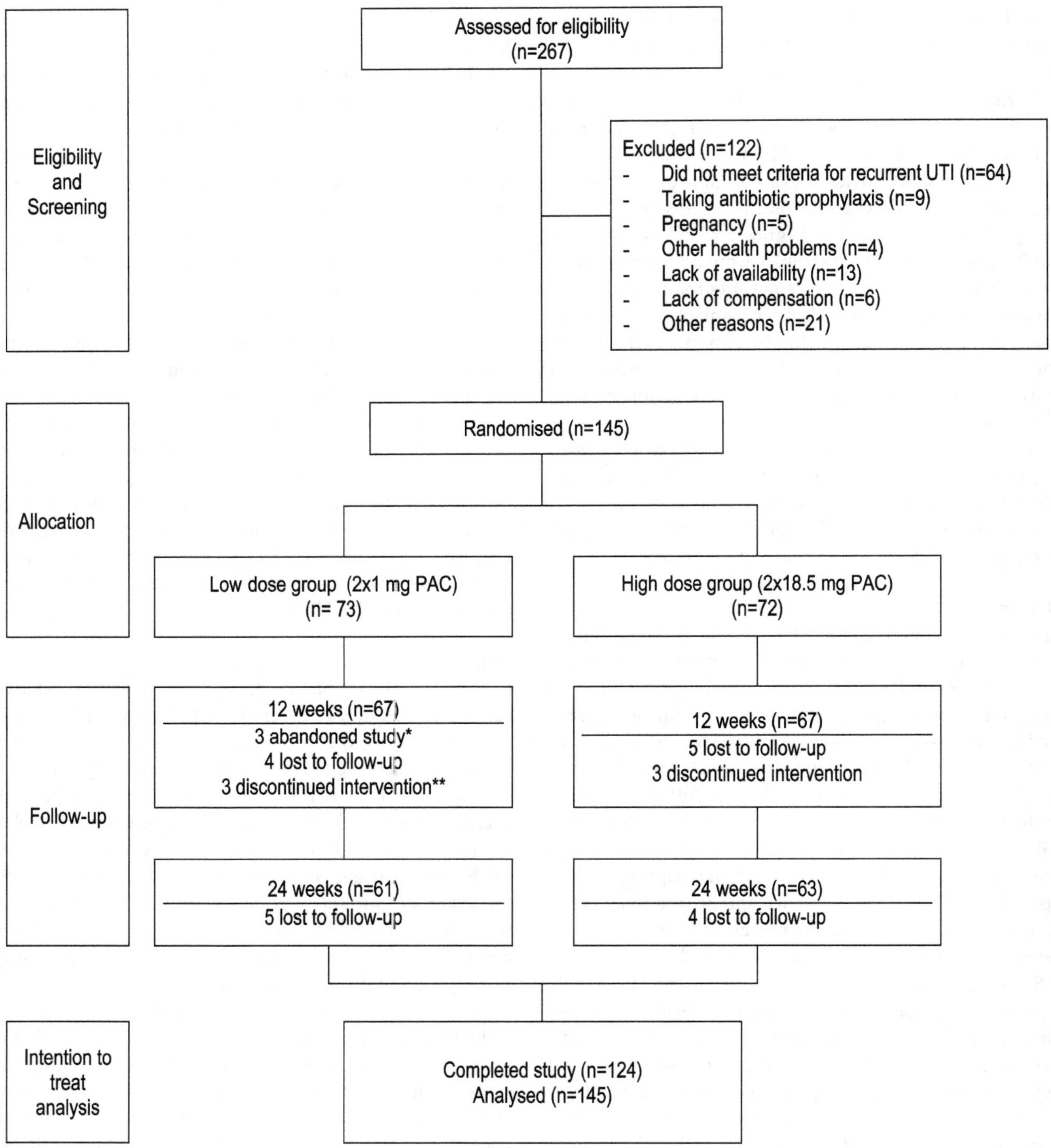

Fig. 1 Participant flow diagram.

*Women who abandoned the study provided a date and specific reason for their cessation of participation in the trial **Women who ceased the intake of cranberry extract capsules, but presented themselves at study visits

Table 2 Baseline demographic characteristics of participants by study arm

Demographic characteristics	Low dose group, 2 × 1 mg PAC (n = 73)	High dose group, 2 × 18.5 mg PAC (n = 72)	*P**
Age (mean ± SD)**,***	32.5 ± 14.2	27.2 ± 8.8	0.009
Age subgroup, years, n (%)			0.028
18–24 years	30 (41.1)	37 (51.4)	
25–44 years	29 (39.7)	31 (43.1)	
> 45 years	14 (19.2)	4 (5.6)	
Age subgroup, years, n (%)			0.003
18–51 years	62 (84.9)	71 (98.6)	
> 51 years	11 (15.1)	1 (1.4)	
Ethnic origin			0.681
Caucasian	65 (89.0)	65 (90.3)	
Non-Caucasian	6 (8.2)	5 (6.9)	
Biracial	2 (2.7)	2 (2.8)	
Marital status			0.230
Single	25 (34.3)	26 (36.1)	
Common law	33 (45.2)	39 (54.2)	
Married	13 (17.8)	7 (9.7)	
Divorced	2 (2.7)	0 (0)	
Has children	21 (28.7)	12 (16.7)	0.082
Living environment			0.998
Urban	50 (68.5)	49 (68.1)	
Suburban	18 (24.7)	18 (25)	
Rural	5 (6.9)	5 (6.9)	
Education			0.814
University	39 (53.4)	42 (58.3)	
College	28 (38.4)	24 (33.3)	
Secondary school	6 (8.2)	6 (8.3)	

*Comparability of numerical and categorical baseline characteristics between groups was assessed with a student's t-test and ANOVA and chi-squared tests, respectively

**Numbers represent frequency (%) unless otherwise indicated

***Significant difference between groups (student t-test, $p = 0.009$)

demographic (Table 2) and clinical (Table 3) characteristics. However, women randomized to the high dose group were significantly younger (mean age 27.2 ± 8.8 years old) than those randomized in the low dose group (mean age 32.5 ± 14.2 years old) (Student t-test, $p = 0.009$).

Symptomatic UTI

A total of 45 symptomatic UTIs were diagnosed in the high dose PAC group compared to 59 in the low dose group. The annualized incidence rate of symptomatic UTI for women receiving 2 × 18.5 mg PACs at 24 weeks was 1.48 (95%CI 1.11–1.99) compared to 1.96 (95%CI 1.52–2.53) in women receiving 2 × 1 mg PACs (Incidence rate ratio (IRR) = 0.76, 95% CI 0.51–1.11; Table 4). UTI-free median was 24.0 weeks in the high dose group compared to 16.6 weeks in the low dose group. The hazard ratio for the difference between the number of subjects who had experienced a first symptomatic UTI by the end of the 24-week period was 0.73 (95% CI 0.45–1.16; Fig. 2).

Univariate Poisson regression analysis for total number of symptomatic UTIs and known risk factors are shown in Table 5. After adjustment for age, only the number of UTI in the 12 months preceding enrolment showed a significant interaction between groups. Among participants with less than 5 UTIs in the 12 months preceding enrolment (n = 97), the age-adjusted annualized incidence rate of UTI in the high dose group was 1.32 (95%CI 0.81–2.13) compared to 2.29 (95%CI 1.66–3.16) in the low-dose group (IRR = 0.57, 95%CI 0.33–0.99) (Table 6).

Symptomatic UTI with pyuria

Data were obtained from women who presented themselves to the research facility in order to provide a urine sample in 70 out of 104 symptomatic UTI episodes. Eighty-one percent of the 70 urine samples obtained presented pyuria as measured by a positive leucocyte esterase dipstick test. No statistically significant reductions in the incidence rate of symptomatic UTI with pyuria were found between treatment groups. In women with less than 5 UTIs in the 12 months prior to enrolment, the daily intake of 2 × 18.5 mg PAC, compared to 2 × 1 mg PAC, was associated with a statistically significant 47% reduction in the age-adjusted incidence rate of symptomatic UTI with pyuria (IRR = 0.54, 95%CI 0.30–0.99), where symptomatic UTI without urine samples were classified as symptomatic UTI with pyuria (Table 7)).

Symptomatic UTI with bacteriuria

Urine culture was performed in 61 of the 70 urine samples collected during symptomatic UTI. A positive culture was confirmed in 49% of the 61 urine samples analyzed during symptomatic UTI. No statistically significant reductions in the age-adjusted incidence rate of symptomatic UTI with bacteriuria were found between groups nor in sub-group analyses in women with less than 5 UTIs in the 12 months prior to enrolment (Table 8).

Compliance, side effects and adherence to double-blind procedures

Compliance based on number of returned capsules at 24 weeks was similar in both groups (92.9% in the high dose group vs 92.7% in the low dose group, student t-test $p = 0.9$). Compliance according to daily intake journals was comparable in both groups, 87.3% in the high dose group and 88.8% in the low dose group (Student t-test, $p = 0.6$). No serious adverse events occurred in either of the study groups. The only reported side

Table 3 Baseline clinical characteristics of participants by study arm

Clinical characteristics	Low dose group, 2 × 1 mg PAC (n = 73)	High dose group, 2 × 18.5 mg PAC (n = 72)	*P* value*
Number of episodes of UTI in the past 6 months**			0.816
1	13 (17.8)	8 (11.1)	
2	34 (46.6)	37 (51.4)	
3	17 (23.3)	16 (22.2)	
4	6 (8.22)	7 (9.7)	
≥ 5	3 (4.11)	4 (5.6)	
Number of episodes of UTI in the past 12 months			0.249
2	13 (17.8)	7 (9.72)	
3	22 (30.1)	29 (40.3)	
4	11 (15.1)	15 (20.8)	
≥ 5	27 (37.0)	21 (26.17)	
Frequency of sexual intercourse (per week)			0.304
≤ 1	22 (30.1)	14 (19.4)	
2–4	34 (46.6)	41 (56.9)	
5–6	10 (13.7)	13 (18.1)	
≥ 7	7 (9.6)	4 (5.6)	
Number of sexual partners			0.256
0	5 (6.9)	1 (1.4)	
1	67 (91.8)	70 (97.2)	
2	1 (1.4)	1 (1.4)	
Stability in sexual relations			0.987
No stability	3 (4.1)	2 (1.4)	
Stable in the past month	7 (9.6)	6 (8.3)	
Stable in the past 6 months	16 (21.9)	15 (20.8)	
Stable in the past year	46 (63.0)	48 (66.7)	
Prefer not to respond	1 (1.4)	1 (1.4)	
New partner in last month	4 (5.5)	5 (6.9)	0.715
Type of Contraception			0.373
Hormonal contraception	43 (58.9)	53 (73.6)	
Spermicide	1(1.4)	0	
Non hormonal IUD	7 (9.6)	4 (5.6)	
Condom	17 (23.3)	11 (15.3)	
None	5 (6.8)	4 (5.6)	
First UTI before age 15	15 (20.6)	16 (22.2)	0.839
Maternal history of UTI	38 (52.1)	43 (59.7)	0.352
Personal history of recurrent UTI***			0.775
< 1 year	4 (8.2)	2 (4.3)	
1–2 years	9 (18.4)	12 (25.5)	
3–5 years	15 (30.6)	15 (31.9)	
6–10 years	14 (28.6)	10 (21.3)	
> 10 years	7 (14.3)	8 (17.0)	
Missing data	24	25	
Hydration (average litres of water per day)***			0.147
Mean ± SD	1.62 ± 0.75	1.81 ± 0.63	
< 1	9 (15.8)	4 (7.0)	
≥ 1–2	30 (52.6)	27 (47.4)	
> 2–3	13 (22.8)	23 (40.4)	
≥ 3	5 (8.8)	3 (7.0)	
Missing data	16	15	

Table 3 (continued)

Clinical characteristics	Low dose group, 2 × 1 mg PAC (n=73)	High dose group, 2 × 18.5 mg PAC (n=72)	*P* value*
Alcohol consumption (per week)***			0.140
<1	7 (12.7)	15 (25.9)	
1–3	28 (50.9)	21 (36.2)	
>4	20 (36.4)	22 (37.9)	
Missing data	18	14	
Tobacco use***			0.448
Smoker	5 (8.8)	3 (5.2)	
Non-smoker	52 (91.2)	55 (94.8)	
Missing data	16	14	

*Comparability of numerical and categorical baseline characteristics between groups was assessed with a student's t-test and ANOVA and chi-squared tests, respectively

**Numbers represent frequency (%) unless otherwise indicated

***Factors questioned during the follow-up period with missing data indicated

Table 4 Incidence of symptomatic UTI at 24 weeks by study arm

	Low dose group, 2 × 1 mg PAC (n=73)	High dose group, 2 × 18.5 mg PAC (n=72)	Incidence rate ratio (95% CI)	*p* value
Subjects reporting symptomatic UTI, episodes, n (%)				
0	34 (46.6)	41 (57.0)		
1	26 (35.6)	21 (29.2)		
2	8 (11.0)	7 (9.7)		
3	4 (5.5)	2 (2.8)		
4	0 (0.0)	1 (1.4)		
5	1 (1.4)	0 (0.0)		
≥1	39 (53.4)	31 (43.1)		
Total symptomatic UTIs, episodes	59	45		
Follow-up, days (mean ± SD)	151 ± 43	154 ± 39		
Total person-days	10,997	11,088		
UTI, annualized incidence density (95% CI)[a]	1.96 (1.52–2.53)	1.48 (1.11–1.99)	0.76 (0.51–1.11)	0.16
UTI, age-adjusted annualized incidence density (95% CI)[b]	2.28 (1.74–2.98)	1.93 (1.36–2.72)	0.85 (0.57–1.26)	0.42

[a] UTI = urinary tract infection

[b] Incidence rate ratios and *P* values for the number of UTIs per woman-year of observation were determined from the generalized linear model with the Poisson distribution specified

effect, dyspepsia, led to a discontinuation of the intervention of one participant in each group. Participants were asked if they were aware of which treatment group they were assigned to in order to validate the effectiveness of blinding procedures. The majority of women in both groups responded that they were unaware of group allocation as show in "Appendix 4".

Discussion

This randomized clinical trial is the first to evaluate the efficacy of a standardized split daily dose of 37 mg cranberry PACs in capsule form on symptomatic UTI. It is of particular interest that this dose was compared to another cranberry extract containing a low concentration of PACs, as often found on the Canadian supplement market to prevent UTI. Our results indicate that the intake of 2 × 18.5 mg PACs daily was associated with a non-statistically significant 24% reduction in the risk of symptomatic UTI compared to a daily dose of 2 × 1 mg PACs during a 24-week follow-up period, similar to the results of a recent meta-analysis [16].

The present study is distinct given that we recruited according to a guideline-based definition of recurrent UTI [17]. Our cohort had a higher mean incidence of UTI prior to study enrolment (mean UTI = 2.4/6 months and 3.9/1 year) compared to similar trials such as Maki

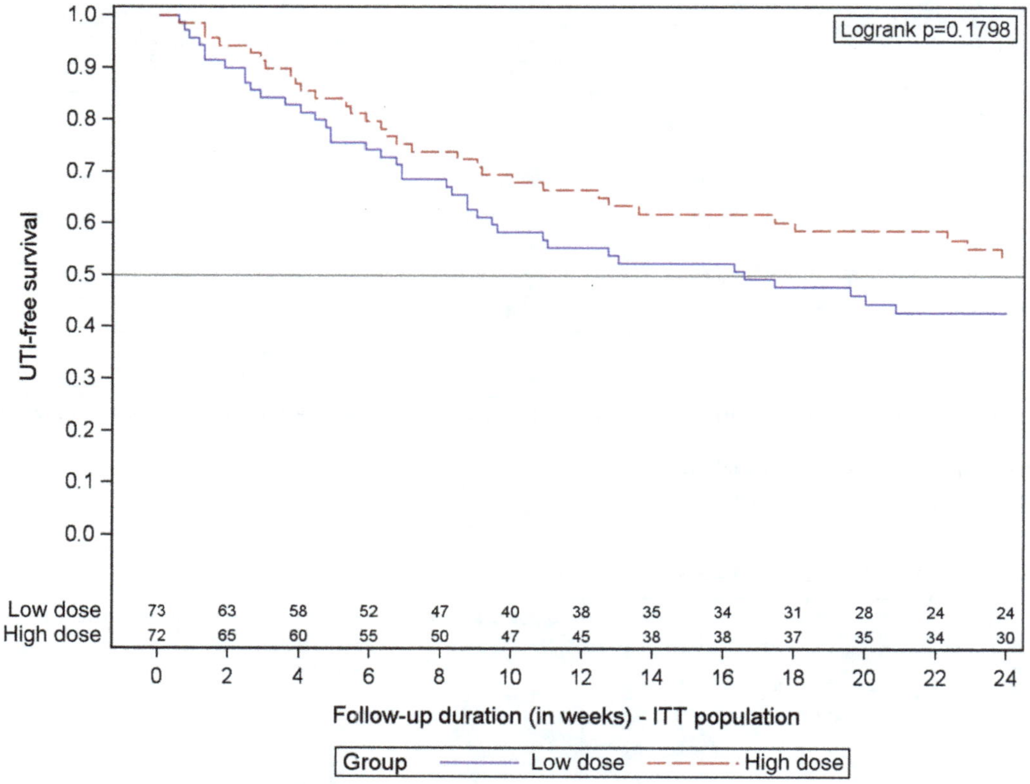

Fig. 2 Kaplan Meier analysis of survival to first UTI by treatment group

Table 5 Univariate poisson regression analysis of total number of symptomatic UTIs and baseline risk factors

Variable	*p* value Incidence rate ratio (95%CI)
Age (ref. = 18–45 years)	*p* = 0.01
45 years and older	1.97 (1.25–3.11)
Number infections past 12 months (ref. < 5)	*p* = 0.02
≥ 5	1.62 (1.1–2.39)
Frequency of sexual intercourse (per week) (ref. < 1)	*p* = 0.12
2–4	0.63 (0.4–0.97)
≥ 5–6	0.78 (0.46–1.32)
Hormonal contraception (ref. = no)	*p* = 0.84
Yes	0.96 (0.65–1.41)
Hydratation (average number of litres of liquid per day) (ref. < 1 L/day)	*p* = 0.19
1–2 L/day	0.57 (0.32–1.02)
≥ 2 L/day	0.66 (0.36–1.18)

et al. [18] (1.65/6 months), Barbosa-Cesnik et al. [19] (1.13 /1 year) or Stothers et al. [20] (2.8/1 year). The proportion of women in the 2 mg PAC group that experienced more than 1 UTI (53.4%) was also greater than the estimated 35% [21] used to calculate our sample size. Considering these key differences with previous reports, we explored if UTI burden at baseline could impact the treatment effect. Statistical analysis confirmed that number of recurrent UTI was indeed a modifying factor. In women who experienced fewer than 5 UTI (mean number = 3.1) in the year prior to enrolment, symptomatic UTIs were significantly reduced by 43%. No significant effect was observed in women with higher past UTI burden.

Table 6 Poisson regression sensitivity analysis of symptomatic UTIs by number of UTI prior to enrolment

	Low dose group, 2 × 1 mg PAC	High dose group, 2 × 18.5 mg PAC	Incidence rate ratio (95% CI) *p* value
Participants with less than 5 UTIs in the 12 months preceding enrolment	n = 46	n = 51	
Number of symptomatic UTI	39	21	
Symptomatic UTI, age-adjusted incidence density (95% CI)[a]	2.29 (1.66–3.16)	1.32 (0.81–2.13)	0.57 (0.33–0.99) $p = 0.048$
Participants with 5 UTIs or more in the 12 months preceding enrolment	n = 27	n = 21	
Number of symptomatic UTI	20	24	
Symptomatic UTI, age-adjusted incidence density (95% CI)[a]	2.23 (1.37–3.61)	3.34 (1.96–5.68)	1.50 (0.81–2.76) $p = 0.195$

[a] Incidence rate ratios and *p* value for symptomatic UTIs per woman-year of observation by number of UTI in the 12 months prior to enrolment (less than 5 UTIs vs greater than 5 UTIs) and adjusted for age group (< 45 years vs ≥ 45 year)

In women experiencing higher level of UTI (> 5), certain factors that were not measured in our study could explain the mitigated response to PAC intake. It is possible that in these women, UTI recurrence may be the result of complex interactions between bacterial urovirulence and a particular host susceptibility (altered gut microbiota, less efficient adaptive immune response) [22–24]. Considering that PACs are poorly absorbed and are difficult to quantify in the urine, future studies should focus on the effect of these molecules on the gut microbiota, a natural reservoir for uropathogenic *Escherichia coli* [22, 25]. Gut microbiota composition and function largely vary between individuals which might explain differences in individual's susceptibility to UTI. This could be mediated by a direct effect (e.g. growth inhibition of pathobiont [26], encroachment of uropathogenic bacteria in the gut) or an indirect effect (microbial metabolism of PAC or potential bioactive urinary metabolites). In order to provide mechanistic insight explaining different levels of recurrence, feces and urine samples are being analysed and results will be published in a future article.

Our study was based on medical practice in Quebec whereby many women receive antibiotics without delaying treatment for several days while awaiting urine culture results. Similarly, Maki et al. [18]. compared daily intake of 41 mg PACs from cranberry juice cocktail compared to a placebo beverage on the incidence of symptomatic UTI during a 24-week follow-up. In our study, pyuria was present in 81% and bacteriuria was confirmed in 49% of the urine samples provided by participants during symptomatic UTI. This corresponds to the similar proportion of 80% of symptomatic UTI with pyuria and 60% with bacteriuria in a total of 106 symptomatic UTI episodes presented by Maki et al. [18].

This study had limitations that could influence our findings. The use of a control dose instead of placebo may explain why we were unable to find a significant reduction in the recurrence of UTI in our cohort with a high UTI burden. A study conducted by Vostavola et al. has shown that 2.8 mg PAC daily can significantly impact the incidence of recurrent UTIs compared to placebo [27]. Moreover, urine cultures were incomplete for a proportion of urine samples provided by symptomatic participants. Urine culture contaminated by improper clean-catch urine technique were excluded from analyses in order to mitigate a risk of detection bias. We also experienced technical issues such as delays in delivery to the microbiology laboratory and improperly stored samples.

Conclusions

The intake of 2 × 18.5 mg PACs daily was associated with a non-statistically significant 24% reduction in the risk of symptomatic UTI compared to a daily dose of 2 × 1 mg PACs during a 24-week follow-up period. In a subset of participating women with a history of less than 5 UTIs per year, the daily consumption of 2 × 18.5 mg PACs resulted in a significant reduction in the rate of symptomatic UTI during the trial period compared to 2 × 1 mg PAC. These findings need to be tested in women with moderate burden of recurrent UTI who may benefit from a preventive treatment with a split dose of 37 mg/day of PACs from cranberry extract, with few associated side effects. Further investigations are also needed to examine dose-dependent impacts of cranberry PACs for the prevention of recurrent UTI and their effects on the microbiota.

Table 7 Incidence of symptomatic UTI with pyuria at 24 weeks by study arm

	Low dose group, 2 × 1 mg PAC	High dose group, 2 × 18.5 mg PAC	Incidence rate ratio (95% CI) *p* value
Symptomatic UTI with pyuria, episodes, n (%)[a]	n=73	n=72	
0	50 (68.5)	53 (73.6)	
1	17 (23.3)	14 (19.4)	
2	5 (6.8)	4 (5.6)	
3	0 (0.0)	0 (0.0)	
4	1 (1.4))	1 (1.4)	
≥1	23 (31.5)	19 (26.4)	
Total symptomatic UTIs with pyuria, episodes	31	26	
Total person-days	10,997	11,088	
Symptomatic UTI with pyuria, annualized incidence density (95% CI)	1.03 (0.72–1.46)	0.86 (0.58–1.26)	0.83 (0.49–1.40) $p=0.49$
Symptomatic UTI with pyuria, age adjusted annualized incidence density (95% CI)	1.24 (0.86–1.77)	1.21 (0.77–1.89)	0.98 (0.57–1.68) $p=0.94$
Subgroup analyses In women with < 5 UTI in past 12 months	n=46	n=51	
Symptomatic UTI with pyuria	21	12	
Symptomatic UTI with pyuria, annualized incidence density (95% CI)	1.05 (0.60–1.50)	0.55 (0.24–0.87)	0.53 (0.26–1.07) $p=0.08$
Symptomatic UTI with pyuria, age-adjusted annualized incidence density (95% CI)	1.27 (0.82–1.95)	0.83 (0.44–1.54)	0.65 (0.31–1.37) $p=0.26$
Symptomatic UTI with pyuria, episodes, n (%)[b]	n=73	n=72	
0	39 (53.4)	45 (62.5)	
1	23 (31.5)	18 (25.0)	
2	6 (8.2)	7 (9.7)	
3	4 (5.5)	1 (1.4)	
4	0 (0.0)	1 (1.4)	
5	1 (1.4)	0 (0.0)	
≥1	34 (46.6)	27 (37.5)	
Total symptomatic UTIs with pyuria, episodes	52	39	
Total person-days	10,997	11,088	
Symptomatic UTI with pyuria, annualized incidence density (95% CI)	1.73 (1.32–2.27)	1.28 (0.94–1.72)	0.74 (0.49–1.13) $p=0.16$
Symptomatic UTI with pyuria, age-adjusted annualized incidence density (95% CI)	2.05 (1.54–2.71)	1.75 (1.22–2.52)	0.86 (0.56–1.32) $p=0.48$
Subgroup analyses In women with < 5 UTI in past 12 months	n=46	n=51	
Symptomatic UTI with pyuria	35	17	
Symptomatic UTI with pyuria, age-adjusted annualizec incidence density (95% CI)	1.75 (1.26–2.20)	0.78 (0.41–1.16)	0.45 (0.25–0.80) $p=0.01$
Symptomatic UTI with pyuria, age-adjusted annualizec incidence density (95% CI)	2.1 (1.50–2.94)	1.14 (0.68–1.92)	0.54 (0.30–0.99) $p=0.047$

[a] Symptomatic UTI episodes without urine sample were considered as no symptomatic UTI with pyuria

[b] Symptomatic UTI episodes without urine sample were considered as symptomatic UTI with pyuria

Table 8 Incidence of symptomatic UTI with bacteriuria at 24 weeks by study arm

	Low dose group, 2 × 1 mg PAC	High dose group, 2 × 18.5 mg PAC	Incidence rate ratio (95% CI) *p* value
Symptomatic UTI with bacteriuria, episodes, n (%)[a]	n=73	n=72	
0	55 (75.3)	63 (87.5)	
1	17 (23.3)	7 (9.7)	
2	1 (1.4)	2 (2.8)	
≥1	18 (24.7)	9 (12.5)	
Total symptomatic UTIs with bacteriuria, episodes	19	11	
Total person-days	10,997	11,088	
Symptomatic UTI with bacteriuria, annualized incidence density (95% CI)	0.63 (0.40–0.99)	0.36 (0.20–065)	0.57 (0.27–1.21) $p=0.14$
Symptomatic UTI with bacteriuria, age-adjusted annualized incidence density (95% CI)	0.76 (0.48–1.21)	0.53 (0.27–1.02)	0.69 (0.32–1.49) $p=0.34$
Subgroup analyses In women with < 5 UTI in past 12 months	n=46	n=51	
Symptomatic UTI with bacteriuria	14	5	
Symptomatic UTI with bacteriuria, annualized incidence density (95% CI)	0.70 (0.42–1.18)	0.23 (0.10–0.55)	0.33 (0.12–0.91) $p=0.03$
Symptomatic UTI with bacteriuria, age-adjusted annualized incidence density (95% CI)	0.85 (0.50–1.43)	0.35 (0.14–0.89)	0.41 (0.14–1.19) $p=0.10$
Subjects reporting symptomatic UTI with bacteriuria, episodes, n %)[b]			
0	42 (57.5)	51 (70.8)	
1	22 (30.1)	15 (20.8)	
2	6 (8.2)	4 (5.6)	
3	3 (4.1)	1 (1.4)	
4	0 (0.0)	1 (1.4)	
≥1	31 (42.5)	21 (29.2)	
Total symptomatic UTIs with bacteriuria, episodes	43	30	
Total person-days	10,997	11,088	
Symptomatic UTI with bacteriuria, annualized incidence density (95% CI)	1.43 (1.06–1.93)	0.99 (0.69–1.41)	0.69 (0.43–1.10) $p=0.12$
Symptomatic UTI with bacteriuria, age-adjusted annualized incidence density (95% CI)	1.71 (1.26–2.33)	1.40 [0.93–2.10)	0.81 (0.50–1.32) $p=0.40$
Subgroup analyses In women with < 5 UTI in past 12 months	n=46	n=51	
Symptomatic UTI with bacteriuria	28	13	
Symptomatic UTI with bacteriuria, annualized incidence density (95% CI)	1.40 (0.97–2.03)	0.60 (0.35–1.03)	0.43 (0.22–0.83) $p=0.01$
Symptomatic UTI with bacteriuria, age-adjusted annualized incidence density (95% CI)	1.70 (1.17–2.46)	0.93 (0.52–1.66)	0.55 (0.28–1.08) $p=0.08$

[a] Symptomatic UTI episodes without urine sample were considered as no symptomatic UTI with uropathogenic bacteriuria > 10^3 CFU/ml

[b] Symptomatic UTI episodes without urine sample were considered as symptomatic UTI with uropathogenic bacteriuria > 10^3 CFU/ml

Appendix 1

See Table 9.

Table 9 Cranberry extract composition in polyphenols

Compound (mg/capsule)	Low dose group	High dose group
PAC[a]	1.00	18.50
PAC oligomers[b]	0.35	4.15
PAC polymers[b]	0.55	6.50
Phenolic acids[c]	0.28	2.30
Anthocyanins[c]	0.11	0.55
Flavonols[c]	0.32	1.65

[a] BL-DMAC equivalent A2

[b] HPLC normal phase fluorescence

[c] HPLC inverse phase

Appendix 2

See Table 10.

Table 10 Reasons for abandoning study

Reason	Low dose group (n = 12)
Moved out of province	1
Too difficult to adhere to capsule intake	1
Family disapproval of study participation	1
No explanation given	9
Reason	High dose group (n = 9)
Too difficult to adhere to capsule intake	3
Health problems not related to capsule intake	2
No explanation given	4

Appendix 3

See Table 11.

Table 11 Reasons for discontinuing intervention

Reason	Low dose group (n = 3)
Too difficult to adhere to capsule intake	1
Dyspepsia	1
No reason	1
Reason	High dose group (n = 3)
No reason	2
Dyspepsia	1

Appendix 4

See Table 12.

Table 12 Adherence to double blind procedures

Perception	Low dose group (n = 73)	High dose group (n = 72)
Intervention dose	21 (29)	17 (24)
Control dose	15 (21)	11 (15)
Don't know	22 (30)	32 (44)
Missing data	15 (21)	12 (17)

Numbers represent frequency (%)

Acknowledgements

We thank Iseult Grenier-Ouellet, Marie-Pier Bernard-Genest and Lydia Tétrault for their assistance in the clinical follow-up of participants during this clinical trial at the Institute of Nutrition and Functional Foods, Laval University. The authors are very grateful to the laboratory and clinical staff and all participants in this study.

Authors' contributions

AB performed recruitment, clinical follow up, interpretation of data, statistical analyses and writing of the manuscript; VL contributed to the design of this study, recruitment, clinical follow up, interpretation of data, statistical analyses and revision of the manuscript; S. Dudonne undertook supervision of the biomarker measures and review of the manuscript; SL and YD contributed to the original concept and design of this study and reviewed the manuscript; DG and VB approved of the final manuscript; S. Dodin contributed to the original concept and design of this study, undertook supervision of the clinical follow-up of participants, and wrote the study grant. All authors read and approved the final manuscript.

Competing interests

Denis Guyonnet and Valerie Bochard are employees of Diana Food Canada. All other authors report no conflict of interest. The authors alone are responsible for the content and writing of the paper.

Author details

[1] CHU de Québec-Laval University Research Center, Québec City, Canada. [2] Department of Social and Preventive Medicine, Faculty of Medicine, Laval University, Québec City, Canada. [3] Institute of Nutrition and Functional Foods, Laval University, Québec City, Canada. [4] Diana Food, Rennes, France. [5] Diana Nova, Paris, France. [6] Department of Obstetrics and Gynecology, Saint-Francois D'Assise Hospital, Laval University, 10 Espinay Road, Québec City G1V 0A6, Canada.

References

1. Czaja CA, Hooton TM. Update on acute uncomplicated urinary tract infection in women. Postgrad Med. 2006;119(1):39–45.
2. Giesen LG, Cousins G, Dimitrov BD, van de Laar FA, Fahey T. Predicting acute uncomplicated urinary tract infection in women: a systematic review of the diagnostic accuracy of symptoms and signs. BMC Fam Pract. 2010;11:78.
3. Jepson RG, Williams G, Craig JC. Cranberries for preventing urinary tract infections. Cochrane Database Syst Rev. 2012;10:CD001321.
4. Gupta K, Chou MY, Howell A, Wobbe C, Grady R, Stapleton AE. Cranberry products inhibit adherence of p-fimbriated *Escherichia coli* to primary cultured bladder and vaginal epithelial cells. J Urol. 2007;177(6):2357–60.

5. Howell AB, Botto H, Combescure C, et al. Dosage effect on uropathogenic *Escherichia coli* anti-adhesion activity in urine following consumption of cranberry powder standardized for proanthocyanidin content: a multicentric randomized double blind study. BMC Infect Dis. 2010;10:94.
6. Lavigne JP, Bourg G, Combescure C, Botto H, Sotto A. In-vitro and in-vivo evidence of dose-dependent decrease of uropathogenic *Escherichia coli* virulence after consumption of commercial *Vaccinium macrocarpon* (cranberry) capsules. Clin Microbiol Infect Off Publ Eur Soc Clin Microbiol Infect Dis. 2008;14(4):350–5.
7. Asma B, Vicky L, Stephanie D, Yves D, Amy H, Sylvie D. Standardised high dose versus low dose cranberry Proanthocyanidin extracts for the prevention of recurrent urinary tract infection in healthy women [PAC-CANN]: a double blind randomised controlled trial protocol. BMC Urol. 2018;18(1):29.
8. Canada H. Licensed natural health products database. http://www.hc-sc.gc.ca/. Published 2008. Accessed 24 Jan 2017.
9. Prior RL, Fan E, Ji H, et al. Multi-laboratory validation of a standard method for quantifying proanthocyanidins in cranberry powders. J Sci Food Agric. 2010;90(9):1473–8.
10. Dudonné SVTV, Forato AF, Dubé P, Roy D, Pilon G. Modulatory effects of a cranberry extract co-supplementation with Bacillus subtilis CU1 probiotic on phenolic compounds bioavailability and gut microbiota composition in high-fat diet-fed mice. PharmaNutrition. 2015;3:89–100.
11. Jenkinson C, Layte R, Jenkinson D, et al. A shorter form health survey: can the SF-12 replicate results from the SF-36 in longitudinal studies? J Public Health Med. 1997;19(2):179–86.
12. Goulet J, Nadeau G, Lapointe A, Lamarche B, Lemieux S. Validity and reproducibility of an interviewer-administered food frequency questionnaire for healthy French-Canadian men and women. Nutr J. 2004;3:13.
13. INESSS. Urinary tract infections in adults. In: Services NIoEiHaS, ed. Quebec; 2017.
14. Gupta K, Hooton TM, Naber KG, et al. International clinical practice guidelines for the treatment of acute uncomplicated cystitis and pyelonephritis in women: A 2010 update by the Infectious Diseases Society of America and the European Society for Microbiology and Infectious Diseases. Clin Infect Dis. 2011;52(5):e103–20.
15. Mogollon JA, Bujold E, Lemieux S, et al. Blood pressure and endothelial function in healthy, pregnant women after acute and daily consumption of flavanol-rich chocolate: a pilot, randomized controlled trial. Nutr J. 2013;12:41.
16. Fu Z, Liska D, Talan D, Chung M. Cranberry reduces the risk of urinary tract infection recurrence in otherwise healthy women: a systematic review and meta-analysis. J Nutr. 2017;147(12):2282–8.
17. Epp A, Larochelle A, Lovatsis D, et al. Recurrent urinary tract infection. J Obstet Gynaecol Can. 2010;32(11):1082–101.
18. Maki KC, Kaspar KL, Khoo C, Derrig LH, Schild AL, Gupta K. Consumption of a cranberry juice beverage lowered the number of clinical urinary tract infection episodes in women with a recent history of urinary tract infection. Am J Clin Nutr. 2016;103(6):1434–42.
19. Barbosa-Cesnik C, Brown MB, Buxton M, Zhang L, Debusscher J, Foxman B. Cranberry juice fails to prevent recurrent urinary tract infection: results from a randomized placebo-controlled trial. Clin Infect Dis. 2011;52(1):23–30.
20. Stothers L. A randomized trial to evaluate effectiveness and cost effectiveness of naturopathic cranberry products as prophylaxis against urinary tract infection in women (structured abstract). Can J Urol. 2002;9(3):1558–62.
21. Foxman B, Barlow R, D'Arcy H, Gillespie B, Sobel JD. Urinary tract infection: self-reported incidence and associated costs. Ann Epidemiol. 2000;10(8):509–15.
22. Foxman B. The epidemiology of urinary tract infection. Nat Rev Urol. 2010;7(12):653–60.
23. Ejrnaes K, Stegger M, Reisner A, et al. Characteristics of *Escherichia coli* causing persistence or relapse of urinary tract infections: phylogenetic groups, virulence factors and biofilm formation. Virulence. 2011;2(6):528–37.
24. Schreiber HLT, Conover MS, Chou WC, et al. Bacterial virulence phenotypes of *Escherichia coli* and host susceptibility determine risk for urinary tract infections. Sci Transl Med. 2017;9:382.
25. Lewis AJ, Richards AC, Mulvey MA. Invasion of host cells and tissues by uropathogenic bacteria. Microbiol Spectr. 2016;4:6.
26. Mena P, González de Llano D, Brindani N, et al. 5-(3′,4′-Dihydroxyphenyl)-γ-valerolactone and its sulphate conjugates, representative circulating metabolites of flavan-3-ols, exhibit anti-adhesive activity against uropathogenic *Escherichia coli* in bladder epithelial cell. J Funct Foods. 2017;29:275–80.
27. Vostalova J, Vidlar A, Simanek V, et al. Are high proanthocyanidins key to cranberry efficacy in the prevention of recurrent urinary tract infection? Phytother Res. 2015;29(10):1559–67.

5

The protective effect of crocin on cisplatin-induced testicular impairment in rats

Behzad Mesbahzadeh[1], Mohammadmehdi Hassanzadeh-Taheri[2,4], Mohadese-sadat Aliparast[3], Pardis Baniasadi[3] and Mehran Hosseini[2,4*]

Abstract

Background: Side effects of cisplatin (CIS) such as testicular toxicity restrict its clinical use. Instead, evidence indicates that crocin (CR) has synergistic anti-cancer potential with CIS and exhibited beneficial effects on CIS-induced hepatorenal damage. The aim of this study was to investigate the protective potential of CR against CIS-induced testicular toxicity in rats.

Methods: Fifty adult male Wistar rats randomly assigned to five equal groups including control, CIS, and CIS plus CR at doses of 6.25 mg/kg (CIS + CR6.25), 25 mg/kg (CIS + CR25), and 100 mg/kg (CIS + CR100). CIS and CIS + CR groups received a single intraperitoneally (i.p.) injection of CIS (7 mg/kg). CR (6.25–100 mg/kg i.p.) injections were started three days before the CIS injection and continued once a day for up to 13 days. On the 14th day, all animals were sacrificed and their blood samples and testes were removed for biochemical and histological analyses.

Results: Compared to the control group, CIS significantly decreased relative testis weight (0.28 vs. 0.39, $p < 0.001$), testosterone level (0.3 vs. 2.31 ng/mL, $p < 0.001$), germinal layer area (25,886 vs. 35,320 μm^2, $p < 0.001$), superoxide dismutase (SOD) (0.9 vs.1.73 U/mg, $p < 0.001$) and increased testicular lipid peroxidation (3.05 vs. 15.35 nmol/mg, $p < 0.001$). CR at 25 mg/kg ameliorated testicular lipid peroxidation and enhanced SOD activity compared to CIS group ($p < 0.05$). Besides, CR treatment at the maximum dose (100 mg/kg) resulted in reversing CIS effects on testis weight, testosterone level, SOD, lipid peroxidation, and germinal layer area.

Conclusions: These findings demonstrated that CR co-treatment could prevent CIS-induced testicular toxicity in rats.

Keywords: Cisplatin, Crocin, Germinal epithelium, Lipid peroxidation, Testis

Background

Cisplatin (CIS) is one of the most important chemotherapeutic agents used to control several types of cancers. Despite its promising anti-cancer potential, CIS can adversely affect liver and kidney functions and induce testicular toxicity [1–5]. Nevertheless, CIS benefits outweigh its disadvantages, and currently, it is one of the most widely used chemotherapeutic agents for hematologic and solid tumor malignancies. The U.S. Food and Drug Administration approved CIS for the treatment of advanced ovarian and testicular cancers as well as bladder carcinoma [6]. However, clinical evidence demonstrates that CIS is used to treat a wide range of malignancies (off-label) [7]. Mechanistically, CIS binds to the purine bases of DNA and leads to strand breaks. Consequently, the damaged DNA, RNA, and proteins activate DNA repair mechanisms that lead to apoptotic or

*Correspondence: mehranhosseiny@yahoo.co.in; mehranhosseiny@bums.ac.ir
[2] Cellular and Molecular Research Center, Birjand University of Medical Sciences, Birjand, Iran
Full list of author information is available at the end of the article

non-apoptotic cell death [8]. Several studies found that CIS causes severe testicular damage through impairment of Leydig cell function (inhibiting testosterone production) and induction of germ cell apoptosis. Besides the DNA damage, excessive production of reactive oxygen species (ROS) is also implicated as one of the main causes of CIS-induced testicular damage [9].

Previous studies revealed that several natural products such as eugenol, curcumin and arjunolic acid could limit CIS-induced testicular damage by reducing oxidative stress and anti-inflammatory properties [10–15]. Considering everything, natural product research is regarded as a powerful approach for developing efficient, safe, and convenient drugs [16]. Hence, there is a great interest in combining antineoplastic drugs with natural products to enhance their efficacy while minimizing side effects through the delivery of lower doses [17]. CIS can be used singly or in combination therapy for induction and neoadjuvant therapy in the clinic. Therefore, it makes CIS a suitable candidate for the combination therapy formula [18].

Crocin (CR) is the main active constituent of saffron (*Crocus sativus*) with a wide range of pharmacological properties such as antidiabetic, anti-inflammatory, antioxidant, antidegenerative, and anti-cancer [19]. Interestingly, recent studies have indicated that CR enhanced chemosensitivity of some cancerous cell lines' to CIS. CR in combination therapy with CIS exhibited synergistic effects by induction of cell cycle arrest and apoptosis [20–22]. These findings indicate that there is no adverse interaction between CR and CIS in combination therapy. On the other hand, some works have shown that CR attenuated CIS-induced liver and kidney damage in rats [23, 24]. Therefore, it is of interest to know whether CR protective effect against CIS-induced testicular damage is still valid or not. This study aimed to investigate the potential protective effect of CR against CIS-induced testicular toxicity in rats.

Methods

Experimental animals

All procedures involving animals were according to the guides and rules in care and use of Laboratory Animals in Scientific Affairs with the Iranian Ministry of Health and Medical Education (2019) based on the 1964 Helsinki declaration and its later amendments or comparable ethical standards. Moreover, the animal experiments were approved by the Birjand University of Medical Sciences ethics committee (permit code: Ir.bums.REC.1398.066) in compliance with the ARRIVE guidelines [25].

Adult male albino rats (Wistar strain) weighing 180–200 g (8-week old) were used in the present study. All animals were housed in polypropylene cages in a temperature-controlled room (24 ± 2 °C) with 30–35% relative humidity and a 12-h light/dark cycle. Besides, rats had *ad libitum* access to water and standard laboratory animal chow (Behparvar Co., IR) during the study period.

Study design and treatments

A total of 50 rats were randomly allocated into the following five equal groups (n = 10): Control group, CIS model group (CIS), CIS plus CR at the dose of 6.25 mg/kg (CIS + Cr6.25), CIS plus CR at the dose of 25 mg/kg (CIS + CR25) and CIS plus CR at the dose of 100 mg/kg (CIS + CR100). The CR doses were selected based on previous studies revealing both protective and anti-cancer potentials. Accordingly, some studies showed that CR exhibited more anti-cancer potential at the lower doses, while others reported testicular or hepatorenal protective efficacies at higher doses [23, 24, 26]. Hence, a wide range of CR doses (6.25–100 mg/kg) were tested in this study.

The control and CIS groups only received intraperitoneal (i.p.) injections of normal saline once a day for 13 consecutive days. The Cr-treated groups (CIS + CR6.25-100) received i.p. injections of CR (Product No. 17,304, Sigma Aldrich, U.S.) dissolved in normal saline at 6.25 mg/kg, 25 mg/kg, and 100 mg/kg doses once a day for 13 consecutive days. On the 3rd day, all groups (except for control) received a single i.p. injection of CIS (PL 04515/0026, Hospira, U.K.) at the dose of 7 mg/kg. The study period and CIS dose were carefully chosen based on previous studies [1, 12, 14].

All animals were weighed on the 14th day and then sacrificed under anesthesia with ketamine-xylazine (65:10 mg/kg i.p.) [27]. Blood samples were collected by cardiac puncture for hormonal assay. Immediately after blood collection, testes were dissected out and weighed. Afterwards, the right testis was fixed in 4% paraformaldehyde solution for histology, while the left testis was kept in liquid nitrogen at −70 °C for antioxidant assay.

Testosterone assessment

Blood samples were centrifuged for 15 min at 3000 rpm, then sera were obtained, and testosterone assay performed using a commercially ELISA kit (Monobind, Inc., U.S.) following the manufacturer's instruction.

Lipid peroxidation assessment

An equal amount (100 mg) of each testis sample was homogenized in 900 μL of 0.1 M phosphate buffered saline (PBS, pH 7.4). Then, centrifuged at 4500 rpm for 15 min at 4 °C and its supernatant was collected. Total protein content was quantified using a commercial protein assay kit (NS-15,073, Navand Salamat, Iran).

Lipid peroxidation in the testicular tissue samples evaluated by the thiobarbituric acid reactive species (TBARS) method. In this method, the level of malondialdehyde (MDA), the main end product of the lipid peroxidation process, is calculated. In brief, 100 μL supernatant was added to 200 μL of 0.67% thiobarbituric acid and 600 μL of 1% O-phosphoric acid and the mixture was placed in a water bath (90 ℃) for 45 min. Then, the reaction was stopped by placing samples on ice and 800 μL N-butanol was added to each sample, vortexed, and the butanol phase was separated by centrifugation at 5000 rpm for 20 min. The supernatant was collected (200 μL) and its absorbance was measured spectophotometrically at 532 nm. Finally, the MDA level was expressed as nmol/mg protein [28].

Measurement of superoxide dismutase (SOD) activity

The SOD activity in the testis homogenates were evaluated by measuring the reduction rate of the water-soluble tetrazolium WST-1 dye. The reaction mixture was prepared by adding 100 μL of 10 mM WST-1 solution, 100 μL of 2 mg/mL catalase, 5 μL of xanthine oxidase (with the final concentration of 4.5 mU/mL) and 45 μL of assay buffer (50 mM Na3PO4, 0.1 mM diethylenetriamine pentaacetic acid, and 0.1 mM hypoxanthine in 20 mL). In brief, 50 μL supernatant and 250 μL of the reaction mixture were added into each well of a 96-well plate and mixed appropriately and incubated for 5 min at room temperature. The absorbance was read at 405 nm, and the SOD activity was expressed in terms of U/mg protein [29].

Histopathological evaluations

Tissue samples of testes were processed for paraffin-embedding by routine histological procedures, and serial Sec. (5 μm thickness) were prepared. The slides were stained with hematoxylin and eosin and analyzed under a light microscope (Euromex-CMEX-10). The quantitative parameters including seminiferous tubule area (μm^2) and germinal layer area (μm^2) were measured using Image J Software (1.44p; National Institute of Health, U.S.) as previously described [30, 31]. Moreover, the coefficient of germinal layer area to seminiferous tubule area was calculated.

To categorize the spermatogenesis efficacy, Johnsen's scoring (JS) system was applied. Briefly, the degree of testicular damages was tested using a 1–10 point's scale ranging from the lowest score of 1, indicating no seminiferous epithelium, to 10, representing complete spermatogenesis and perfect tubules (Table 1) [31]. All the evaluations were done blindly.

Table. 1 Johnsen score description

Johnsen score	Description
10	Complete spermatogenesis and perfect tubules
9	Slightly impaired spermatogenesis, many late spermatids, disorganized epithelium
8	Less than five spermatozoa per tubule, few late spermatozoa
7	No spermatozoa, no late spermatids, many early spermatids
6	No spermatozoa, no late spermatids, few early spermatids
5	No spermatozoa, no late spermatids, many spermatocytes
4	No spermatozoa and spermatids, few spermatocytes
3	Spermatogonia only
2	No germinal cell, Sertoli cells only
1	No seminiferous epithelium

Statistical analysis

Data were expressed as mean ± standard deviation. Analyzes were performed using SPSS software, version 22. The homogeneity of data was checked by Shapiro–Wilk test. The differences between groups were determined with ANOVA and Dunnett's T3 post hoc tests. Statistical significance was inferred at $p < 0.05$.

Results

Effects on body and testicular weight changes

The means of body weight, testis weight and relative testicular weight (testis weight/ body weight) of the studied groups are presented in Table 2. The CIS-treated animals exhibited lower body-weight, absolute and relative testicular weights compared to the control group ($p < 0.001$ all). Compared to the CIS group, CR treatment could significantly prevent body weight loss ($p = 0.04$), testicular weight loss ($p < 0.001$), and fall of relative testicular weight ($p < 0.001$) only at the maximum dose (100 mg/kg) in CIS-treated rats. However, these parameters were still statistically lower than normal ranges.

Effects on the serum testosterone

A significant reduction ($p < 0.001$) in serum testosterone concentration was observed in the CIS-treated group compared to the control group (0.3 ± 0.19 vs. 2.31 ± 0.4 ng/mL, $p < 0.001$). CR treatment at doses up to 25 mg/kg could not prevent serum testosterone reduction in CIS-treated animals (Fig. 1). However, CR administration at the dose of 100 mg/kg caused a significant increase in serum testosterone level compared to the CIS-treated group (1.70 ± 0.13 vs. 0.3 ± 0.19 ng/mL, $p < 0.001$).

Table. 2 Effects of crocin treatment (6.25–100 mg/kg) on body weight, absolute and relative testis weights

Groups	Body weight (g)	Testis weight (g)	Relative testis weight(testis weight /body weight)*100
Control	201.62±7.97	1.23±0.10	0.61±0.06
CIS (7 mg/kg)	187.98±4.59***	0.65±0.05***	0.35±0.02***
CIS+CR6.25 mg/kg	186.00±6.26***	0.73±0.10***	0.39±0.05***
CIS+CR25 mg/kg	185.38±2.13***	0.70±0.09***	0.38±0.05***
CIS+CR100 mg/kg	195.40±4.75#	0.94±0.09**,###	0.48±0.04***,###

Values are expressed as mean±standard deviation (n=10). CIS: cisplatin; CR: crocin; CIS+CR6.25-100: cisplatin (7 mg/kg) injected groups treated with 6.25–100 mg/kg crocin. *$p<0.05$, **$p<0.01$ and ***$p<0.001$ in comparison with the normal control group. #$p<0.05$, ##$p<0.01$ and ###$p<0.001$ in comparison with the CIS group

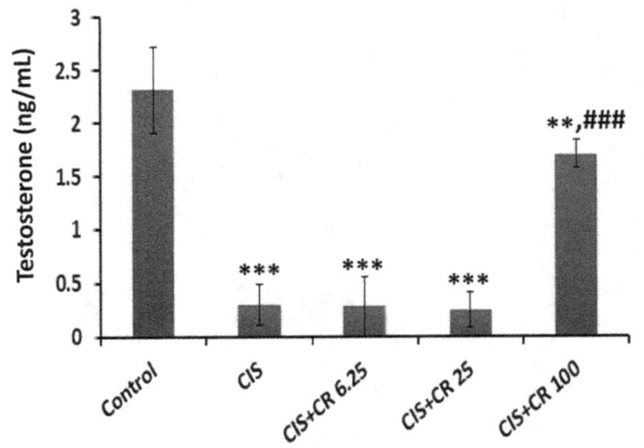

Fig. 1 Effects of crocin treatment on plasma testosterone .Values are expressed as mean±standard deviation (n=10). CIS: cisplatin; CR: crocin; CIS+CR6.25-100: CIS (7 mg/kg) injected animals treated with 6.25–100 mg/kg CR. **$p<0.01$ and ***$p<0.001$ in comparison with the normal control group. ###$p<0.001$ in comparison with the CIS group

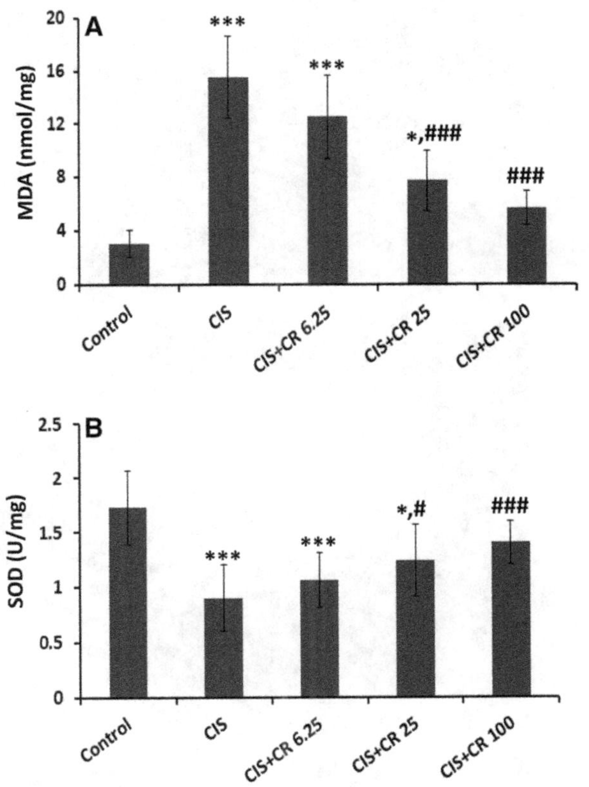

Fig. 2 Effects of crocin treatment on testis lipid peroxidation (**A**) and superoxide dismutase (**B**). Values are expressed as mean±standard deviation (n=10). MDA: malondialdehyde; SOD: superoxide dismutase; CIS: cisplatin; CR: crocin; CIS+CR6.25-100: CIS (7 mg/kg) injected animals treated with 6.25–100 mg/kg CR. *$p<0.05$ and ***$p<0.001$ in comparison with the normal control group. #$p<0.05$, and ###$p<0.001$ in comparison with the CIS group

Meanwhile, the testosterone level in the CIS+Cr100 group was still lower than the control group ($p=0.003$).

Effects on MDA and SOD

The testicular MDA level of CIS-treated rats was statistically higher than their counterparts in the control group (15.53±3.07 vs. 3.05±1.05 nmol/mg, $p<0.001$) (Fig. 2A). CR treatment at the doses of 25 mg/kg and 100 mg/kg could significantly keep MDA concentration lower than the CIS group (7.70±2.29 in CIS+CR 25 mg/kg and 5.63±1.27 nmol/mg protein in CIS+CR100 mg/kg). CR treatment could keep the MDA level close to the normal level only at the 100 mg/kg dose so that there was no significant difference between CIS+CR100 and control groups ($p=0.403$).

CIS administration significantly suppressed the SOD activity in the testis tissue compared to the control group (0.9±0.3 vs. 1.73±0.34 U/mg, $p<0.001$) (Fig. 2B). CR treatment at the doses of 25 mg/kg and 100 mg/kg could significantly enhance the SOD activity compared to the CIS group ($p<0.05$ and $p<0.001$ respectively).

Testis histopathology

In the control group, histological examination of testis samples revealed the normal structure of seminiferous tubules in which different phases of spermatogenic cells were evident. In the germinal layer, proliferating germ cells including spermatogonia, Sertoli cells, primary spermatocytes and spermatids were radially arranged toward the lumen (Fig. 3A). However, CIS-treated rats' seminiferous tubules showed extensive shrinkage, disruption in spermatogenesis, increased tubular lumen caused by sloughing of germinal epithelium (Fig. 3B, C). In the CIS-treated animals germinal layer area and its coefficient to seminiferous area were markedly reduced ($p < 0.001$) compared to the control group (Table 3). CR treatment could not completely restore the CIS-related damage at doses of 6.25 mg/kg (Fig. 3D) and 25 mg/kg

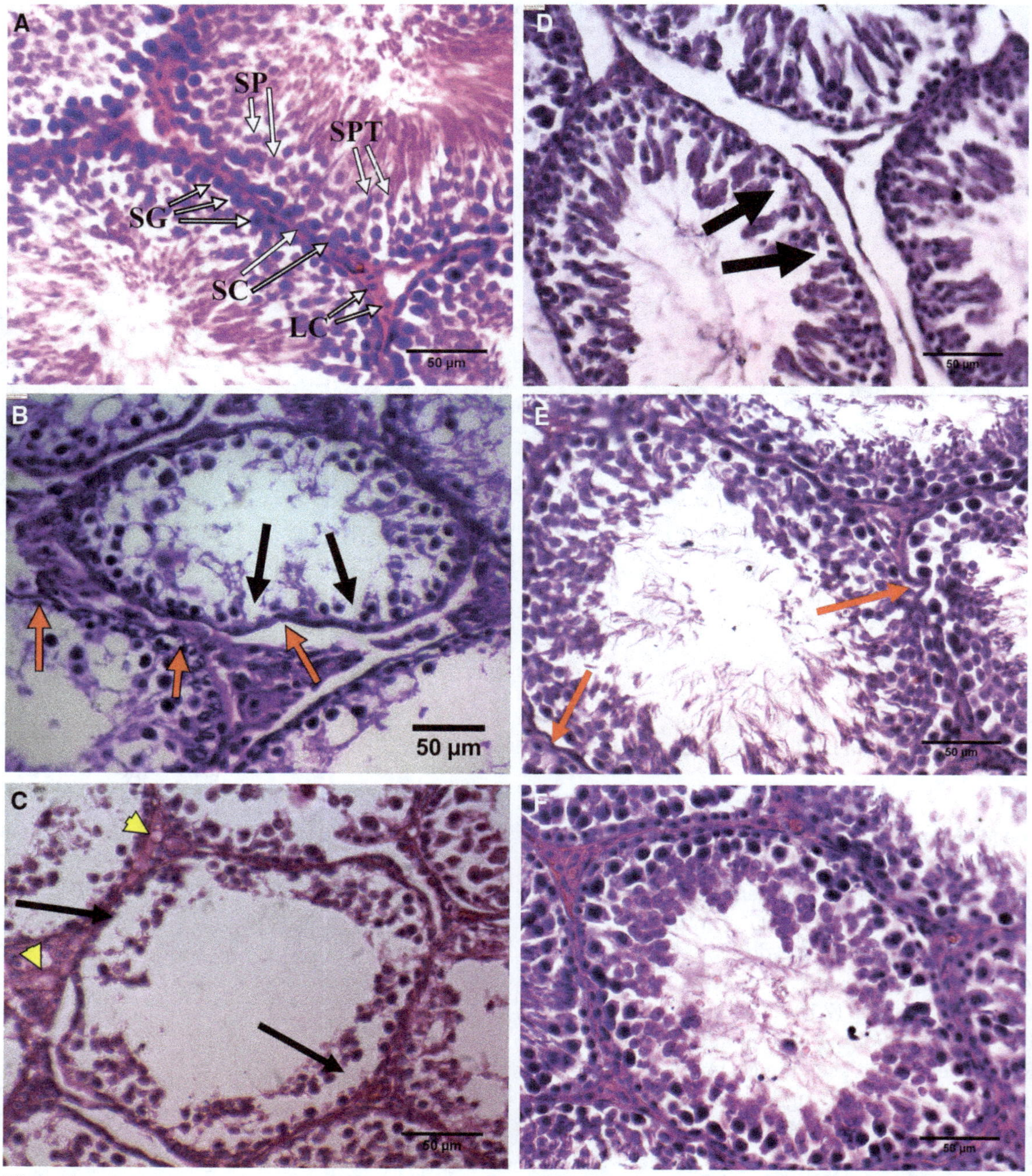

Fig. 3 Effects of crocin treatment on the testis histology of cisplatin-treated rats. Light microscope photomicrograph of the testicular tissue of the control group (**A**) cisplatin (**B, C**) and cisplatin plus crocin at the doses of 6.25 mg/kg (**D**), 25 mg/kg (**E**) and 100 mg/kg (**F**). SG: spermatogonium; SP: spermatocyte; SPT: spermatid; SC: Sertoli cell; LC: leydig cell. Red arrows mark extensive shrinkages, black arrows indicate sloughing of germinal epithelium and yellow arrowheads show vacuolation. Sections were stained with Hematoxylin and eosin (400X, bars = 50 µm)

Table 3 Effects of crocin (6.25–100 mg/kg) on the seminiferous tubule area and germinal layer area

Groups	SA (μm^2) × 10^3	EA area (μm^2) × 10^3	EA/SA * 100
Control	44.61 ± 8.10	35.32 ± 4.75	81.93 ± 8.89
CIS (7 mg/kg)	43.08 ± 2.94	25.89 ± 4.70***	59.08 ± 12.07**
CIS + CR6.25 mg/kg	42.53 ± 5.03	22.56 ± 4.18***	56.35 ± 8.19**
CIS + CR25 mg/kg	43.31 ± 5.12	23.96 ± 3.80***	59.48 ± 13.78**
CIS + CR100 mg/kg	44.83 ± 6.61	33.59 ± 6.40#	69.38 ± 10.98*,#

Values are expressed as mean ± standard deviation (n = 10). CIS: cisplatin; CR: crocin; CIS + CR 6.25–100: cisplatin (7 mg/kg) injected groups treated with 6.25–100 mg/kg crocin; SA: seminiferous tubule area; EA: germinal layer area. *$p < 0.05$, **$p < 0.01$ and ***$p < 0.001$ in comparison with the normal control group. #$p < 0.05$, ##$p < 0.01$ and ###$p < 0.001$ in comparison with the CIS group

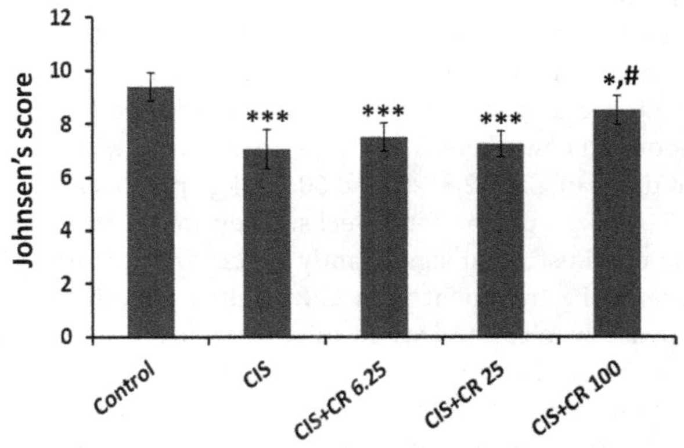

Fig. 4 Johnsen's scoring of testicular damage and spermatogenesis in the studied groups. Each bar indicates mean ± standard deviation. CIS: cisplatin; CR: crocin; CIS + CR6.25-100: cisplatin (7 mg/kg) injected animal treated with 6.25–100 mg/kg crocin. *$p < 0.05$ and ***$p < 0.001$ in comparison with the normal control group. #$p < 0.05$ in comparison with the CIS group

(Fig. 3E); however, at 100 mg/kg it preserved the overall structure of seminiferous tubules close to normal condition (Fig. 3F).

While there was no difference between the studied groups in the seminiferous area, a significant reduction in the germinal layer area and its coefficient to seminiferous area was observed in the CIS group compared to the control group ($p < 0.001$). Treatment with CR at the maximum dose (100 mg/kg) efficiently improved the germinal epithelium in comparison with the CIS group ($p < 0.05$). The germinal layer area to seminiferous area coefficient reveals more reliable details regarding germinal layer changes. Accordingly, 81% of the seminiferous area was filled with germinal epithelium in the control group, while this rate decreased to 59% in the CIS group. This decrease is statistically significant ($p = 0.003$). Treatment with CR at doses of 6.25 mg/kg and 25 mg/kg could not inhibit germinal epithelium loss in CIS-treated animals. Administration of CR at the dose of 100 mg/kg prevented germinal epithelium disruption and kept germinal layer area around 69% of the seminiferous area, which was statistically higher than the CIS group ($p = 0.02$). Nevertheless, the germinal layer area coefficient in the CIS + CR100 group was still lower than the control group ($p = 0.04$).

The results of JS of spermatogenesis are shown in Fig. 4. The control group exhibited the maximum score (mean score = 9.7), whereas CIS-treated rats had a significantly lower score (mean score = 7.6, $p < 0.001$). CR treatment could never keep spermatogenesis at the normal level at any dose. A slight improvement was observed only in the CIS + CR100 group (mean score = 8.5), which was statistically higher than the CIS group score (mean score = 7.6, $p = 0.03$).

Discussion

Chemotherapy is often accompanied by some side effects depending on several factors such as chemotherapy duration, dose, patient's age, etc. [32]. Testicular toxicity is one of the most critical challenges in cancer chemotherapy leading to the emergence of a new medical discipline called oncofertility. The oncofertility aims to preserve the fertility of patients who received chemotherapy or radiotherapy. Testicular toxicity is one of the most important chemotherapy side effects restricting the use and efficacy of antineoplastic drugs, such as CIS. In the present study, the protective efficacy of CR was tested on CIS-induced testicular damage in rats. The results demonstrated that Cr, a natural product with anti-cancer efficacy, attenuated CIS-induced testicular damage in rats.

Testicular relative weight is a good indicator of normal spermatogenesis, frequently measured in reproductive studies [30]. CIS administration (7 mg/kg) significantly reduced the relative testicular weight in the current study, which is consistent with previous reports [10, 12, 33]. CR treatment only at the maximum dose (100 mg/kg) significantly prevented testicular relative weight loss in CIS-treated rats. These results go beyond previous reports, showing that CR has increased the testicular weight in nicotine/paraquat-induced mice testicular damage [34, 35].

The production of testosterone and sperms is the primary function of the testis [36]. Consequently, testosterone measurement is considered as a marker indicating optimal testicular function. In this study, CIS administration caused a severe drop in serum testosterone levels, which is in line with previous studies' findings [13, 37]. The results showed that CR had no significant effect on testosterone reduction in CIS-treated rats at doses of 6.25–25 mg/kg, whereas it could attenuate testosterone reduction significantly at the dose of 100 mg/kg. These results are consistent with the findings reported by Salahshoor and coworkers. They have treated mice with different doses of CR (12.5, 25, and 50 mg/kg i.p.) plus nicotine (2.5 mg/kg i.p.) for four weeks. They found that nicotine administration significantly reduced testosterone in mice, while treatment with CR resulted in testosterone increase in nicotine-treated mice only at the maximum dose (50 mg/kg) [35].

Seminiferous tubules are responsible for about 80% of the total testicular volume. In the cross-section, the lumen of the seminiferous tubule is lined by Sertoli cells. It contains spermatozoa in various stages of development, from spermatogonia near the base of tubules to progressively mature forms (spermatocytes, spermatids, and spermatozoa) arranged towards the center of the lumen [36]. The most common pathological feature observed concerning the testicular toxicity is the germinal epithelium's loosening [38, 39]. Therefore, quantitative assessment of germinal epithelium area or its diameter has been performed in different studies [1, 30, 31, 36]. It is well-demonstrated that CIS affects testicular germinal epithelium by both cytotoxic effect and induction of apoptosis [40]. The results indicate that CIS administration did not significantly affect the seminiferous area, but it caused a significant decrease in the germinal layer area. Germinal epithelial atrophy is generally accompanied by seminiferous tubule degeneration. Besides, it is observed in the early stage of testicular damage; whereas, seminiferous atrophy is considered an irreversible and end-stage change of testicular damage [41]. The maximum CR dose (100 mg/kg) could prevent germinal epithelium loss in CIS-treated rats in the present study. To our knowledge, no study has been yet investigated the impact of CR treatment on testicular morphology in CIS-induced reproductive damaged animals. However, there are studies in which CR has been investigated on other testicular damage. In the Bayatpour and colleagues' study, diabetic rats were treated with saline or CR (20 mg/kg i.p.) for 60 days. They reported that untreated diabetic rats exhibited significant testicular damage, but the CR treatment caused a significant prevention in germinal epithelium sloughing [42]. Contrary to Bayatpour and coworkers' study [42], we found that CR cannot influence germinal layer loss in CIS-treated rats at doses up to 25 mg/kg. It is important to highlight that in the mentioned study, CR was administrated for 60 days while only 13 injections of CR were performed in the current study. In line with germinal epithelium damage, spermatogenesis evaluated using the JS system was significantly decreased in CIS and CIS + CR6.25 and CIS + CR25 groups compared to the control group. CR treatment significantly increased the JS compared to the CIS group only at 100 mg/kg. A recent study demonstrated that 60 days of CR administration (20 mg/kg i.p.) to Wistar rats that simultaneously received high-fat diet plus streptozotocin could effectively prevent spermatogenesis impairment by increasing the JS [43].

Mechanistic studies demonstrated that impairment in oxidant-antioxidant balance and lipid peroxidation play a pivotal role in CIS-induced testicular damage [44]. Another promising finding was that CR could effectively attenuate testicular MDA levels as well as enhance SOD activity in CIS-treated rats at 25 mg/kg and 100 mg/kg doses. This result is in line with earlier studies wherein testicular lipid peroxidation has been decreased with CR treatments [34, 45].

Conclusions

In conclusion, the present study's findings demonstrated that CR partially attenuated some of the CIS-related pathological effects on testicular tissue because of its antioxidant property. Numerous studies have shown that CR has anti-cancer efficacy on a wide range of cancer cells. Moreover, CR not only does not interfere with cisplatin but also has synergistic effects. Some studies have also reported the protective effects of crocin on renal, hepatic, and gastrointestinal side effects of chemotherapy drugs. Therefore, it is suggested that CR might be used as a potent therapeutic agent combined with CIS to reduce testicular damage caused by CIS.

Abbreviations

CIS: Cisplatin; CR: Crocin; PBS: Phosphate buffered saline; TBARS: Thiobarbituric acid reactive species; MDA: Malondialdehyde; SOD: Superoxide dismutase; JS: Johnsen's scoring.

Acknowledgements

The authors are thankful to Ms. Gholizadeh for her help in providing cisplatin.

Authors' contributions

BM and MHT conceived the idea of the study and contributed to the data interpretation. MA and PB performed the experiments and MH designed animal experiment, analyzed the data and wrote the manuscript draft. All authors read and approved the final manuscript.

Competing interests

The authors declare that they have no competing interests.

Author details

[1]Department of Physiology, School of Allied Medical Sciences, Birjand University of Medical Sciences, Birjand, Iran. [2]Cellular and Molecular Research Center, Birjand University of Medical Sciences, Birjand, Iran. [3]Student Research Committee, Birjand University of Medical Sciences, Birjand, Iran. [4]Present Address: Department of Anatomical Sciences, Faculty of Medicine, Birjand University of Medical Sciences, Birjand, Iran.

References

1. Jahan S, Munawar A, Razak S, Anam S, Ain QU, Ullah H, Afsar T, Abulmeaty M, Almajwal A. Ameliorative effects of rutin against cisplatin-induced reproductive toxicity in male rats. BMC Urol. 2018;18:107.
2. Ekinci Akdemir FN, Albayrak M, Çalik M, Bayir Y, Gülçin İ. The protective effects of p-coumaric acid on acute liver and kidney damages induced by cisplatin. Biomedicines. 2017;5:18.
3. Ekinci-Akdemi RF, Bi Ngöl Ç, Yıldırım S, Kandemi RF, Küçükler S, Sağlam YS. The investigation of the effect of fraxin on hepatotoxicity induced by cisplatin in rats. Iran J Basic Med Sci. 2020; 23:1382–1387.
4. Kilic K, Sakat MS, Akdemir FNE, Yildirim S, Saglam YS, Askin S. Protective effect of gallic acid against cisplatin-induced ototoxicity in rats. Braz J Otorhinolaryngol. 2019; 85:267–274.
5. Sakat MS, Kilic K, Akdemir FNE, Yildirim S, Eser G, Kiziltunc A.The effectiveness of eugenol against cisplatin-induced ototoxicity. Braz J Otorhinolaryngol. 2019; 85:766–773.
6. Pillai G. Nanotechnology toward treating cancer. A comprehensive review. In: Mohapatra SS, Ranjan S, Dasgupta N, Mishra RK, Thomas S, editors. Applications of targeted nano drugs and delivery systems. Amsterdam: Elsevier; 2019. p. 221–56.
7. Armstrong DK, Bundy B, Wenzel L, Huang HQ, Baergen R, Lele S, Copeland LJ, Walker JL, Burger RA. Intraperitoneal cisplatin and paclitaxel in ovarian cancer. N Engl J Med. 2006; 354:34–43.
8. Riddell IA. Cisplatin and oxaliplatin: our current understanding of their actions. Met Ions Life Sci. 2018;5:18.
9. Wang T-E, Lai Y-H, Yang K-C, Lin S-J, Chen C-L, Tsai P-S. Counteracting cisplatin-induced testicular damages by natural polyphenol constituent honokiol. Antioxidants (Basel). 2020;9:723.
10. Afsar T, Razak S, Almajwal A. Acacia hydaspica ethyl acetate extract protects against cisplatin-induced DNA damage, oxidative stress and testicular injuries in adult male rats. BMC Cancer. 2017;17:1–14.
11. Amin A, Hamza AA. Effects of Roselle and Ginger on cisplatin-induced reproductive toxicity in rats. Asian J Androl. 2006;8:607–12.
12. Ilbey YO, Ozbek E, Cekmen M, Simsek A, Otunctemur A, Somay A. Protective effect of curcumin in cisplatin-induced oxidative injury in rat testis: mitogen-activated protein kinase and nuclear factor-kappa B signaling pathways. Hum Reprod. 2009; 24:1717–25.
13. Soni KK, Zhang LT, You JH, Lee SW, Kim CY, Cui WS, Chae HJ, Kim HK, Park JK. The effects of MOTILIPERM on cisplatin induced testicular toxicity in Sprague–Dawley rats. Cancer cell Int. 2015;15:1–11.
14. Sherif IO, Abdel-Aziz A, Sarhan OM. Cisplatin-induced testicular toxicity in rats: the protective effect of arjunolic acid. J Biochem Mol Toxicol. 2014; 28: 515-21.11.
15. Ekinci Akdemir FN, Yildirim S, Kandemir FM, Aksu EH, Guler MC, Kiziltunc Ozmen H, Kucukler S, Eser G. The antiapoptotic and antioxidant effects of eugenol against cisplatin-induced testicular damage in the experimental model. Andrologia. 2019; 51:e13353.
16. Cragg GM, Pezzuto JM. Natural products as a vital source for the discovery of cancer chemotherapeutic and chemopreventive agents. Med Princ Pract. 2016; 25:41–59.
17. Zhang Y, Li H, Zhang J, Zhao C, Lu S, Qiao J, Han M. The combinatory effects of natural products and chemotherapy drugs and their mechanisms in breast cancer treatment Phytochem Rev. 2020;19:1179–97.
18. Liu G-Y, Lv X, Wu Y-S, Mao M-J, Ye Y-F, Yu Y-H, Liang H, Yang J, Ke L-R, Qiu W-Z et al. Effect of induction chemotherapy with cisplatin, fluorouracil, with or without taxane on locoregionally advanced nasopharyngeal carcinoma: a etrospective, propensity score-matched analysis. Cancer Commun (Lond). 2018; 38: 21.
19. Cerdá-Bernad D, Valero-Cases E, Pastor J-J, Frutos MJ. Saffron bioactives crocin, crocetin and safranal. effect on oxidative stress and mechanisms of action. Crit Rev Food Sci Nutr. 2020. https://doi.org/10.1080/10408398.2020.1864279.
20. Chen S, Zhao S, Wang X, Zhang L, Jiang E, Gu Y, Shangguan AJ, Zhao H, Lv T, Yu Z. Crocin inhibits cell proliferation and enhances cisplatin and pemetrexed chemosensitivity in lung cancer cells. Transl Lung Cancer Res. 2015;4:775–83.
21. Mollaei H, Hoshyar R, Abedini MR, Safaralizadeh R. Crocin enhances cisplatin-induced chemosensitivity in human cervical cancer cell line. Int J Cancer Manag. 2019;12: e94909
22. Vali F, Changizi V, Safa M. Synergistic apoptotic effect of crocin and paclitaxel or crocin and radiation on MCF-7 cells, a type of breast cancer cell line. Int J Breast Cancer. 2015;2015:e139349.
23. Naghizadeh B, Mansouri SMT, Mashhadian NV: Crocin attenuates cisplatin-induced renal oxidative stress in rats. Food Chem Toxicol. 2010;48:2650–5.
24. Sun Y, Yang J, Wang L, Sun L, Dong Q. Crocin attenuates cisplatin-induced liver injury in the mice. Hum Exp Toxicol. 2014;33:855–62.
25. Percie du Sert N, Ahluwalia A, Alam S, Avey MT, Baker M, Browne WJ, Clark A, Cuthill IC, Dirnagl U, Emerson M. Reporting animal research. Explanation and elaboration for the ARRIVE guidelines 2.0. PLoS Biol. 2020; 18:e3000411.
26. Sun Y, Xu H-J, Zhao Y-X, Wang L-Z, Sun L-R, Wang Z, Sun X-F. Crocin exhibits antitumor effects on human leukemia HL-60 cells in vitro and in vivo. Evid Based Complement Altern Med. 2013;2013:e690164.
27. Hassanzadeh-Taheri M, Hassanpour-Fard M, Doostabadi M, Moodi H, Vazifeshenas-Darmiyan K, Hosseini M. Co-administration effects of aqueous extract of turnip leaf and metformin in diabetic rats. J Tradit Complement Med. 2018;8:178–83.
28. Moodi H, Hosseini M, Abedini MR, Hassanzadeh-Taheri M, Hassanzadeh-Taheri M. Ethanolic extract of Iris songarica rhizome attenuates methotrexate-induced liver and kidney damages in rats. Avicenna J Phytomed. 2020;10:372–83.
29. Ataie Z, Mehrani H, Ghasemi A, Farrokhfall K. Cinnamaldehyde has beneficial effects against oxidative stress and nitric oxide metabolites in the brain of aged rats fed with long-term, high-fat diet. J Funct Foods. 2019; 52:545–551.
30. Hassanzadeh-Taheri M, Hosseini M, Dorranipour D, Afshar M, Moodi H, Salimi M. The Oleo-Gum-Resin of Commiphora myrrha ameliorates male reproductive dysfunctions in streptozotocin-induced hyperglycemic rats. Pharm Sci. 2019;25:294–302.
31. Hassanzadeh-Taheri M, Jahani F, Hassanzadeh-Taheri M, Doostabadi M, Doostabadi H, Hosseini M. The impacts of yoghurt butter oil on rat testicular morphology and sexual hormones in a 150-day study. Comp Clin Path. 2018;27:959–65.
32. Hoshyar R, Sebzari A, Balforoush M, Valavi M, Hosseini M. The impact of Crocus sativus stigma against methotrexate-induced liver toxicity in rats. J Complement Integr Med. 2019;17:e2019-0201.
33. Eid AH, Abdelkader NF, Abd El-Raouf OM, Fawzy HM, El-Denshary ES. Carvedilol alleviates testicular and spermatological damage induced by cisplatin in rats via modulation of oxidative stress and inflammation. Arch Pharm Res. 2016; 39:1693–702.
34. Sadat Kamali F, Shahrooz R, Najafi G, Razi M. Ameliorative effects of crocin on paraquat-induced oxidative stress in testis of adult mice: an experimental study. Int J Reprod Biomed. 2019;17:807–18.
35. Salahshoor MR, Khazaei M, Jalili C, Keivan M. Crocin improves damage induced by nicotine on a number of reproductive parameters in male mice. Int J Fertil Steril. 2016;10:71–8.
36. Hassanzadeh-Taheri M, Hosseini M. Comments on "The improvement effects of *Gordonia bronchialis* on male fertility of rats with diabetes mellitus induced by Streptozotocin". Pharm Sci. 2020;26:93–5.
37. Tian M, Liu F, Liu H, Zhang Q, Li L, Hou X, et al. Grape seed procyanidins extract attenuates Cisplatin-induced oxidative stress and testosterone synthase inhibition in rat testes. Syst Biol Reprod Med. 2018;64: 246–59.
38. Catlin NR, Willson CJ, Creasy DM, Rao DB, Kissling GE, McIntyre BS, et al. Differentiating between testicular toxicity and sexual immaturity in ortho-phthalaldehyde inhalation toxicity studies in rats and mice. Toxicol Pathol. 2018;46:753–63.
39. Serki E, Vazifeshenas Darmiyan K, Ezi S, Bayat J, Shahamat, Farhad, Ghiravani Z, et al. Effects of colostrum on sperm parameters, sex hormones and testes histopathological changes in diabetic rats. JMUMS. 2016;26:83–94.
40. Mohammadnejad D, Abedelahi A, Soleimani-Rad J, Mohammadi-Roshandeh A, Rashtbar M, Azami A. Degenerative effect of Cisplatin on testicular germinal epithelium. Adv Pharm Bull. 2012;2:173–7.
41. Creasy D, Bube A, Rijk Ed, Kandori H, Kuwahara M, Masson R, et al. Proliferative and nonproliferative lesions of the rat and mouse male reproductive system. Toxicol Pathol. 2012;40:40S-121S.
42. Bayatpoor ME, Mirzaee S, Mohammadi MT. Effect of crocin on spermatogenesis in streptozotocin-induced diabetic rats. *JMUMS*. 2018; 28: 24–35.

43. Mirzaee S, Bayatpoor ME, Shahyad S, Mohammadi MT, Bahari Z. The protective effects of Crocin on testopathy in fat-fed and streptozotocin-treated diabetic rats: an experimental study. Int J Reprod Biomed. 2019;17:89–98.
44. Liu Z, Sun Y, Su L, Sun Y, Kong S, Chang X, et al. Effects of cisplatin on testicular enzymes and Sertoli cell function in rats. Fundam Toxicol Sci. 2015; 2:137–45.
45. Bakhtiary Z, Shahrooz R, Ahmadi A, Zarei L. Evaluation of antioxidant effects of crocin on sperm quality in cyclophosphamide treated adult mice. Vet Res Forum. 2014;5:213–8.

6

Preoperative hydronephrosis is a predictive factor of ureteral stenosis after flexible ureteroscopy: A propensity scores matching analysis

Yuefan Shen, Anping Xiang and Sihai Shao*

Abstract

Objectives: Ureteral stenosis is a serious complication of flexible ureteroscopy. How to predict the possibility of stricture before surgery is an important topic. This research retrospectively studied the influence of preoperative hydronephrosis on ureteral stenosis after flexible ureteroscopy, to explore whether the preoperative hydronephrosis could predict postoperative ureteral stenosis.

Methods: We conducted a retrospective study on patients who received flexible ureteroscopy in our hospital for upper ureteral calculi from January 2015 to June 2018. Patients were followed-up for 36 months after surgery, and intraoperative and postoperative complications were recorded. We divided patients into the mild hydronephrosis group and moderate to severe hydronephrosis group. Preoperative clinical baseline data of the patients were adjusted by propensity matching score analysis. Differences of intraoperative ureteral injury, operative time, postoperative ureteral stricture, and SFR one month after surgery was statistically analyzed. Kaplan–Meier's method and Log-rank test were used to compare the differences in the cumulative incidence of ureteral stenosis between the two groups. Cox regression was used to compare the hazard ratio of ureteral stenosis between the two groups.

Results: A total of 447 patients with 469 sides surgery were included, including 349 sides in the mild hydronephrosis group and 120 sides in the moderate to severe hydronephrosis group. Twenty-nine patients with 30 sides developed ureteral stenosis. Before and after propensity, the incidence of ureteral stricture matching analysis was 6.4% and 8%, respectively. There were statistical differences in ureteral stricture and injury, but the statistical differences in SFR and operation time were inconsistent. Kaplan–Meier showed a significant difference in the cumulative incidence of ureteral stenosis between the two groups.

Conclusions: Patients with moderate to severe hydronephrosis before surgery were more likely to have an intraoperative ureteral injury and postoperative ureteral stricture after FRUS. Preoperative hydronephrosis is an important predictor of ureteral stricture.

Keywords: Ureteral stenosis, Flexible ureteroscopy, Upper ureteral stones, Hydronephrosis, Propensity scores matching analysis

Background

With the development of the flexible ureteroscope technical, the FRUS has gradually become an choice for upper ureteral calculi. Guidelines of EAU [1] suggested that "percutaneous nephrolithotomy is considered for ureteral stone larger than 15 mm with stone impaction." However, in practical work, the indications for flexible uretero-

*Correspondence: kipling21@sina.com
Department of Urology, The First People's Hospital of Huzhou, No.158 Guangchanghou Road, Huzhou, Zhejiang Province, China

scope are gradually relaxed. Some doctors prefer a flexible ureteroscope because it is more minimally invasive. The FRUS presents several advantages over percutaneous nephrolithotomy, including reduced post-operational pain, lower risk of hemorrhage and shorter hospitalization time. It is more acceptable to patients. Nevertheless, further minimally invasive does not always mean better. As the number of FRUS increased, so did the complication of surgeries. Ureteral stenosis is a rare and severe complication after FRUS. It eventually requires reoperation, causing physical pain and financial burden to the patients. Early ureteroscopy studies reported ureteral stricture rates around 0.30%-23.81%, mostly in rigid and semi-rigid ureteroscopy studies [2]. Some scholars have studied the risk factors of ureteral stenosis, and believe that stone burden, stone impaction and operation time are important factors [3]. "Stone impaction" has been mentioned in the EAU guideline and many other literatures [1, 4, 5]. In recent years, research has shown that thickness of the renal parenchyma and ureteral wall on CT are related to stone impaction [6, 7]. In addition, few studies have investigated how to judge "stone impaction." In clinical diagnosis and treatment, we find that the degree of hydronephrosis is closely related to ureteral injury and stricture irrespective of the stone size. The degree of hydronephrosis may represent the severity of stone impaction, which may be another predicator for ureteral stricture. We undertake a retrospective study to evaluate this hypothesis.

Methods

Patients

From January 2015 to June 2018, 688 patients underwent flexible ureteroscopy for upper ureteral stone treatment at our institution. Most of them were patients with high stone burden unsuitable for SWL, or patients with ureteral calculi before unsuccessful SWL. The clinical data were obtained by reviewing medical records. The inclusion and exclusion criteria were like following.

Inclusion criteria: (1) patients with upper ureteral calculi above the level of iliac vessels, including calculi at the ureteropelvic junction; (2) double J tubes were placed one to two weeks before surgery.

Exclusion criteria: (1) previous history of ipsilateral upper ureteral calculi surgery [8], including ureteroscopy, percutaneous nephrolithotomy, laparoscopy or open surgery; (2) preoperative ureteral stricture; (3) patients with too much missing data; (4) urinary malformation; (5) neurogenic bladder; (6) orthotopic neobladder history.

We selected patients with mild hydronephrosis as the case group, and patients with moderate to severe hydronephrosis as the control group. The primary outcome was ureteral stenosis. The secondary outcome was operative time, intraoperative ureteral injury and stone clearance rate one month after surgery.

Definition of terms in this paper

Onset time: the onset time was days from the onset of symptoms until the date of surgery.

Calculi size and hydronephrosis: these values were obtained from the CTU. The width of the renal pelvis less than 2 cm was considered mild hydronephrosis, while that larger than 2 cm was considered moderate to severe hydronephrosis.

Stone burden calculation: maximum length $\times$ maximum width $\times \pi \times 0.25 (\pi = 3.14)$.

Stone removal: KUB indicates residual stone ≤ 4 mm.

FRUS procedure

All the patients finished CTU before operation to exclude ureteral stenosis. Double J tubes were placed preoperatively for one to two weeks to dilate the ureter. All patients received general anesthesia. The surgeon used a Ureteroscope (Wolf 6/7.5 or 8/9.8) to remove the stent, and then found the ureteral orifice. A guidewire was introduced via which a rigid ureteroscope was passed through the ureteral orifice. The middle and lower sections of the ureter were explored by a ureteroscope. After the endoscope was removed, an access sheath (F12, Cook Company) was placed into the ureter along the guide wire, and a flexible ureteroscope (8.5/9.9F, Olympus) was placed at the inferior end of the stones. The stones were fragmented by 200 μm Holmium laser with power of 0.8–1.2 J and frequency of 15–25Hz. Postoperatively, an F6 Double-J stent was placed routinely. Antibiotic was used to prevent infection for 24–48 h. The Double J tube was removed 15–60 days later according to the situation.

Postoperative follow-up

All patients were followed up in the outpatient department. They underwent KUB one month after surgery, and B-ultrasound of the urinary system three months, six months, one year, two years and three years after Double J tube removed. If there was no aggravation of hydronephrosis, we defined it as no ureteral stenosis. If B-ultrasound indicated gradual aggravation of hydronephrosis, CTU would be performed to determine the cause of obstruction.

Postoperative complications

Ureteral injury was classified according to Ureteroscopic Lesion Scale (PULS) [9]. Postoperative complications were graded according to the Clavien–Dindo grading system [10].

Statistical analysis

Data were collected retrospectively, entered into an Excel 16 software, and analyzed with the IBM SPSS 25. The independent sample *t*-test (continuous variable) or chi-square test (categorical variable) were used for comparing surgical outcomes and characteristics of the two groups. The clinical baseline characteristics of patients were adjusted by 1:1 propensity matching. After propensity scores matching analysis, paired sample T test (continuous variable) or McNEMA test (categorical variable) were adopted to compare the clinical characteristics of the two groups. The Kaplan–Meier method was applied to estimate cumulative incidence, and log-rank test was constructed to compare the differences between the two groups. A Cox proportional-hazards model was used to evaluate the hazard ratio for ureteral stricture in both groups.

Results

A total of 688 patients with upper ureteral calculi underwent flexible ureteroscope in our hospital. There were 659 cases of non-stricture and 29 cases of strictures. Sixty-one patients had been missing operation time data; Thirty-two patients had been missing other important data. The patients excluded for other reasons were shown in Fig. 1. A total number of 469 sides surgical procedures for 447 patients were included in our retrospective analysis. 349 sides were mild hydronephrosis, and 120 sides were moderate to severe hydronephrosis. The average age of patients was 50.43 ± 12.14 years, the mean time since onset was 46.80 ± 55.34 days, the mean BMI was 24.05 ± 3.65, and the mean stone burden was 86.66 ± 46.76 mm^2. Before propensity matching, there were significant differences in age, onset time, renal colic and stone burden between the two groups. A total of 75 pairs of patients were obtained after 1:1 propensity matching, and all baseline characteristics were balanced between the two groups (Table 1). After surgery, twelve patients (13 sides of strictures) were lost to follow up, including 8 patients (9 sides of strictures) with confirmed stenosis. They were transferred to other hospitals. Data were not available for the remaining 4 patients with non-stenosis due to review at other hospitals. The differences of observational outcomes before and after propensity matching are shown in Table 2. A total of 29 patients had ureteral stenosis on 30 sides after operation. The stenosis rate before and after the propensity matching was 6.4% and 8%, respectively. There were significant differences before and after propensity matching. Although the SFR and operation time reached statistical significance

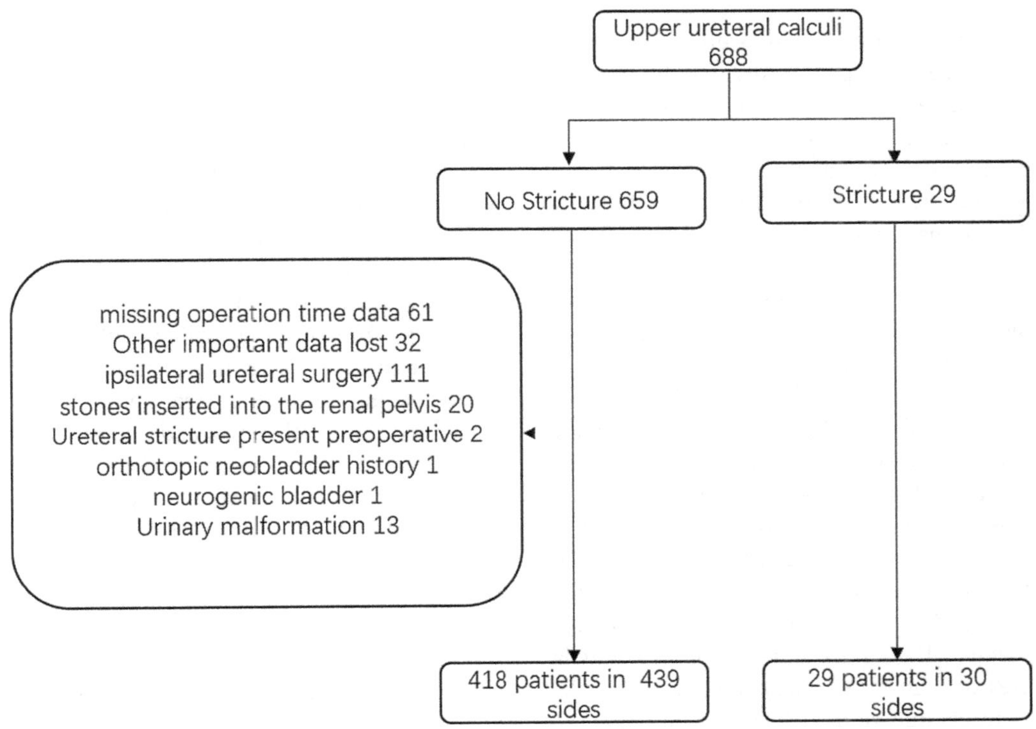

Fig. 1 Patient selection

Table 1 Patient baseline characteristics

	Before propensity matching			After propensity matching		
	Mild hydronephrosis	Moderate and severe hydronephrosis	*P* value	Mild hydronephrosis	Moderate and severe hydronephrosis	*P* value
	N=349	N=120		N=75	N=75	
Age (year)	49.58±12.03	52.91±12.18	0.010	52.00±10.54	53.29±11.94	0.483
Male (%)	69.1%	69.2%	0.982	68.0%	66.7%	1.000
BMI	23.97±3.53	24.27±4.00	0.475	24.43±3.21	24.26±3.95	0.779
Disease time (days)	41.95±45.41	60.88±75.81	0.011	46.63±42.26	43.00±41.59	0.596
Renal colic (%)	65.6%	31.7%	0.000	34.7%	37.3%	0.804
Fever (%)	4.6%	7.5%	0.220	8.0%	8.0%	1.000
SWL (%)	20.9%	19.2%	0.682	24.0%	21.3%	0.815
Stone burden (mm^2)	78.65±41.93	109.89±52.17	0.000	97.94±39.36	99.75±39.86	0.675

Table 2 Patient observational outcomes

	Before propensity matching			After propensity matching		
	Mild hydronephrosis	Moderate and severe hydronephrosis	*P* value	Mild hydronephrosis	Moderate and severe hydronephrosis	*P* value
	N=349	N=120		N=75	N=75	
Ureteral stenosis	2.3%	18.3%	0.000	0	16.0%	0.000
Ureteral injury (≥grade2)	5.2%	42.5%	0.000	5.3%	37.3%	0.000
Operation time	67.75±33.62	83.29±37.89	.000	74.90±31.29	80.12±37.53	0.383
SFR	88.5%	78.3%	.006	77.3%	80.0%	0.839

before propensity matching, there were no clinically significant differences after propensity matching.

The median follow-up time of both groups was 36 months. The mean follow-up time of mild hydronephrosis group and moderate to severe hydronephrosis group was 35.26±4.32 months and 30.88±10.87 months, respectively. Figure 2 showed that the cumulative incidence of ureteral stenosis was higher in the moderate to severe hydronephrosis group before propensity matching [HR 8.72; 95% CI 3.88–19.60; $P=0.000$]. When baseline clinical characteristics were matched, moderate to severe hydronephrosis group was associated with a significantly higher risk of ureteral stenosis (HR 69.86;95% CI 0.67–7279.84; $P=0.073$).

The incidence of ureteral injury was higher in the moderate to severe hydronephrosis group, most of which were grade 1–2. There were only 4 cases of grade 3 injuries, among which 3 cases had ureteral strictures, and no injury above grade 4. Data for postoperative complications were collected. There were 2 cases of low fever (Clavien1), 12 cases of high fever (body temperature > 38.5) with urinary tract infection (Clavien2), 66 cases of residual stones (Clavien3a), 29 cases of ureteral stricture requiring reoperation (Clavien3b), and 1 case of postoperative sepsis requiring intensive care (Clavien 4). Long-term follow-up revealed 2 cases of asymptomatic severe hydronephrosis (Clavien3b).

Twenty-nine patients had postoperative stenosis, of which 21 underwent reoperation in our hospital. Two patients accepted nephrectomy due to severe hydronephrosis. Eleven patients were cured after partial ureterectomy and ureteral end-to-end anastomosis. One person was cured after ureteral balloon dilation. Four patients had ureteral laser incision, and after failure, they went to other hospitals for further treatment. Three patients were placed with ureteral stents, and one of them had ureteral recanalization after removal of the stents. The other two patients did not improve the hydronephrosis, so they went to other hospitals for further treatment.

Discussion

The main results of our research were as follows. First, the incidence of stenosis in moderate to severe hydronephrosis group was higher than that in the mild hydronephrosis group. Second, in the moderate to severe hydronephrosis group, the incidence of intraoperative

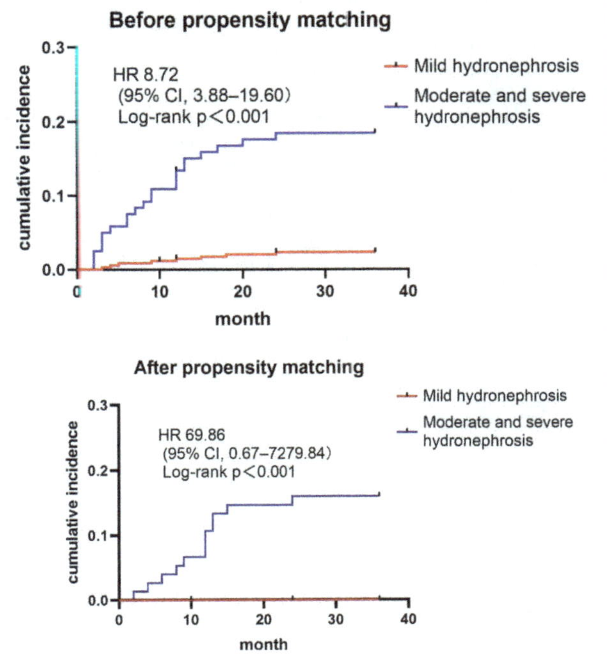

Fig. 2 Kaplan–Meier cumulative event curves of ureteral stenosis before and after propensity score-matching. Adjusted risks of mild hydronephrosis relative to Moderate and severe hydronephrosis are shown

ureteral injury was higher; the duration of operation was longer, and the postoperative SFR was lower. However, there was no difference in the SFR and operation time between groups after adjusting for baseline. Third, the Kaplan–Meier cumulative event curve showed that incidence of ureteral stricture was higher in the moderate to severe hydronephrosis group.

There are several studies on the risk factors of ureteral stricture. In a prospective study, AMR E. Darwish et al. included variables such as stone burden, stone impaction, operative time, and double J tube placement time. Logistic regression analysis found that stone impaction was associated with ureteral stricture. There were only 4 cases of Ureteral stricture in the article [3]. Xeng Inn Fam et al. explored the risk factors for ureteral stricture after ureteroscopy in the treatment of impaction calculi. The variables included ureteral perforation, mucosal injury, stone impaction, impaction time, stone size, impaction location, etc., but they failed to find any predictive factors. However, there were only 5 cases of Ureteral stricture [11]. Both above two studies used Logistic regression analysis to correct other factors, but the sample size and the number of stenosis cases were small, which affected power and statistical analysis. In our study, 29 patients with ureteral stenosis were included. Patients were grouped according to hydronephrosis. We got 75 pairs of matched patients through propensity matching. Sample size was expanded as far as possible to improve the accuracy of statistical results.

There are many speculations about the mechanism of ureteral stenosis after Ureteroscopic surgery, such as stone impaction, access sheath injury, large stone burden, intraoperative ureteral perforation and the surgeon's experience [2, 12]. Daniel A Wollin et al. designed an in vitro model to study the water temperature at different perfusion rates during holmium laser lithotripsy. The authors found that, even with high laser power, adequate irrigation could still maintain a relatively stable temperature. With the decrease of the perfusion velocity, the laser-induced temperature could be significantly increased in spite of lower laser power. This condition might cause ureteral tissue damage [13]. Shiulian Chen et al. included eight studies with a total of 1760 patients in a meta-analysis. The results showed that the incidence of ureteral stenosis after holmium laser lithotripsy was higher than pneumatic lithotripsy. The authors believed that this issue demanded further research [14]. In actual practice, we find that if the calculi cannot be pushed during the operation, ureteral stricture is more likely to happen postoperatively. If the ureteral stone is pushed into the renal pelvis after a brief time holmium laser lithotripsy, there is almost no postoperative ureteral stenosis. This is consistent with Daniel A Wollin's model. The above studies show that stone impaction and ureteral injury may be causal. The key is how to predict stone impaction before surgery. Stone impaction is a vague concept, which is difficult to judge only by preoperative clinical manifestations. The thickening of the ureteral wall on CT may reveal stone impaction and the stone wrapping by polyps, which can predict postoperative stenosis [6]. In our practice, we found that the degree of hydronephrosis was associated with postoperative stenosis, which might be another indicator to predict postoperative stenosis after FRUS. This point was confirmed by our retrospective study.

Our study has some limitations. First, this is a single-center retrospective study with a limited sample size. Surgical equipment and techniques are restricted by the center. Randomized controlled studies will be ideal, but studies of postoperative complications may be difficult to achieve. Propensity matching can be an effective tool to reduce potential bias and baseline differences in a retrospective study. Second, after propensity scores matching analysis, there is no statistical difference of the operation time and SFR, possibly because the patients with ipsilateral ureteral calculi and large renal stones account for a sizeable proportion, which prolongs the operative time and reduces SFR. However, an extended version of exclusion criteria may include a relatively small number of patients, which may reduce the strength of the conclusions in this paper. Third, the author did not participate in all the operations and could only evaluate the patient's condition according to the medical records and imaging. So intraoperative details may be omitted. Fourth, Patients are lost to follow-up and the missing data may affect our results.

Conclusions

Preoperative moderate to severe hydronephrosis is a predictor of postoperative ureteral stricture. Patients with moderate to severe hydronephrosis have an increased risk of complications such as ureteral injury and postoperative stricture after FURS. The prevalence of ureteral stricture has increased over time. Clinicians may choose the appropriate surgical procedure based on the preoperative degree of hydronephrosis.

Abbreviations

FURS: Flexible ureteroscopy; SWL: Extracorporeal shock wave lithotripsy; BMI: Body mass index; CTU: Computed tomography urography; KUB: X-ray of kidney ureter bladder; SFR: Stone-free rate; HR: Hazard ratio; CI: 95% Confidence interval.

Authors' contributions

SS contributed to the conception of the study; AX collected information and followed up patients, YS performed the data analyses and wrote the manuscript. All authors read and approved the final manuscript.

Competing interests

The authors declare that they have no competing interests.

References

1. Türk (Chair) AN C, Petřík A, Seitz C, Skolarikos (Vice-chair) A, Somani B, Thomas K, Gambaro G; members of the EAU–ESTRO–ESUR–IOG urolithiasis guidelines panel: EAU–ESTRO–ESUR–SIOG guidelines on urolithiasis. 2021. https://uroweb.org/guideline/urolithiasis/#3.
2. Dong H, Peng Y, Li L, Gao X. Prevention strategies for ureteral stricture following ureteroscopic lithotripsy. Asian J Urol. 2018;5(2):94–100.
3. Darwish AE, Gadelmoula MM, Abdelkawi IF, Abdellatif AM, Abdel-Moneim AM, Hammouda HM. Ureteral stricture after ureteroscopy for stones: a prospective study for the incidence and risk factors. Urol Ann. 2019;11(3):276–81.
4. Srougi V, Padovani GP, Marchini GS, Vicentini FC, Mazzucchi E, Srougi M. Outcomes of surgical treatment of ureteral strictures after laser ureterolithotripsy for impacted stones. Can J Urol. 2015;22(6):8079–84.
5. Shao Y, Wang DW, Lu GL, Shen ZJ. Retroperitoneal laparoscopic ureterolithotomy in comparison with ureteroscopic lithotripsy in the management of impacted upper ureteral stones larger than 12 mm. World J Urol. 2015;33(11):1841–5.
6. Yoshida T, Inoue T, Omura N, Okada S, Hamamoto S, Kinoshita H, Matsuda T. Ureteral wall thickness as a preoperative indicator of impacted stones in patients with ureteral stones undergoing ureteroscopic lithotripsy. Urology. 2017;106:45–9.
7. Qin C, Yin H, Du Y, Li Q, Liu H, Xu T. Predicting ureteral status below the ureteral calculi in patients undergoing ureteroscopic lithotomy. Acta Radiol. 2021; 284185120988092.
8. May PC, Hsi RS, Tran H, Stoller ML, Chew BH, Chi T, Usawachintachit M, Duty BD, Gore JL, Harper JD. The morbidity of ureteral strictures in patients with prior ureteroscopic stone surgery: multi-institutional outcomes. J Endourol. 2018;32(4):309–14.
9. Schoenthaler M, Buchholz N, Farin E, Ather H, Bach C, Bach T, Denstedt JD, Fritsche HM, Grasso M, Hakenberg OW, et al. The Post-Ureteroscopic Lesion Scale (PULS): a multicenter video-based evaluation of inter-rater reliability. World J Urol. 2014;32(4):1033–40.
10. Öğreden E, Oğuz U, Demirelli E, Benli E, Sancak EB, Gülpinar MT, Akbaş A, Reşorlu B, Ayyildiz A, Yalçin O. Categorization of ureteroscopy complications and investigation of associated factors by using the modified Clavien classification system. Turk J Med Sci. 2016;46(3):686–94.
11. Fam XI, Singam P, Ho CC, Sridharan R, Hod R, Bahadzor B, Goh EH, Tan GH, Zainuddin Z. Ureteral stricture formation after ureteroscope treatment of impacted calculi: a prospective study. Korean J Urol. 2015;56(1):63–7.
12. Ulvik Ø, Harneshaug JR, Gjengstø P. Ureteral strictures following ureteroscopic stone treatment. J Endourol. 2021;35(7):985–90.
13. Wollin DA, Carlos EC, Tom WR, Simmons WN, Preminger GM, Lipkin ME. Effect of laser settings and irrigation rates on ureteral temperature during holmium laser lithotripsy, an in vitro model. J Endourol. 2018;32(1):59–63.
14. Chen S, Zhou L, Wei T, Luo D, Jin T, Li H, Wang K. Comparison of holmium: YAG laser and pneumatic lithotripsy in the treatment of ureteral stones: an update meta-analysis. Urol Int. 2017;98(2):125–33.

7

Transplant-associated penile Kaposi sarcoma managed with single agent paclitaxel chemotherapy

Matthew A. Anderson[1*], Tracey Ying[1,2,3], Kate Wyburn[1,2,3], Peter M. Ferguson[3,4], Madeleine C. Strach[5], Peter Grimison[3,5], Steve Chadban[1,2,3] and David M. Gracey[1,2,3]

Abstract

Background: Kaposi's sarcoma is an uncommon complication in renal transplant patients, and typically presents with cutaneous lesions on the lower extremities. Penile involvement has been reported only rarely. Management of cutaneous-limited disease is primarily reduction of immunosuppression and conversion to an mTOR-inhibitor, whereas the treatment of disseminated disease in transplant patients is more variable.

Case presentation: A 75-year-old male, originally from Somalia, received a deceased-donor kidney transplant for diabetic and hypertensive nephropathy. Seven months post-transplant he presented with lower limb lesions, oedema and bilateral deep vein thromboses. He then developed a fast-growing painful lesion on his penile shaft. A biopsy of this lesion confirmed KS, and a PET scan demonstrated disseminated disease in the lower extremities, penis and thoracic lymph nodes. His tacrolimus was converted to sirolimus, and his other immunosuppression was reduced. He was treated with single agent paclitaxel chemotherapy in view of his rapidly progressing, widespread disease. The penile lesion completely resolved, and the lower extremity lesions regressed significantly. His kidney allograft function remained stable throughout treatment.

Conclusion: This case illustrates a rare presentation of an uncommon post-transplant complication and highlights the need for a high index of suspicion of KS in transplant patients presenting with atypical cutaneous lesions. It serves to demonstrate that the use of single agent paclitaxel chemotherapy, switch to an mTORi and reduction in immunosuppression where possible produces excellent short-term outcomes, adding to the body of evidence for this management strategy in disseminated Kaposi's sarcoma.

Keywords: Kaposi sarcoma, Transplant, Renal, Malignancy, Therapy, Chemotherapy, Immunosuppression, Sirolimus

Background

Kaposi Sarcoma (KS) is a low-grade multi-centric tumour composed of endothelium-lined vascular spaces and spindle cells [1]. It was initially described in 1872 by Moritz Kaposi, and remained an uncommon phenomenon until 1979, when it was first recognised in solid organ transplant patients [2]. The incidence in kidney transplant recipients has since been reported to be as high as 500-times that of the general population [3]. Its pathogenesis derives from reactivation of human herpesvirus-8 (HHV-8) in the setting of immunosuppression. KS classically presents as angiomatous cutaneous lesions on the lower limbs. Disseminated disease with visceral involvement is uncommon and carries a poorer prognosis. The optimal management of disseminated disease in the transplant setting is not well defined.

*Correspondence: matthew.anderson@health.nsw.gov.au
[1] Department of Renal Medicine and Renal Transplant, Royal Prince Alfred Hospital, Missenden Rd, Camperdown, NSW, Australia
Full list of author information is available at the end of the article

Case presentation

The case was a 75-year-old male of Somali heritage, who received a deceased donor kidney transplant for presumed diabetic and hypertensive nephropathy. The donor was marginal but immunologically low-risk, being a 4/6 HLA mismatch with a single weak class II donor-specific antibody. At the time of transplant, he received our unit's standard induction immunosuppression with basiliximab and methylprednisolone, then commenced maintenance immunosuppression with tacrolimus, everolimus, and prednisone. A denovo mTOR inhibitor (mTORi) was chosen in place of mycophenolate mofetil due to the recipients older age, pre-existing leukopenia and known vascular disease in the donor. The transplant was complicated by delayed graft function necessitating haemodialysis on day one. A renal biopsy on day nine demonstrated borderline acute T-cell mediated rejection; as such, the everolimus was replaced with mycophenolate mofetil. The graft function subsequently improved to a baseline creatinine of 170 μmol/L (eGFR 34 ml/min) with minimal proteinuria (albumin: creatinine ratio 2.6 mg/mmol). A protocol biopsy at eight weeks showed no features of rejection.

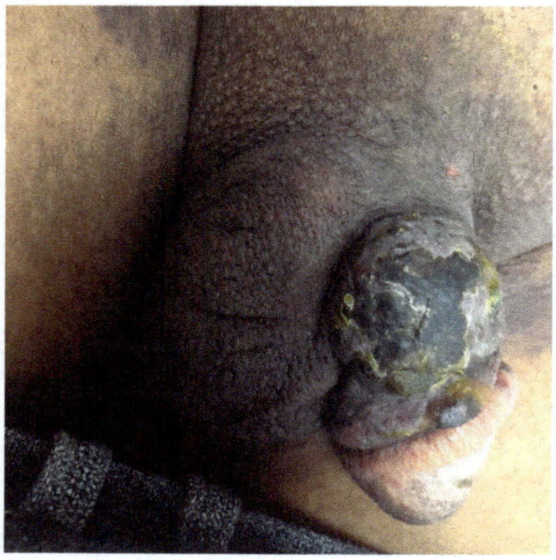

Fig. 1 Painful rapidly growing penile lesion in a renal allograft recipient 7 months post-transplant

Seven months post-transplant the recipient presented with bilateral lower limb pain and swelling, and dark macular skin lesions on his legs. He underwent a duplex ultrasound which demonstrated bilateral proximal deep vein thromboses. Anticoagulation with apixaban was commenced. Soon after he presented with a painful papular lesion on his penile shaft, which began as a small macule and had grown rapidly (Fig. 1). There was no associated exudate or surrounding erythema, nor associated urinary symptoms. Two small satellite lesions had also erupted on the glans of the penis. The patient was referred for a biopsy.

A biopsy of the penile lesion demonstrated diffuse involvement of the dermis by nodules of mitotically active spindled cells, with irregular slit-like spaces, which stained positive for HHV-8, diagnostic of KS (Fig. 2).

A PET scan demonstrated diffusely increased metabolism in the skin and subcutaneous tissues of the feet and lower legs, and over the surface of the penis. There was also abnormally increased metabolism in the paratracheal lymph nodes, with no increased metabolism in the

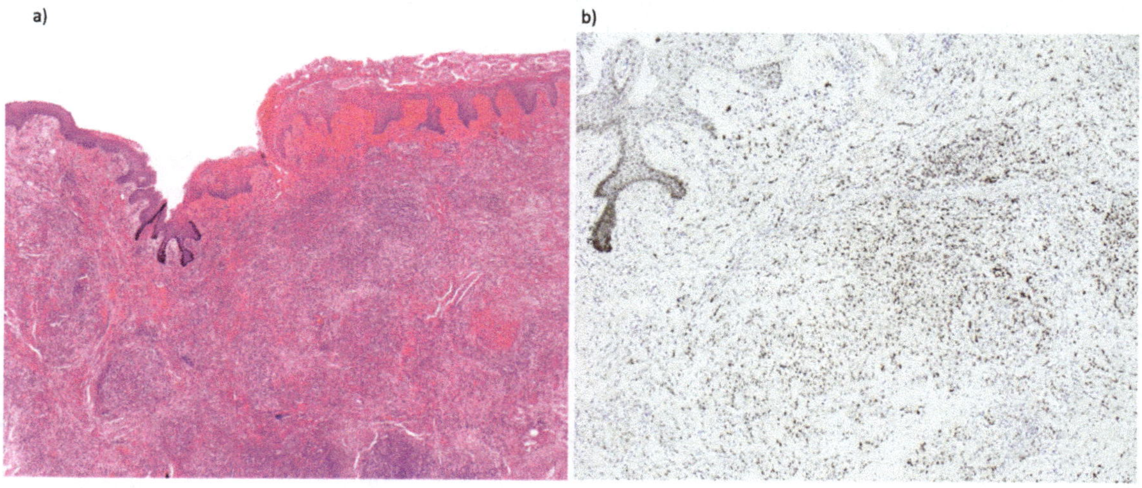

Fig. 2 Biopsy of penile lesion biopsy demonstrating: **a** diffuse infiltration of the stroma by spindled cells forming slit-like anastomosing spaces containing erythrocytes (40× magnification), and **b** immunohistochemistry staining for human herpesvirus-8 (HHV-8) (100× magnification)

inguinal, femoral, pelvic or abdominal nodes nor visceral organs (Fig. 3a).

In view of the rapidly progressive disseminated disease, the recipient commenced weekly single-agent paclitaxel chemotherapy with a plan for twelve weeks in total. His immunosuppression was reduced, with the mycophenolate ceased, prednisone dose tapered to 5 mg daily, and the tacrolimus switched to sirolimus, with a dose of 1.5 mg daily maintaining a level of 5-8 μg/L.

The recipient responded well to chemotherapy and reduced immunosuppression. After four weeks of paclitaxel the penile lesion resolved completely with no

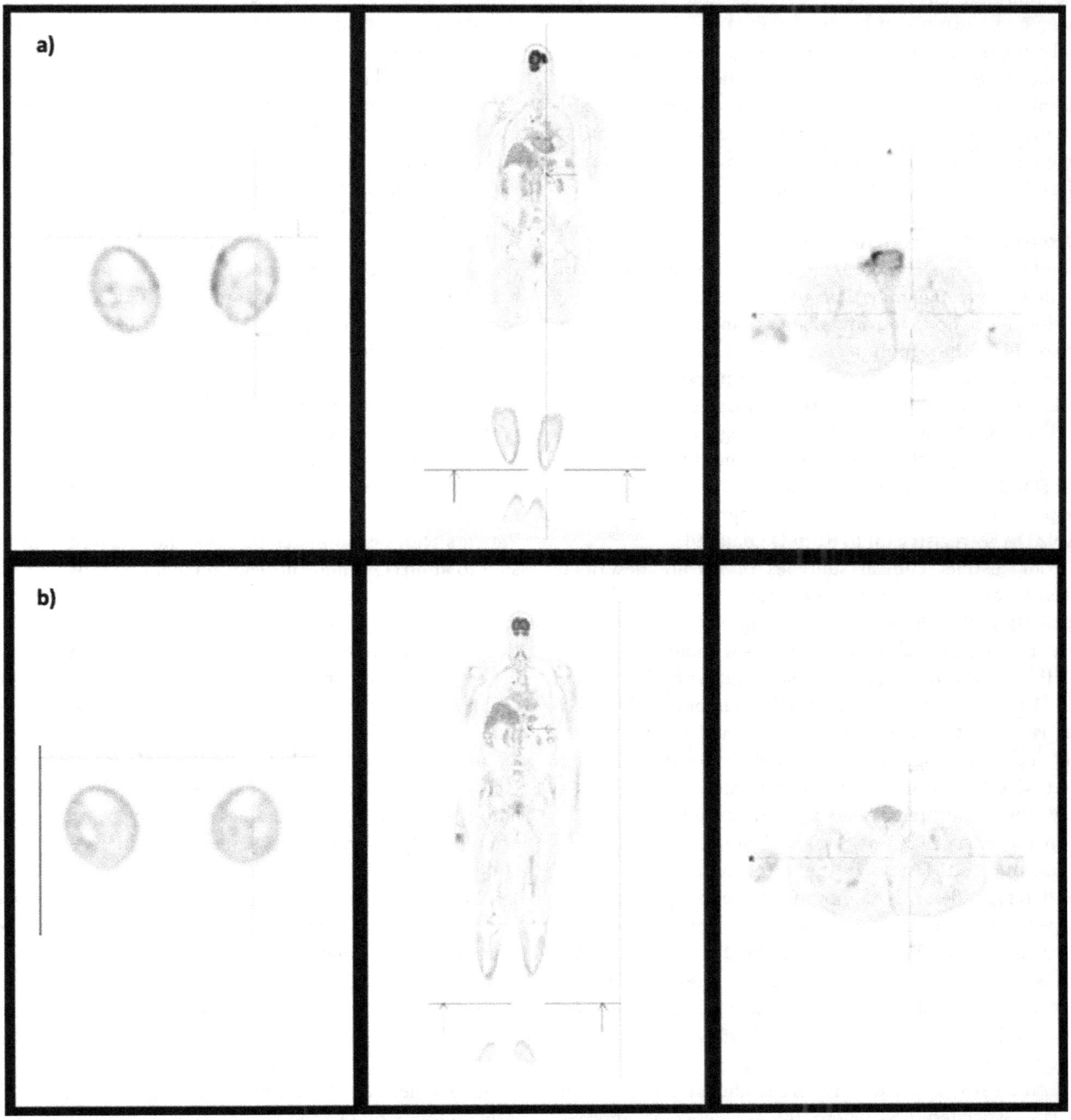

Fig. 3 **a** FET scan at diagnosis demonstrating diffusely increased metabolism in the skin and subcutaneous tissues of the feet, lower legs and over the surface of the penis, as well as abnormally increased metabolism in the paratracheal lymph nodes (middle image, arrow). **b** PET scan after three months of therapy demonstrating decreased metabolism of the skin and subcutaneous tissues of the lower limbs, absence of previously identified increased metabolism in the penile shaft, and reduced but ongoing increased metabolism in the right paratracheal node (arrow)

residual scarring, and the lower limb lesions significantly regressed. A progress PET scan (Fig. 3b) demonstrated decreased metabolism of the skin and subcutaneous tissues of the lower limbs, and absence of previously identified increased metabolism in the penile shaft. There was ongoing increased metabolism in the right paratracheal node. The only complication of chemotherapy was a grade 1 peripheral neuropathy. On most recent review, 11 months following the initial presentation, there has been no recurrence of Kaposi sarcoma.

Throughout the treatment the patient's transplant function remained stable, with no evidence of rejection despite the reduction in immunosuppression. He is now 18 months post-transplant, with the most recent pathology demonstrating a creatinine of 162 µmol/L, with no proteinuria (ACR 1.3 mg/mmol).

Discussion and conclusions

Solid organ transplant is associated with an increased risk of de novo malignancy, with registry data demonstrating an incidence up to fourfold higher than the general population [4] [5] [6]. Immunosuppression is hypothesised to have a carcinogenic effect through impaired immunosurveillance mechanisms and direct damage to host DNA, as well as the potentiation of proto-oncogenic viruses [7].Of all post-transplant malignancies, KS has by far the highest standardised incidence ratio compared to the general population, with reported ratios ranging from 22 in the ANZDATA registry [8] to 61 in US data [9].

Four distinct clinical subtypes of KS are described: classic; organ-transplant associated; epidemic (AIDS-related); and endemic (a unique aggressive subtype that occurs in equatorial African patients without HIV).

HHV-8 has been causally associated with all forms of KS [10]. The seroprevalence of HHV8 in population studies is highest in the Mediterranean and Central Africa [11, 12]. Paralleling this, transplant recipients of African and Mediterranean origin are consistently identified to have the highest rates of KS post-transplant [9].

In more than 90% of cases, KS presents as angiomatous cutaneous lesions in the lower extremities. Associated lymphedema is common, and often precedes the appearance of cutaneous lesions. Disseminated visceral involvement occurs in approximately 25% of kidney transplant-associated KS, with higher rates seen in liver and heart transplant recipients [13] [14]. The most frequently implicated extra-cutaneous sites are the lymph nodes, gastrointestinal tract and lungs.

Genital KS is rare and reported almost exclusively in AIDS-associated KS, where the incidence is approximately 3% [15]. Only a single case report of penile KS in a transplant patient is reported in the literature [16]. In that case, the KS was cutaneous-limited (confined to the glans of the penis), and the patient was treated with reduction in immunosuppression and conversion to mTORi; however, they sustained subsequent graft loss due to acute rejection.

Reduction in immunosuppression is the cornerstone of management in transplant-associated KS and is often adequate in treating cutaneous-limited disease. However, any reduction in immunosuppression must be balanced with the risk of allograft loss from rejection. Switching the more oncogenic immunosuppressants (particularly calcineurin inhibitors) for an mTORi has become a commonly accepted management strategy. The efficacy of this approach was demonstrated in a 2005 case series of 15 patients, where cessation of cyclosporine and commencement of sirolimus was associated with complete resolution of cutaneous KS in all patients, with no reports of graft dysfunction [1].

The management of disseminated KS in transplant recipients is not well described in the literature. In 2019 a retrospective analysis was published describing the management strategies of 145 organ transplant recipients with KS across different European centres [17]. Of these patients, 51% had disseminated disease at diagnosis. Their first-line management was highly variable, with 95% of patients having a reduction in immunosuppression, 28% being converted to an mTORi, and 16% receiving chemotherapy [14 anthracycline, 1 paclitaxel] in addition to immunosuppression regimen alteration. Patients with disseminated disease who received conversion to an mTORi and short-term chemotherapy had the best response rates.

There are no guidelines recommending which chemotherapeutic agent to use in disseminated transplant-associated KS. Treatment decisions are typically based off safety and efficacy data extrapolated from AIDS-related and classic KS cohorts with disseminated disease. In a 2020 update on therapy for Kaposi sarcoma, bleomycin and vinblastine were identified as the most widely employed single-agent therapies [18]. However, they are often poorly tolerated, particularly in elderly patients, and their use is limited by potential toxicity. Taxanes (paclitaxel and docetaxel) and liposomal doxorubicin are better tolerated and have been found to be efficacious in disseminated KS, and thus are being used more often in this setting [19, 20]. There are also reports of responses to anti-programmed-cell-death-protein immune checkpoint inhibitors, however their safety in renal transplant recipients has not been established [21].

Management of KS in transplant recipients is particularly complex due to the risk of rejection and graft loss with immunosuppression reduction, and the increased risk of infection when already immunosuppressed patients are treated with chemotherapy. Outcomes for disseminated disease have traditionally been poor. In 1997 Penn reported a mortality rate of 57% in those with disseminated disease (22). In a 2005 South African retrospective analysis of 21 transplant patients with KS, six had disseminated disease, three died rapidly, while the other three survived but suffered allograft loss due to acute rejection.

In summary, we present a case of a very rare manifestation of KS in a kidney transplant recipient. Penile lesions in immunosuppressed men should prompt consideration for KS and early referral for biopsy. Given the rarity of this disease, trials in this area are not feasible. There are no clear guidelines for optimal management of disseminated KS in transplant patients, and prognosis for allograft function and mortality are poor. This case serves to demonstrate that treatment with single agent taxane chemotherapy, switch to an mTORi, and reduction in immunosuppression where possible produced excellent short-term outcomes, and thus should be considered as a potential management strategy in similar patients.

Abbreviations

KS: Kaposi sarcoma; HHV-8: Human herpesvirus 8; HLA: Human leukocyte antigen; mTOR: Mammalian target of rapamycin; mTORi: Mammalian target of rapamycin inhibitor; eGFR: Estimated glomerular filtration rate; ACR: Albumin:creatinine ratio; DVT: Deep vein thrombosis; PET: Positron emission tomography; ANZDATA: Australian and New Zealand Dialysis and Transplant Registry; AIDS: Acquired immunodeficiency syndrome; HIV: Human immunodeficiency virus.

Acknowledgements

Dr Francesca Watts (Anatomical Pathology Registrar, Royal Prince Alfred Hospital) for her assistance in procuring the histology images.

Authors' contributions

MA collected the data and wrote the article. TY, DG, MS, PG and SC provided substantive assistance in revising the report. KW, MS and PG provided guidance with conception and design of the report and assisted in acquisition and analysis of references. PF performed testing of the biopsy sample and analysed the data. All authors have reviewed the final draft and approved the article.

Competing interests

The authors all declare that they have no competing interests.

Author details

[1]Department of Renal Medicine and Renal Transplant, Royal Prince Alfred Hospital, Missenden Rd, Camperdown, NSW, Australia. [2]Kidney Node, Charles Perkins Centre, University of Sydney, Camperdown, NSW, Australia. [3]Central Clinical School, Faculty of Medicine, University of Sydney, Camperdown, NSW, Australia. [4]Department of Tissue Pathology, Royal Prince Alfred Hospital, Missenden Rd, Camperdown, NSW, Australia. [5]Department of Medical Oncology, Chris O'Brien Lifehouse, Camperdown, NSW, Australia.

References

1. Stallone G, Schena A, Infante B. Sirolimus for Kaposi's sarcoma in renal-transplant patients. N Eng J Med. 2005;352(13):1317–23. https://doi.org/10.1056/NEJMoa042831.
2. Penn I. Kaposi's sarcoma in recipients of renal transplants; report of 20 cases. Transplantation. 1979;27(1):8–11. https://doi.org/10.1097/00007890-197901000-00003.
3. Harwoord AR, Osoba D, Hofstader SL, et al. Kaposi's sarcoma in recipients of renal transplants. Am J Med. 1979;67(5):759–65. https://doi.org/10.1016/0002-9343(79)90731-9.
4. Stewart JH, Vajdic CM, Van Leeuwen MT, et al. The pattern of excess cancer in dialysis and transplantation. Nephrol Dial Transplant. 2009;24(10):3225–31. https://doi.org/10.1093/ndt/gfp331.
5. Vadjic CM, McDonald SP, McCredie MRE, et al. Cancer incidence before and after kidney transplantation. JAMA. 2006;296(23):2823–31. https://doi.org/10.1001/jama.296.23.2823.
6. Au EH, Chapman JR, Craig JC. Overall and site-specific cancer mortality in patients on dialysis and after kidney transplant. J Am Soc Nephrol. 2019;30(3):471–80. https://doi.org/10.1681/ASN.2018090906.
7. Billups K, Neal J, Salyer J. Immunosuppressant-driven de novo malignant neoplasms after solid-organ transplant. Prog Transplant. 2015;25(2):182–8. https://doi.org/10.7182/pit2015826.
8. Webster AC, Peng A, Kelly PJ. *ANZDATA 35th Annual Report 2012. Chapter Ten, Cancer Report.* Adelaide: Australian and New Zealand Dialysis and Transplant Registry; 2012:10-1-9.
9. Engels EA, Pfeiffer RM, Fraumeni JF, et al. Spectrum of cancer risk among US solid organ transplant recipients. JAMA. 2011;306(17):1891–901. https://doi.org/10.1001/jama.2011.1592.
10. Sing N. Human herpesviruses-6,-7 and -8 in organ transplant recipients. Clin Mocrobiol Infect. 2000;6(9):453–9.
11. Whitby D, Luppi M, Barozzi P. Human Herpesvirus 8 Seroprevalence in Blood Donors and Lymphoma Patients From Different Regions of Italy. J Natl Cancer Inst. 1998;90:395–7. https://doi.org/10.1093/jnci/90.5.395.
12. Dollard SC, Butler LM, Graves AM, et al. Substantial regional differences in human herpesvirus 8 seroprevalence in sub-Saharan Africa: insights on the origin of the "Kaposi's sarcoma belt." Int J Cancer. 2010;127(10):2395–401. https://doi.org/10.1002/ijc.25235.
13. Moosa MR. Kaposi's sarcoma in kidney transplant recipients: a 23 year experience. Q J Med. 2005;98(3):205–14. https://doi.org/10.1093/qjmed/hci028.
14. Farge D. Kaposi's sarcoma in organ transplant recipients: the collaborative transplantation research group of Ile de France. Eur J Med. 1993;2(6):339–43 (**PMID: 8252179**).
15. Micali G, Nasca MR, Pasquale RD, et al. Primary Kaposi's sarcoma of the penis: report of a case and review. J Eur Acad Dematol Venerol. 2003;17(3):320–3. https://doi.org/10.1046/j.1468-3083.2003.00747.
16. Imko-Walczuk B, Kuelbowicz M, Malyszko J. Kaposi sarcoma in the genital area in a kidney transplant patient: a case report and literature review. Transplant Proc. 2016;48(5):1843–8. https://doi.org/10.1016/j.transproced.2016.01.070.
17. Deylon J, Rabate C, Euvrad S, et al. Management of Kaposi sarcoma after solid organ transplantation: a European study. J Am Acad Dematol. 2019;81(2):448–55. https://doi.org/10.1016/j.jaad.2019.03.028.
18. Dupin N. Update on oncogenesis and therapy for Kaposi sarcoma. Curr Opin Oncol. 2020;32(2):122–8. https://doi.org/10.1097/CCO.0000000000000601.
19. Dennis D, Regnier-Rosencher E, Kamkimel N, et al. First line treatment with paclitaxel for non-HIV related Kaposi sarcoma: experience in ten cases. Br J Dermatol. 2016;174:905–90. https://doi.org/10.1111/bjd.14237.
20. Gill PS, Wernz J, Scadden DT, et al. Randomised phase III trial of liposomal daunorubicin versus doxorubicin, bleomycin and vincristine in AIDS-related Kaposi sarcoma. J Clin Oncolo. 1996;14:2453–64. https://doi.org/10.1200/JCO.1996.14.8.2353.
21. Deylon J. PD1 blockade with pembrolizumab in classic and endemic Kaposi sarcoma: a multicentre phase II study. ESMO Virtual Congress 2020. Abstract 1077M. Ann Oncol. 2020;31(4):672–710. https://doi.org/10.1016/annonc/annonc280.
22. Penn I. Kaposi's sarcoma in transplant recipients. Transplantation. 1997;64(5):669–73. https://doi.org/10.1097/00007890-199709150-00001.

8

Current antibiotic resistance patterns of rare uropathogens: Survey from Central European Urology Department 2011–2019

Jan Hrbacek[1*], Pavel Cermak[2] and Roman Zachoval[1]

Abstract

Background: While the resistance rates of commonly detected uropathogens are well described, those of less frequent Gram-negative uropathogenic bacteria have seldom been reported. The aim of this study was to examine the resistance rates of less frequent uropathogenic Gram-negatives in a population of patients treated in a Department of Urology of a tertiary referral centre in Central Europe over a period of 9 years.

Methods: Data on all positive urine samples from urological in- and out-patients were extracted form the Department of Clinical Microbiology database from 2011 to 2019. Numbers of susceptible and resistant isolates per year were calculated for these uropathogens: *Acinetobacter* spp. ($n = 74$), *Citrobacter* spp. ($n = 60$), *Enterobacter* spp. ($n = 250$), *Morganella morganii* ($n = 194$), *Providencia* spp. ($n = 53$), *Serratia* spp. ($n = 82$) and *Stenotrophomonas maltophilia* ($n = 27$). Antimicrobial agents selected for the survey included: ampicillin, amoxicillin/clavulanic acid, piperacillin/tazobactam; cefuroxime, cefotaxime, ceftazidime and cefepime; ciprofloxacin and ofloxacin; gentamicin and amikacin; ertapenem, meropenem and imipenem; trimethoprim-sulfamethoxazole (co-trimoxazole), nitrofurantoin and colistin.

Results: Penicillin derivatives have generally poor effect except piperacillin/tazobactam. Cefuroxime is not efficient unlike cefotaxime (except against *Acinetobacter* spp. and *S. maltophilia*). Susceptibility to fluoroquinolones is limited. Amikacin is somewhat more efficient than gentamicine but susceptibilities for both safely exceed 80%. Nitrofurantoin shows virtually no efficiency. Cotrimoxazole acts well against *Citrobacter* spp., *Serratia* spp. and it is the treatment of choice for *S. maltophilia* UTIs. Among carbapenems, ertapenem was less efficient than meropenem and imipenem except for *S. maltophilia* whose isolates were mostly not suceptible to any carbapenems.

Conclusions: Uropathogenic microorganisms covered in this report are noteworthy for their frequently multi-drug resistant phenotypes. Knowledge of resistance patterns helps clinicians choose the right empirical antibiotic treatment when the taxonomical assignment of the isolate is known but sensitivity results are pending.

Keywords: Urinary tract infections, Drug resistance, Bacterial, Anti-infective agents, Urinary, Acinetobacter, Citrobacter, Enterobacter, Morganella, Providencia, Serratia, Stenotrophomonas

Background

With approximately 150–250 million cases occurring globally per year [1, 2], urinary tract infections (UTIs) represent some of the most common infectious diseases in humans. Gram-negative enteric bacteria such as *Escherichia coli*, *Klebsiella* spp. and *Proteus* spp. are their most common causative agents. UTIs occur more frequently among women than in men: 50% of females

*Correspondence: jan.hrbacek@ftn.cz
[1] Department of Urology, 3rd Faculty of Medicine, Charles University and Thomayer University Hospital, Videnska 800, 140 59 Prague, Czech Republic
Full list of author information is available at the end of the article

will experience at least one UTI in their lifetime [3]. Recurrences are common and besides associated morbidity, UTIs put pressure on health care systems, too. While the cost of treatment of a single UTI episode is insignificant, their frequent incidence means they consume a non-negligible part of the health care budget: in France alone, the expense for adult female UTIs amounted to 58 million euro in 2012 [4]. Complicated UTIs are even more costly: one episode of a complicated UTI costs between 4028 and 7740 euro [5] depending on the health care system.

Antimicrobial resistance (AMR) has become a major concern threathening many an advance of medicine in the twenty-first century. Uropathogenic microorganisms are no exception to this: rates of AMR among Enterobacteriaceae are increasing globally, albeit with temporal and spatial differences [6–15]. Antibiotic consumption is a primary driver for the spread of AMR as evidenced on local and country levels [16, 17]. For instance, southern European states exhibit higher AMR rates than northern ones. Of note, four top antibiotic prescribers in Europe (Greece, Cyprus, France and Italy) belong among south European countries [18].

International guidelines for UTI treatment are freely available; yet, poor antibiotic prescription remains common. Thirty percent of primary care antibiotic prescriptions were inadequate in a report from the United States [19]. Appropriate antibiotic treatment was reported in 68% of adult cystitis cases and only 46% of pyelonephritis cases in another survey [20].

One of the ways to improve the quality of antibiotic prescribing is antibiotic stewardship including the monitoring of local antimicrobial susceptibility patterns [6]. While AMR patterns of the commonest causative uropathogenic agents—*E. coli*, *Klebsiella* spp., *Proteus* spp., *Pseudomonas aeruginosa* etc. have been widely reported, less attention has been devoted to microbes at the bottom of the prevalence ladder. These microorganisms constitute only a small fraction of UTI etiological agents but frequently display a multi-drug resistant phenotype, presenting a therapeutic challenge [21, 22]. Furthermore, they often have the ability to survive in hostile environments such as dry surfaces, nutrient-poor aqueous solutions [23, 24] and require a particularly attentive nursing care.

The aim of this retrospective observational study was to report the AMR patterns for seven less frequent causative agents of UTIs in a Central European tertiary referral centre Department of Urology over a period of nine years.

Methods

Similar to our previous related work [25], urinary cultures from the Department of Clinical Microbiology electronic database between January 2011 and December 2019 were searched for those caused by the following genera: *Acinetobacter*, *Citrobacter*, *Enterobacter*, *Morganella*, *Providencia*, *Serratia* and *Stenotrophomonas*. Urine cultures may have originated from spontaneously voided midstream samples, aseptic catheterisation during theatre procedures, indwelling catheters, suprapubic catheters, nephrostomy tubes and uretero-ileostomies. Because of the small prevalence of these uropathogens, inpatient and outpatient samples were included in the analysis. Duplicates were eliminated, allowing only one isolate of a given pathogen per patient per year. Prevalence of uropathogenic organisms and their antimicrobial susceptibility patterns (including trends where appropriate) were analysed.

Culture methods and susceptibility testing

The method used for culture and susceptibility testing has been described elsewhere [25]. Briefly, uncentrifuged urine was inoculated with a 0.01 ml loop on blood and UriSelect chromogenic agar (Bio-Rad, Berkeley, CA, USA) in a semi-quantitative dilution method. Urine diluted in saline (1:10) was inoculated with a 0.01 mL and 0.001 mL loop on Columbia blood agar (Bio-Rad, Berkeley, CA, USA) and UriSelect chromogenic agar. Agar plates were incubated at 37 °C for 20–24 h. Microorganisms were identified by their phenotypical characteristic and using the semi-automatic system MIKROLATEST ID (Erba-Lachema, Brno, Czech Republic).

Antibiotic susceptibility testing was performed by the disc diffusion method on Mueller–Hinton agar (Bio-Rad, Berkeley, CA, USA) and by the MIC dilution method (TRIOS MIC, Prague, Czech Republic until 2017, then MICRO-LA-TEST ATB (MIC) Erba-Lachema, Brno, Czech Republic). EUCAST MIC breakpoint tables were used. Intermediate results were excluded from this analysis. The cut-off used for significant bacterial presence was 10^5 colony-forming units/mL (10^3 for aseptically catheterised urine specimens).

This survey covers the following antimicrobial agents: ampicillin, amoxicillin/clavulanate and piperacillin/tazobactam; cefuroxime, cefotaxime, ceftazidime and cefepime; ciprofloxacin and ofloxacin; gentamicin and amikacin; ertapenem, meropenem and imipenem; trimethoprim-sulfamethoxazole (co-trimoxazole), nitrofurantoin and colistin.

Cochrane-Armitage test was used to assess statistical significance of trends. Statistical analyses were performed in XLSTAT 2020.1.3 (Addinsoft, New York, USA). Alpha level of 0.05 was considered significant.

Results

From a total of 15,909 positive urine cultures (duplicates excluded) between 1 January 2011 and 31 December 2019, the pathogens surveyed in the present study were detected in 740 samples (4.65%, range 3.33–6.03% of all positive urine cultures per year, no evidence for trend in incidence rate [p = 0.23]) from 607 patients. Of these, 466 (76.8%) were males and 141 (23.2%) were females. Mean age (interquartile range) was 70.3 (64–77) and 69.2 (59–76) for men and women, respectively. Two-thirds of urine samples (n = 482) originated from out-patients and 258 from in-patients (see Additional file 2: Table S7 for details). *Enterobacter* spp. was the most prevalent uropathogen during the study period (n = 250, 33.8%) followed by *Morganella morganii* (n = 194, 26.2%). The isolates identified included *Acinetobacter* spp. (n = 74), *Citrobacter* spp. (n = 60, including *C. braakii* (n = 1), *C. freundii* (n = 2), *C. koseri* (n = 23)), *Enterobacter* spp. (n = 250, including *E. aerogenes* (n = 3), *E. cloacae* (n = 12)), *Morganella morganii* (n = 194), *Providencia* spp. (n = 53, including *P. alcalifaciens* (n = 2), *P. rettgeri* (n = 11), *P. stuartii* (n = 32)), *Serratia* spp. (n = 82, including *S. ficaria* (n = 4), *S. marcescens* (n = 10), *S. odorifera* (n = 1)) and *Stenotrophomonas maltophilia* (n = 27).

There was no trend in the yearly prevalence of individual uropathogens (Fig. 1). Trends in resistance rates were computed for *Enterobacter* spp. and *M. morganii* where the number of isolates was sufficient to justify such analysis (Additional file 1: Table S1–S6).

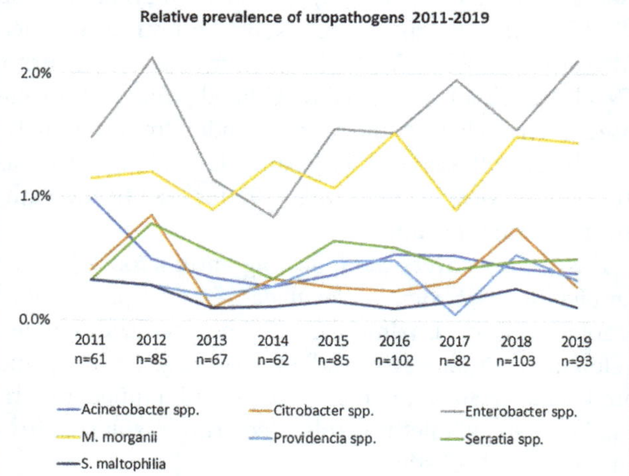

Fig. 1 Prevalence of uropathogens during the study period (relative proportions of all positive urine samples)

Antimicrobial resistance

Penicillin derivatives

Cumulative resistance rates calculated for the entire study period exceeded 80% for ampicillin and amoxicillin/clavulanic acid for all uropathogens. Piperacillin/tazobactam resistance did not exceed 10% in *Citrobacter* spp. and *Providentia* spp.; it was 16.7%, 15.4% and 13.6% for *Acinetobacter* spp., *Serratia* spp. and *M. morganii*, respectively. Table 1 summarizes resistance rates for the entire study period. Additional file 1: Table S1 gives details on the yearly number of isolates over the study period and their resistance rates to penicillins.

Cephalosporines

All uropathogens were resistant (> 50%) to second-generation cephalosporine, cefuroxime. *Citrobacter* spp. susceptibility to 3rd generation cephalosporines, cefotaxime and ceftazidime approximated 5%. *Serratia* spp. was reasonably susceptible to ceftazidime and cefepime. *Providentia* spp. retained good susceptibility to cefepime. See Additional file 1: Table S2, for details on cephalosporine resistance rates.

Fluoroquinolones

Resistance rates of all uropathogens to ciprofloxacin exceeded 20% and approximated 60% in the case of *S. maltophilia*. Resistance rates to ofloxacin were somewhat lower but never less than 15%. Additional file 1: Table S3 presents details on fluoroquinolone resistance rates.

Aminoglycosides

Citrobacter spp. and *Serratia* spp. resistance to gentamicin was just above 6%. Resistance rates of the other uropathogens to gentamicin varied between 12.4% and 33.3%. All but *Acinetobacter* spp. and *S. maltophilia* retained good susceptibility to amikacin (see Additional file 1: Table S4 for details).

Carbapenems

While *Citrobacter* spp. and *Providentia* spp. retained good suceptibility (< 10%) to all carbapenems, resistance rates to ertapenem exceeded 10% in all other bacteria examined. *S. maltophilia* resistance rate to all three carbapenems was above 60%; Additional file 1: Table S5 gives a detailed overview.

Colistin, nitrofurantoin and cotrimoxazole

Colistin had poor effect on the pathogens surveyed in this report and their resistance rates exceeded 30% except *Citrobacter* spp. (28.6%). Resistance rate to nitrofurantoin approached 100% for all but *Citrobacter*

Table 1 Cumulative resistance rates (2011–2019) of seven uropathogens to different antimicrobial agents

	ampicillin	amoxiillin/clavulanic acid	piperacillin/tazobactam	cefuroxime	cefotaxime	ceftazidime	cefepime	ciprofloxacin	ofloxacin	gentamicin	amikacin	ertapenem	meropenem	imipenem	colistin	nitrofurantoin	cotrimoxazole
Acinetobacter spp.			16.7%			30.6%	22.9%	30.6%	17.7%	12.5%	11.1%	36.1%	5.6%	5.6%	33.3%		25.7%
Citrobacter spp.		49.1%	6.3%	50.0%	5.3%	5.2%	11.8%	23.5%	15.4%	6.8%	5.9%	6.3%	0.0%	5.9%	28.6%	38.6%	10.2%
Enterobacter spp.			27.9%		20.2%	15.3%	18.8%	31.5%	12.4%	17.0%	1.8%	10.3%	1.8%	1.8%	34.5%		22.3%
Morganella morganii			13.6%		16.3%	13.7%	14.3%	34.4%	26.1%	12.4%	4.3%	13.2%	1.1%	1.1%			27.5%
Providencia spp.			8.0%		19.1%	15.2%	3.8%	37.0%	35.9%	33.3%	0.0%	0.0%	0.0%	0.0%	50.0%		33.3%
Serratia spp.			15.4%		18.9%	8.0%	2.6%	24.4%	25.4%	6.5%	7.5%	10.5%	0.0%	0.0%			15.6%
Stenotrophomonas maltophilia										27.3%	23.5%						13.0%

Numbers refer to the percentage of resistant isolates of a pathogen to a particular antibiotic during the study period. Colour coding: green = resistance rate < 20%; yellow = resistance rate 20–50%; red = resistance rate > 50%

spp. (38.6%). Cotrimoxazole resistance rates fluctuated between 10 and 30%. Cotrimoxazole was, however, the antibiotic *S. maltophilia* had the highest susceptibility to (Additional file 1: Table S6).

Discussion

The uropathogens described in this report taken all together represent 5% of all positive urinary cultures from our urology department during the nine-year study period. Their low incidence likely explains the paucity of data in the literature on their prevalence and resistance patterns compared to other Gram-negative causative agents of UTIs. Some authors report resistance patterns for groups of these bacteria only [1, 26]; others focus on a single species within a genus [27, 28]. This is where discrepancies between our and other authors' resistance data may stem from, apart from true differences in antimicrobial resistance observed across the world [6–15]. General informaion on the microorganisms covered in this report that is relevant to the topic is summarised in Table 2.

In the present study, *Acinetobacter* resistance rate exceeded 30% for most antibiotics including ertapenem. It retained > 90% susceptibility to meropenem and imipenem and its resistance rates to piperacillin/tazobactam, ofloxacin and both aminoglycosides were within the clinically useful range of < 20% (Table 1). Thus, our Acinetobacter isolates were much more susceptible to most antimicrobials (except colistin) in comparison to a Spanish study from 2018 [29].

There is a limited amount of data on antimicrobial susceptibility of *Citrobacter* in clinical urinary isolates; Jiménez-Guerra et al. report a 10-year resistance patterns in urine samples (n = 65) from a tertiary Spanish hospital. Their resistance rates oscillate in line with ours except our three-fold and 5.5-fold higher resistance rate to cefepime and nitrofurantoin, respectively [28]. Of note, solely *C. freundii* was included in the Spanish study which may account for this difference. Fajfr et al. report on *Citrobacter* spp. (n = 97) resistance rates for ampicillin, ciprofloxacin and cotrimoxazole similar to our data [27].

Enterobacter, the most frequent pathogen in our study, retained extremely good susceptibility (> 90%) to amikacin, meropenem and imipenem only; clinically useful susceptibility rates were seen for ceftazidime, cefepime, ofloxacin, aminoglycosides and ertapenem. Cefepime resistance has shown a decreasing trend but this may be related to small numbers of *Enterobacter* isolates in the first half of the study period (Additional file 1: Table S2). A study from Asia–Pacific region reported similar resistance rates for cefepime and ertapenem; other antibiotics had different resistance profiles [15]. In comparison to a geographically closer Jiménez-Guerra et al. report [28], our *Enterobacter* strains were less resistant to imipenem (1.8% vs. 8%) and more resistant to ciprofloxacin (31% vs. 19%). The inclusion of only a particular species

Table 2 Summary of clinically relevant characteristics of the microorganisms covered in this work

Acinetobacter spp.	Originally presumed to be of little pathogenicity, *Acinetobacter* has emerged as a troublesome etiological agent of hospital-acquired infections worldwide. This strictly aerobic Gram-negative coccobacillus is able to accumulate diverse mechanisms of resistance leading to phenotypes resistant to most commercially available antibiotics. The mechanisms implicated in *Acintetobacter* spp. resistance include (1) decreased expression of bacterial porins, hindering the passage of beta-lactams into the periplasmic space (where they can attach to penicillin-binding proteins); (2) over-expression of bacterial efflux pumps, causing decreased concentration of beta-lactams (as well as quinolones and other antibiotics) in the periplasmic space; (3) mutations in *gyrA* and *parC* genes causing resistance to fluoroquinolones; (4) expression of aminoglycoside-modifying enzymes leading to resistance to this class of antibiotics; (5) chromosomally encoded inducible AmpC beta-lactamases conferring resistance to cephalosporins. Finally, *Acinetobacter* spp. acquired (plasmid-mediated) serine- and metallo-beta-lactamases confer resistance to carbapenems [23, 32].
	Nosocomial UTIs are less frequent (most common *Acinetobacter*-related infection being ventilator-associated pneumonia) and are commonly diagnosed in elderly patients in ICU's, mostly men with indwelling catheters [23]. *Acinetobacter* survives for long periods on wet and dry surfaces and several studies have documented extensive contamination of the environment in the vicinity of colonised patients: bed linen, bed curtains, sink traps and hospital floor [23].
Citrobacter spp.	*Citrobacter*, *Enterobacter* and *Serratia* are facultative anaerobic non-spore forming Gram-negative rods sometimes referred to as "CES" group and described together, due to the traits they share: (1) their biochemical characteristics; (2) prevalence and resistance patterns (observation corroborated by our data); (3) various intrinsic and acquired resistance mechanisms; and (4) the fact of being frequently associated with complicated UTIs, disease recurrence and prolonged treatment. Because of their AmpC beta-lactamase production, some authors group them with *Pseudomonas* spp. and indole-positive *Proteus* spp. to complete so-called "SPICE" group [33].
	Citrobacter spp. is also one of the microorganisms implicated in the "purple urine bag syndrome", a conspicuous phenomenon of dubious clinical significance [34].
Enterobacter spp.	The genus Enterobacter comprises of 22 species and is considered an opportunistic pathogen. While its pathogenicity and virulence remain rather unclear, its resistance mechanisms have been extensively studied. The production of beta-lactamase is a major mechanism of resistance to beta-lactams; *E. aerogenes* expresses AmpC beta-lactamase (cephalosporinase) that confers resistance to 1st generation cephalosporins but is inducible during treatment with a 3rd generation cephalosporin, leading again to resistance. Aminoglycosice-modifying enzymes are responsible for resistance to aminoglycosides and a mutation in one of their genetic determinants (*aac-6'-Ib*) leads to a fluoroquinolone-resistant phenotype. A change in porin expression in the presence of imipenem leads to a decreased penetration of beta-lactams into *E. aerogenes* and bacterial efflux pumps remove fluoroquinolones and tetracyclines from *Enterobacter* spp. isolates [35]. Enterobacter is an opportunistic nosocomial pathogen: in a report from Taiwan, *E. cloacae* hospital outbreak has been described, attributale to a contaminated ureteroscope [36].
Serratia spp.	Originally presumed a non-pathogenic microorganism and even used a tracer in medical experiments, *Serratia* has established itself as an accepted clinical pathogen with widely prevalent multi-antibiotic resistant strains [37]. In urology wards, nosocomial outbreaks of *S. liquefaciens* and *S. marcescens* have been described related to cystometry appliance and urine bottles, respectively [37, 38]. Indeed, urine-measurement containers, urinometers, urine-collecting basins and urinals as well as cystoscopy suite have been found to be reservoirs of *S. marcescens* [37].
Morganella spp. and *Providencia* spp.	*Morganella* and *Providencia* are sometimes (together with *Proteus*) grouped under the tribe *Proteae*. Originally not considered frank pathogens, they have emerged as importang causative agents of hospital-acquired infections in different organ systems [39]. Their common characteristics include (1) strong urease production; (2) frequent association with complicated UTIs, prolonged treatment and disease recurrence; (3) intrinsic resistance to nitrofurantoin and colistin (as confirmed by our data) and to tetracycline; (4) intrinsically decreased susceptibility to imipenem (not observed on our data); and (5) production of various beta-lactamases including AmpC [26].
	Providencia frequently colonizes indwelling catheters; in a case-series (n = 14) of *Providencia* bacteraemia, UTI was identified as the source in 36% of cases and 71% of patients had an indwelling urinary catheter [40].
	M. morganii, *P. stuartii* and *P. rettgeri* are among the causative microorganisms of the purple-urine bag syndrome (see above).
S. maltophilia	*S. maltophilia* intrinsic resistance mechanisms (low membrane permeability, chromosomally encoded multidrug resistance efflux pumps, beta-lactamases, antibiotic-modifying enzymes etc.) were suggested to have been acquired in non-human natural environments and not being due solely to clinical use of antibiotics. Its survival is facilitated by wet surfaces and aqueous solutions with minimal nutrients (e.g. drinking water, treated water, dialysate effluent) [24].

(*E. cloacae*) in the Spanish study may account for these differences.

Our *Serratia* spp. isolates exhibited highest resistance rates to ampicillin, amoxicillin/clavulanic acid, 2nd generation cephalosporins, colistin and nitrofurantoin, in line with its characteristics described in the literature [1]. Gajdács and Urbán [1] report on the cumulative resistance rates (n = 1132 in- and out-patients combined) of CES pathogens (Citrobacter, Enterobacter, Serratia) which are very close to our population (n = 392 in- and out-patients combined): 28.8% versus 20.2%, 13.3% versus 17.0% and 19.1% versus 18.0%, for ciprofloxacin, gentamicin and cotrimoxazole, respectively.

Providencia spp. had been presumed to be more resistant to antimicrobial drugs than *Morganella* spp. [26], but neither our nor others' data [26] support this general assumption. *Providencia* spp. retained very good susceptibility to piperacillin/tazobactam and cefepime and no resistant strains were isolated to amikacin and all carbapenems. No report on urinary isolates AMR rates for

Providencia was found in the literature. For *M. morganii*, Jiménez-Guerra et al. report twice lower resistance rates to ciprofloxacin and cotrimoxazole and ten times higher resistance to imipenem (11% vs. 1.1%) [28] when compared to our data. *M. morganii* resistance rates for some of the relevant antibiotics (specifically cefotaxime, ceftazidime, amikacin and ertapenem) showed statistically significant increasing trends. Interestingly, resistance to cotrimoxazole was decreasing (Additional file 1: Table S2, S4–S6).

Although the majority of infections caused by *S. maltophilia* are respiratory tract infections [24, 30]—it is the least prevalent uropathogen in the present study—its significance as causative agent of UTIs should not be underestimated; not for its prevalence but more so for its far-reaching resistance. In our study, *S. maltophilia* resistance rate exceeded 50% for all antibiotics tested (including carbapenems); only aminoglycosides and cotrimoxazole showed more favourable resistance profiles. Its resistance to cotrimoxazole was in fact among the lowest in the present survey, despite a (statistically non-significant) increasing trend in our and others' data [31].

The limitations of the present report that need to be acknowledged include (1) the combination of both in- and out-patients in the analysis; due to small numbers of isolates cultured from urinary samples, the authors did not find further division of the study population feasible (interested readers can find the division into in- and out-patients in Additional file 2: Table S7); (2) the impossibility to distinguish between community and hospital-acquired infections as the dates of urine cultures could not be linked to admission and discharge dates of each in-patient episode; (3) lack of identification of isolates down to species level. It might also be insightful to discriminate urine samples representing asymptomatic bacteriuria as opposed to a clinically symptomatic UTI but the nature of our retrospective data would not allow for this. Our report lacks information on fosfomycin due to the fact this agent has not been used in our health care system and therefore not tested in the microbiology laboratory.

To our knowledge, this report is one of the few in the literature systematically describing prevalence and resistance patterns of uropathogens covered herein. Similarity of our resistance data to those originating from not-so-distant regions (in instances where a direct comparison was possible) suggests that our data are applicable in a wider geographic area and not just in our own institution.

Monitoring of antibiotic resistance patterns is an important contribution to (1) providing a better service to patients by the likely best choice of antimicrobial empirical treatment; (2) economically rational allocation of resources in healthcare; and (3) the prevention of the global rapid spread of antibiotic resistance, a phenomenon that jeopardises many advances in medicine and surgery achieved over the last century. The knowledge of most efficiently acting antimicrobial agents (piperacilin/tazobactam, carbapenems) should however not lead to their indiscriminate use as empirical treatment—perhaps with the exception of the gravest clinical scenarios.

Conclusions

The uropathogens described in this report are important microorganisms not for their prevalence but for their high resistance rates to a majority of commonly used antibiotics. Penicillin derivatives have generally poor effect except piperacillin/tazobactam. Cefuroxime is not efficient unlike cefotaxime, ceftazidime and cefepime (except against *Acinetobacter* spp. and *S. maltophilia*). Susceptibility to fluoroquinolones is limited. Amikacin is somewhat more efficient than gentamicine but susceptibilities for both safely exceed 80%. Nitrofurantoin shows virtually no efficiency. Cotrimoxazole acts well against *Citrobacter* spp., *Serratia* spp. and it is the treatment of choice for *S. maltophilia* UTIs. Among carbapenems, ertapenem was less efficient than meropenem and imipenem except for *S. maltophilia* whose isolates were mostly not suceptible to any carbapenems.

Abbreviations

AMR: Antimicrobial resistance; CES: Citrobacter, Enterobacter, Serratia; EUCAST: The European Committee on Antimicrobial Susceptibility Testing; ICU: Intensive care unit; MIC: Minimal inhibitory concentration; SPICE: Serratia, Pseudomonas, indole-positive Proteus, Citrobacter, Enterobacter; UTI: Urinary tract infection.

Authors' contributions

JH: Conceptualization, Formal Analysis, Funding acquisition, Investigation, Methodology, Project administration, Visualization, Writing—original draft, Writing—review and editing; PC: Resources, Validation, Writing—review and editing; RZ: Data curation, Supervision, Writing—review and editing. All authors read and approved the final manuscript.

Competing interests

The authors declare that they have no competing interests.

Author details

[1] Department of Urology, 3rd Faculty of Medicine, Charles University and Thomayer University Hospital, Videnska 800, 140 59 Prague, Czech Republic. [2] Department of Clinical Microbiology, Thomayer University Hospital, Videnska 800, Prague 14059, Czech Republic.

References

1. Gajdács M, Urbán E. Resistance trends and epidemiology of Citrobacter—Enterobacter—Serratia in urinary tract infections of inpatients and outpatients (RECESUTI): a 10-year survey. Medicina (B Aires). 2019;55(285):1–13.
2. Zowawi HM, Harris PNA, Roberts MJ, Tambyah PA, Schembri M, Pezzani MD, et al. The emerging threat of multidrug-resistant Gram-negative bacteria in urology. Nat Rev Urol. 2015;12:570–80. https://doi.org/10.1038/nrurol.2015.199.
3. Schaeffer A, Schaeffer E. Infections of the urinary tract. In: Wein A, Kavoussi L, editors. Campbell-Walsh Urology. 10th ed. 2012. p. 258–60.

4. François M, Hanslik T, Dervaux B, Le Strat Y, Coignard B, Souty C, et al. The economic burden of urinary tract infections in women visiting general practices in France: a cross-sectional survey. BMC Health Serv Res. 2016;16(1):1–10. https://doi.org/10.1186/s12913-016-1620-2.
5. Vallejo-Torres L, Pujol M, Shaw E, Wiegand I, Vigo JM, Stoddart M, et al. Cost of hospitalised patients due to complicated urinary tract infections: a retrospective observational study in countries with high prevalence of multidrug-resistant Gram-negative bacteria: The COMBACTE-MAGNET, RESCUING study. BMJ Open. 2018;8(4):1–9.
6. Bonkat G, Bartoletti R, Bruyère F, Cai T, S.E. G, Köves B, et al. Urological infections [Internet]. 2020 [cited 2020 Sep 17]. https://uroweb.org/guideline/urological-infections/.
7. Cullen IM, Manecksha RP, Mccullagh E, Ahmad S, Kelly FO, Flynn RJ, et al. The changing pattern of antimicrobial resistance within 42 033 Escherichia coli isolates from nosocomial, community and urology patient-specific urinary tract infections, Dublin, 1999–2009. BJUI Int. 2011;109(109):1198–206.
8. Iacchini S, Sabbatucci M, Gagliotti C, Rossolini GM, Moro ML, Iannazzo S, et al. Bloodstream infections due to carbapenemas eprocucing Enterobacteriaceae in Italy: results from nationwide surveillance, 2014 to 2017. Eurosurveillance. 2019;24(5):66.
9. Lob SH, Nicolle LE, Hoban DJ, Kazmierczak KM, Badal RE, Sahm DF. Susceptibility patterns and ESBL rates of *Escherichia coli* from urinary tract infections in Canada and the United States, SMART 2010–2014. Diagn Microbiol Infect Dis. 2016;85(4):459–65.
10. Guyomard-Rabenirina S, Malespine J, Ducat C, Sadikalay S, Falord M, Harrois D, et al. Temporal trends and risks factors for antimicrobial resistant Enterobacteriaceae urinary isolates from outpatients in Guadeloupe. BMC Microbiol. 2016;16:121. https://doi.org/10.1186/s12866-016-0749-9.
11. Sierra-Díaz E, Hernández-ríos CJ, Bravo-cuellar A. Antibiotic resistance: microbiological profile of urinary tract infections in Mexico. Circ Circ. 2019;87:176–82.
12. Okeke IN, Laxminarayan R, Bhutta ZA, Duse AG, Jenkins P, Brien TFO, et al. AMR Resistance in developing countries. Lancet Infect Dis. 2005;5(August):481–93.
13. Fasugba O, Mitchell BG, Mnatzaganian G, Das A, Collignon P, Gardner A. Five-year antimicrobial resistance patterns of urinary *Escherichia coli* at an Australian Tertiary Hospital: time series analyses of prevalence data. PLoS ONE. 2016;11(10):1–14.
14. Hyun M, Noh CI, Ryu SY, Kim HA. Changing trends in clinical characteristics and antibiotic susceptibility of *Klebsiella pneumoniae* bacteremia. Korean J Intern Med. 2018;33:595–603.
15. Karlowsky JA, Hoban DJ, Hackel MA, Lob SH, Sahm DF. Antimicrobial susceptibility of Gram-negative ESKAPE pathogens isolated from hospitalized patients with intra-abdominal and urinary tract infections in Asia-Pacific countries: SMART 2013–2015. J Med Microbiol. 2017;66(1):61–9.
16. Klein EY, Van Boeckel TP, Martinez EM, Pant S, Gandra S, Levin SA, et al. Global increase and geographic convergence in antibiotic consumption between 2000 and 2015. Proc Natl Acad Sci USA. 2018;115(15):E3463–70.
17. Stapleton PJ, Lundon DJ, McWade R, Scanlon N, Hannan MM, O'Kelly F, et al. Antibiotic resistance patterns of Escherichia coli urinary isolates and comparison with antibiotic consumption data over 10 years, 2005–2014. Ir J Med Sci. 2017;186(3):733–41.
18. Kandil H, Cramp E, Vaghela T. Trends in antibiotic resistance in urologic practice. Eur Urol Focus. 2016;2(4):363–73. https://doi.org/10.1016/j.euf.2016.09.006.
19. Fleming-Dutra K, Hersh AL, Shapiro DJ. Prevalence of inappropriate antibiotic prescriptions among US ambulatory care visits, 2010–2011. JAMA. 2016;315(17):1865–73.
20. Chardavoyne PC, Kasmire KE. Appropriateness of Antibiotic Prescriptions for urinary tract infections. West J Emerg Med. 2020;21(3):633–9.
21. Harris PNA, Wei JY, Shen AW, Abdile AA, Paynter S, Huxley RR, et al. Carbapenems versus alternative antibiotics for the treatment of bloodstream infections caused by Enterobacter, Citrobacter or Serratia species: a systematic review with meta-analysis. J Antimicrob Chemother. 2016;71(2):296–306.
22. Thaden JT, Pogue JM, Kaye KS. Role of newer and re-emerging older agents in the treatment of infections caused by carbapenem-resistant Enterobacteriaceae. Virulence. 2017;8(4):403–16. https://doi.org/10.1080/21505594.2016.1207834.
23. Bergogne-Bérézin E, Towner KJ. Acinetobacter spp as nosocomial pathogens: microbiological, clinical, and epidemiological features. Clin Microbiol Rev. 1996;9(2):148–65.
24. Brooke JS. *Stenotrophomonas maltophilia*: an emerging global opportunistic pathogen. Clin Microbiol Rev. 2012;25(1):2–41.
25. Hrbacek J, Cermak P, Zachoval R. Current antibiotic resistance trends of uropathogens in central europe: survey from a tertiary hospital urology department 2011–2019. Antibiotics. 2020;9(9):1–11.
26. Gajdács M, Urbán E. Comparative epidemiology and resistance trends of proteae in urinary tract infections of inpatients and outpatients: a 10-year retrospective study. Antibiotics. 2019;8(91):1–13.
27. Fajfr M, Louda M, Paterová P, Rysková L, Pacovský J, Košina J, et al. The susceptibility to fosfomycin of Gram-negative bacteria isolates from urinary tract infection in the Czech Republic: data from a unicentric study. BMC Urol. 2017;17(1):1–6.
28. Jiménez-Guerra G, Borrego-Jiménez J, Gutiérrez-Soto B, Expósito-Ruiz M, Navarro-Marí JM, Gutiérrez-F, et al. Evolución de la sensibilidad a los antibióticos de Enterobacter cloacae, Morganella morganii, Klebsiella aerogenes y Citrobacter freundii causantes de infecciones del tracto urinario: un estudio de vigilancia epidemiológica de 11 años. Enferm Infecc Microbiol Clin. 2019. https://doi.org/10.1016/j.eimc.2019.07.010.
29. Jiménez-Guerra G, Heras-Cañas V, Gutiérrez-Soto M, Aznarte-Padial M del P, Expósito-Ruiz M, Navarro-Marí JM, et al. Urinary tract infection by acinetobacter baumannii and pseudomonas aeruginosa: evolution of antimicrobial resistance and therapeutic alternatives. J Med Microbiol. 2018;67(6):790–7.
30. de Lemos MC, de Paixao EF, de Souza Santos MAR. *Stenotrophomonas maltophilia* isolates in a tertiary care hospital in Northeastern Brazil. Braz J Hea Rev. 2019;2(4):3373–84.
31. Nyc O, Matejková J. *Stenotrophomonas maltophilia*: significant contemporary hospital pathogen—review. Folia Microbiol Praha. 2010;55(3):286–94.
32. Munoz-Price S, Weinstein RA. Acinetobacter infection. N Engl J Med. 2008;358(12):1271–81.
33. Moy S, Sharma R. Treatment outcomes in infections caused by "SPICE" (Serratia, Pseudomonas, Indole-positive Proteus, Citrobacter, and Enterobacter) organisms: Carbapenem versus Noncarbapenem Regimens. Clin Ther. 2017;39(1):170–6.
34. Chassin-Trubert CA-M. Síndrome de la bolsa de orina púrpura: un fenómeno inusual y muy llamativo. Rev Med Chile. 2014;142:1482–4.
35. Davin-Regli A, Pagès J. Enterobacter aerogenes and Enterobacter cloacae; versatile bacterial pathogens confronting antibiotic treatment. Front Microbiol. 2015;6:392.
36. Chang C-L, Su L-H, Lu C-M, Tai F-T, Huang Y-C, Chang K-K. Outbreak of ertapenem-resistant Enterobacter cloacae urinary tract infections due to a contaminated ureteroscope. J Hosp Infect. 2013;85(2):118–24.
37. Mahlen SD. Serratia infections: from military experiments to current practice. Clin Microbiol Rev. 2011;24(4):755–91.
38. Su L, Ou JT, Leu H, Chiang P, Chiu Y, Chia J, et al. Extended epidemic of nosocomial urinary tract infections caused by *Serratia marcescens*. J Clin Microbiol. 2003;41(10):4726–32.
39. O'Hara CM, Brenner FW, Miller JM. Classification, identification, and clinical significance of Proteus, Providencia, and Morganella. Clin Microbiol Rev. 2000;13(4):534–46.
40. Choi HK, Kim YK, Kim HY, Park JE, Uh Y. Clinical and microbiological features of Providencia bacteremia: experience at a tertiary care hospital. Korean J Intern Med. 2015;30:219–25.

9

The prevalence of premature ejaculation and its relationship with polygamous men: A cross-sectional observational study at a tertiary hospital in Somalia

Abdikarim Hussein Mohamed*, Hussein Ali Mohamud and Adem Yasar

Abstract

Background: Premature ejaculation (PE) is the most common and prevalent sexual disorder among men. To the best of our knowledge, this is the first study aimed at evaluating the relationship of PE among polygamous men.

Method: Over a 1-year period, a cross-sectional observational study was carried out among 202 married men who visited the urology polyclinic due to different clinical conditions and contributed by completing a standardized structured questionnaire regarding their sociodemographic data, as well as sexual and past medical history.

Results: In our study, the prevalence of PE was 37.1%; half of the monogamous men (50%) complained of PE, while 22% of men with two wives, 20% of men with three wives, and 12% of men with four wives complained of PE ($p < 0.0001$, 95% CI 0.122–1.920). Seventy percent of erectile dysfunction (ED) patients had PE concurrence ($p < 0.0001$, 95% CI 0.057–5.543). Regarding frequency of sexual intercourse, 48% of patients who complained of PE performed sexual intercourse less than two times/week, while two-thirds of the participants who did not complain of PE had sexual intercourse two to four times/week ($p < 0.0001$, 95% CI 0.203–0.568). Among the men who reported ED, 42% had one wife, 21.5% had two wives, 40% had three wives, and 12.5% had four wives ($p < 0.029$, 95% CI 0.417–0.962).

Conclusions: We report that polygamous men have a lower incidence of premature ejaculation and higher sexual satisfaction than monogamous men. There is a significant association between ED and PE, showing a complex and bidirectional relationship between the two conditions. The new taxonomic entity called loss of control of erection and ejaculation (LCEE) views the two sexual symptoms as deeply interrelated. The study results indicate that a sexual intercourse frequency of two or more times per week significantly lowers the risk of PE.

Keywords: Premature ejaculation, Polygamy, Erectile dysfunction, Sexual partners

Background

Premature ejaculation is the most common and prevalent sexual disorder among men, affecting 30% to 50% of the male population [1]. Premature ejaculation is the inability to sufficiently delay ejaculation before or within 60 s of satisfactory sexual intercourse which results in negative sexual effects as defined by the International Society for Sexual Medicine (ISSM) [2]. Waldinger et al. [3] advocated a new classification of premature ejaculation in addition to the two former lifelong PE and acquired PE (APE), i.e., natural variable PE (NVPE) and premature-like ejaculatory dysfunction (PLED).

PE has a significant psychosocial effect that leads to a low quality of life for both partners [4]. Men with PE

*Correspondence: abdikarimgabeyre@gmail.com
Mogadishu Somalia Turkish Training and Research Hospital, Mogadishu, Somalia

frequently feel shame and embarrassment with inferiority feelings, dissatisfaction, and feelings of being incapable of satisfying their partner which raises the risk of depression [5].

Tsai et al. [6] reported that erectile dysfunction is the leading risk factor for about 36% to 50% of PE. ED and PE should not be considered to be separate entities because of their complex and bidirectional relationship between the two conditions. Colonnello et al. [7] introduced a new taxonomic entity called loss of control of erection and ejaculation (LCEE), as the first definition of a disorder that views the two sexual symptoms as deeply interrelated, and helps the assessment of concomitant presence of PE and ED, and to improve both PE diagnosis and management. Kempeneers et al. reported that PE decreases with age due to sexual experience and relationship maturation with a partner. Premature ejaculation is associated with anxiety, early and limited sexual practice, poor health status, weak sexual desire, lower frequency of sexual intercourse, diabetes, chronic prostatitis, metabolic syndrome, and drinking habits [8].

Several studies have focused on the impact of premature ejaculation and depression [9] and female sexual satisfaction for men with premature ejaculation [10]. Regarding premature ejaculation among polygamous men (i.e., marrying more than one woman at the same time), no previous studies in the literature have evaluated the impact of polygamy on PE. The main objective of this study was to investigate the relationship between premature ejaculation among polygamous men. In addition, there are no previous studies that have evaluated the prevalence of PE among Somalian men.

Method

Over a 1-year period, a non-interventional cross-sectional observational study was carried out among married men who visited the urology polyclinic due to different clinical conditions. Men with one or more female sexual wives and having regular sexual intercourse for the last six months were included in the study. Men with diabetes, taking benign prostate hyperplasia (BPH) medications, or who had undergone a prostate operation, and men using antipsychotic drugs were excluded from the study. The diagnostic criterion of premature ejaculation was as defined according to the International Society for Sexual Medicine (ISSM) definition criteria. A total of 202 men were selected for the study and contributed by completing a standardized structured questionnaire that collected data on sociodemographic characteristics (age, number of partners), frequency of sexual intercourse per week and the coexistence of erectile dysfunction, sexual satisfaction, the intravaginal ejaculatory latency time (IELT) reported by the patient, and the premature ejaculation diagnostic tool (PEDT).

The intravaginal ejaculatory latency time (IELT) is the average time between vaginal entrance and ejaculation estimated by the patient. An IELT of <2 min was considered to be PE. A premature ejaculation diagnostic tool (PEDT) that consisted of five questions was used to assess for all of the participants a diagnosis of premature ejaculation. A score of <8 equals no PE, a score of 9 or 10 means probable PE, and a score of >11 indicates PE [4]. The coexistence of erectile dysfunction was measured using the International Index of Erectile Function (IIEF) questionnaire, i.e., a validated questionnaire that contains 15 items (five domains), of which 6 items assess erectile function. A score of <22 was considered to be the coexistence of ED (LCEE) [11]. To prevent the underestimation of the seriousness of the condition or its effect on the relationship of the partners, absolute PE that is generalized occurring irrespective of partners or relative that is situational or confined to a partner were considered true PE.

This study was approved by the Clinical Research Ethics Committee of the Mogadishu Somali Turkish Training and Research Hospital (approval number MSTH/4410). All methods were performed in accordance with the relevant guidelines and regulations. Participants were informed about the purpose of the study, and written informed consent for participation was obtained from all of the participants.

A univariate descriptive analysis was used for data analysis and expressed as the mean ± standard deviation (SD). The chi-square test and cross-tabulations were also used. A bivariate analysis was used to determine the correlation between premature ejaculation and sexual partners, sexual frequency, age, erectile dysfunction, and sexual satisfaction. The binary logistic regression model used variables that displayed significance in the bivariate analysis and the 95% confidence interval was also calculated. A p value of <0.05 was considered to be statistically significant. The statistical analyses were accomplished using IBM SPSS for Windows version 23.

Results

In this cross-sectional observational study, there was a total of 202 married men who completed the questionnaire. The mean age of the participants was 39.76 ± 12.04 years and the prevalence of PE was 37.1%. The assessment with a premature ejaculation diagnostic tool (PEDT) revealed that 25% of the participants had PE, while 12% had probable PE, and 63% had no PE.

In this study, the participants were categorized into four age groups, i.e., 20–29 years (21.8%), 30–39 years (34.2%), 40–49 years (21.8%), and over 50 years (22.3%).

There was no statistically significant association between age groups and PE ($p=0.251$, 95% CI 1.443–26.881).

Regarding sexual partners, 56.4% (114 of 202 participants) had one wife, 32.2% (65/202) had two wives, 7.4% (15/202) had three wives, and 4% (8/202) had four wives. Half of the monogamous men (50%) complained of premature ejaculation; among polygamous men, 22% who had two wives, 20% who had three wives, and 12% who had four wives complained of PE. There was a statistically significant correlation between the number of sexual partners and PE ($p<0.0001$, 95% CI 0.122–1.920) (Table 1).

Regarding the frequency of sexual intercourse per week, 58 (28.7%) men performed sexual intercourse one time or less per week (1, 2, and 3 times per month), 117 men performed sexual intercourse two to four times per week, and 27 men performed sexual intercourse more than four times per week. We noted a statistically significant difference in the number of sexual partners and frequency of sexual intercourse per week ($p=0.016$) (Table 2). On the one hand, among the participants who complained of PE, 48% (36 participants) performed sexual intercourse one time or less per week, 33 participants performed sexual intercourse from two to four times per week, and only six participants performed sexual intercourse more than four times per week. On the other hand, among the participants without PE, two-thirds (84 participants) performed sexual intercourse from two to four times per week, 21 participants performed sexual intercourse more than four times per week, while 17% performed sexual intercourse one time or less per week. There was a statistically significant correlation between the frequency of sexual intercourse per week and PE ($p<0.0001$, 95% CI 0.203–0.568).

Thirty-four percent of the participants had ED; 48 out of 69 of the participants with ED had PE concurrence (LCEE), while 36% with PE had no coexistence with ED. A statistically significant association between ED and PE was revealed throughout the study ($p<0.0001$, 95% CI 0.057–5.543); 42% of men with one wife, 21.5% of men

Table 2 Frequency of sexual intercourse per week among sexual partners

Sexual Partners	Sexual frequencies per week			*p* value
	≤ 1time/week	2–4 times/week	>4 times/week	
1 Wife	41	63	10	$p<0.016$
2 Wife	14	38	13	
3 Wife	3	8	4	
4 Wife	0	8	0	

A *p* value of < 0.05 was considered to be statistically significant

Table 1 Correlation between variables and patients with and without PE

Variables	No. patients (202)	With PE (75)	Without PE (127)	*p* value	95% CI
Age groups	39.76 ± 12.04			0.251	0.066–4.229
20–29	44 (21.3%)	19	25		
30–39	69 (34.2%)	27	42		
40–49	44 (21.8%)	14	30		
>50	45 (22.3%)	15	30		
Sexual partners	1.58 ± 0.79			< 0.0001	0.122–1.920
1 Wife	114 (56.4%)	57	57		
2 Wife	65 (32.2%)	14	51		
3 Wife	15 (7.4%)	3	12		
4 Wife	8 (4%)	1	7		
Sexual frequency/week	2.64 ± 1.75			< 0.0001	0.298–5.193
≤ 1 time/week	58 (28.7%)	36	22		
2–4 times/week	117 (57.9%)	33	84		
>4 times/week	27 (13.4%)	6	21		
ED				< 0.0001	0.057–5.543
Yes	69 (34.2%)	48	21		
No	133 (65.8%)	27	106		
Sexual satisfaction				< 0.0001	0.038–5.517
Normal	127 (62.9%)	13	114		
Low	75 (37.1%)	62	13		

A *p* value of < 0.05 was considered to be statistically significant

Table 3 Distribution of erectile dysfunction among sexual partners

Sexual partners	ED		*p* value	95% CI
	Yes	No		
1 Wife	48	66	0.029	0.417–0.962
2 Wife	14	51		
3 Wife	6	9		
4 Wife	1	7		

A *p* value of < 0.05 was considered to be statistically significant

Table 4 Association of intravaginal ejaculatory latency time (IELT) and sexual partners

Sexual partners	IELT			*p* value
	< 1 min	1–2 min	> 2 min	
1 Wife	37	19	58	$p < 0.0001$
2 Wife	6	8	51	
3 Wife	2	1	12	
4 Wife	1	0	7	

A *p* value of < 0.05 was considered to be statistically significant

with two wives, 40% of men with three wives, and 12.5% of men with four wives reported ED ($p < 0.029$, 95% CI 0.417–0.962) (Table 3).

The mean self-reported intravaginal ejaculatory latency time (IELT) was 4.99 ± 2.15 min; IELTs of < 1 min, 1–2 min, and > 2 min accounted for 22.8%, 13.9%, and 63.4%, respectively. There was a significant correlation between sexual partners and IELT ($p < 0.001$) (Table 4).

Discussion

Due to the lack of a standardized definition, diagnostic tools, and the social hypersensitivity of the disease, the results of studies on the risk factors of PE are still controversial. A multicenter cross-sectional study by Zhang et al. [12] investigated the risk factors of PE and reported that ED, weak sexual desire, lower frequency of sexual intercourse, diabetes, chronic prostatitis, primary married status, lower body mass index, higher age, education level, monthly income, office work, drinking habits, and decreased force of ejaculation were significantly associated with PE. There are no previous studies in the literature that have evaluated the impact of polygamy in PE. Our study indicated that there is a statistically significant difference between the number of sexual partners and PE. Polygamous men have a lower incidence of premature ejaculation and higher sexual satisfaction than monogamous men. Potential reasons include increased sexual experience, relationship maturation, increased sexual intercourse frequency, and psychosexual comfort.

Existing studies regarding the association between age and premature ejaculation are limited. Our study reported no statistically significant association between age groups and PE which was compatible with a multicenter internet-based survey from the Korean Andrological Society in young and middle-aged men that noted no significant differences among PE according to age categories [13]. In contrast to our findings, Kempeneers et al. [8] reported that PE decreased with age due to sexual experience and relationship maturation with a partner.

Sexual frequency is a risk factor of PE and has a clear impact. According to the existing literature, there is no approved frequency of sexual intercourse that lowers or prevents PE. In our study, we acknowledged that a lower frequency of sexual intercourse was significantly related to a higher incidence of PE, which was consistent with a 10-year interval web-based survey on the prevalence and risk factors of PE (The Korean Internet Sexuality Survey (KISS) 2016) by Song, W. H. et al. similarly reported that a low frequency of sexual intercourse per month was related to PE [14]. The study results indicate that a sexual intercourse frequency of two or more times per week significantly lowers the risk of PE.

In our study, the prevalence of PE was 37.1%, which was higher than that reported in previous studies [4, 15, 16]. A study by Karabakan et al. [17], in young Turkish men, revealed a low prevalence of approximately 9.2% PE. The Global Online Sexuality Survey among Arabic Males (GOSS-AR-M) published a much higher prevalence of approximately 83.7% PE [18]. A higher PE rate (40.6%) as compared with our study was also reported in a cross-sectional study conducted at a primary care clinic [19]. The prevalence of PE varies among studies due to the lack of a universally accepted definition and diagnostic tools, as well as the social hypersensitivity of the disease, and the various methods of data collection and analysis.

Several studies have evaluated the association between PE and ED and their co-occurrence, and they have shown a complex relationship between the two diseases. A large, randomized study of 4997 heterosexual men with regular sexual intercourse, aged 18–65 years from nine Asia–Pacific countries, presented that more than 30% of PE patients have concomitant ED, which was in agreement with our findings [20]. Tsai et al. [6] reported that erectile dysfunction is the leading risk factor for about 36% to 50% of PE. A new taxonomic entity called loss of control of erection and ejaculation (LCEE) was introduced by Colonnello et al. [7] that sights the two sexual symptoms as deeply interrelated, and helps the assessment of concomitant presence of PE and ED, and to improve both PE diagnosis and management. A systemic review and meta-analysis of 18 articles, for a total of 57,229 patients, of which 12,144 (21.2%) patients had PE, reported a bidirectional relationship between PE and ED; the presence of PE was associated with a significant increase in ED risk (odds ratio 3.68 (2.61, 5.18), $p < 0.0001$) [21]. Consistent with these studies, in this study, we reported that men with PE have a two-fold risk of developing ED due to anxiety, interpersonal distress, and partner dissatisfaction. In our study, the prevalence of ED was higher in PE patients (64%). Premature ejaculation places a significant burden on an individual and their partner associated with psychological distress and dissatisfaction. Xi et al. reported that when diagnosing erectile dysfunction in patients with PE, SHIM has a sensitivity of about 100% while has a specificity only about 36%; meanwhile, the IIEF-EF is has a higher sensitivity and specificity of about 100% and 77.2% respectively. The authors of this study suggested that the cutoff of SHIM and IIEF-EF should be lowered when assessing erectile function among PE population (SHIM at 17.5 and IIEF-EF at 24.5, respectively). Larger trials are needed to further validate and to expose about the relationship between PE and ED and its association in monogamous and polygamous families. This study mainly focuses the relationship between PE and polygamy compared to monogamous men, and to the best of our knowledge, this is the first study aimed at evaluating the relationship of PE among polygamous men [22].

Neurophysiological, psychosocial, and cognitive factors are some of the mechanisms that involve the pathophysiology of the disease [23]. The coexistence of PE and ED should be carefully evaluated and should not be considered to be separate entities that would increase treatment failure rates [24].

Strengths and limitations

The limitations of this study include the following: (1) the number of the selected participants is small; however, finding men with more than one wife is challenging; (2) the substantial exclusion criteria, although the study intended to examine the influence of polygamy on PE; (3) the lack of information on women, and the validity of erectile function assessment questionnaires in premature ejaculation patients. Further studies are needed to address the relationship between PE and the position of sexual intercourse (missionary vs. non-missionary), and the age of wives.

Conclusions

In this study, we report that polygamous men have a lower incidence of premature ejaculation and higher sexual satisfaction than monogamous men. There is a significant association between ED and PE, showing a complex and bidirectional relationship between the two conditions. The new taxonomic entity called loss of control of erection and ejaculation (LCEE) views the two sexual symptoms as deeply interrelated. The study results indicate that a sexual intercourse frequency of two or more times per week significantly lowers the risk of PE.

Abbreviations

PE: Premature ejaculation; ED: Erectile dysfunction; LPE: Lifelong PE; APE: Acquired PE; NVPE: Natural variable PE; PLED: Premature-like ejaculatory dysfunction; ISSM: International Society for Sexual Medicine; IELT: Intravaginal ejaculatory latency time; PEDT: Premature ejaculation diagnostic tool; IIEF: International Index of Erectile Function; SD: Standard deviation.

Author contributions

Study concept, design, and interpretation, A.H.M., H.A.M., and A.Y.; drafting of the manuscript, A.H.M., H.A.M., and A.Y. All authors read and approved the final manuscript.

Competing interests

The authors declare no conflict of interest associated with this publication.

References

1. Gao J, Zhang X, Su P, Shi K, Tang D, Hao Z, et al. Prevalence and impact of premature ejaculation in outpatients complaining of ejaculating prematurely: using the instruments of intravaginal ejaculatory latency time and patient-reported outcome measures. Int J Impot Res. 2014;26(3):94–9.
2. Gillman N, Gillman M. Premature ejaculation: aetiology and treatment strategies. Med Sci. 2019;7(11):102.
3. Gao J, Zhang X, Su P, Peng Z, Liu J, Xia L, et al. The impact of intravaginal ejaculatory latency time and erectile function on anxiety and depression in the four types of premature ejaculation: a large cross-sectional study in a chinese population. J Sex Med. 2014;11(2):521–8.
4. Hanafy S, Hamed AM, Hilmy Samy MS. Prevalence of premature ejaculation and its impact on the quality of life: results from a sample of Egyptian patients. Andrologia. 2019;51(8):1–5.
5. Abdo CHN. The impact of ejaculatory dysfunction upon the sufferer and his partner. Transl Androl Urol. 2016;5(4):460–9.
6. Tsai WK, Chiang PK, Lu CC, Jiann BP. The comorbidity between premature ejaculation and erectile dysfunction—a cross-sectional internet survey. Sex Med. 2019;7(4):451–8. https://doi.org/10.1016/j.esxm.2019.06.014.
7. Colonnello E, Ciocca G, Limoncin E, Sansone A, Jannini EA. Redefining a sexual medicine paradigm: subclinical premature ejaculation as a new taxonomic entity. Nature Reviews Urology. 2021;18(2):115–27.
8. Kempeneers P, Andrianne R, Bauwens S, Georis I, Pairoux JF, Blairy S. Functional and psychological characteristics of belgian men with premature ejaculation and their partners. Arch Sex Behav. 2013;42(1):51–66.
9. Karakeci A, Korkmaz S, Karakoc O, Karakoc U, Firdolas A, Pirincci F. Effect of premature ejaculation on depression and sexual functions in female partners: a report from Eastern Turkey. Niger J Clin Pract. 2019;22(11):1553–63.
10. Verze P, Arcaniolo D, Imbimbo C, Cai T, Venturino L, Spirito L, et al. General and sex profile of women with partner affected by premature ejaculation: results of a large observational, non-interventional, cross-sectional, epidemiological study (IPER-F). Andrology. 2018;6(5):714–9.
11. Tang DD, Li C, Peng DW, Zhang XS. Validity of premature ejaculation diagnostic tool and its association with International Index of Erectile Function-15 in Chinese men with evidence-based-defined premature ejaculation. Asian J Androl. 2018;20:19–23.
12. Zhang J, Li F, Li H, Zhang Z, Yang B, Li H. Clinical features of and couple's attitudes towards premature ejaculation: a multicenter cross-sectional study. Aging Male. 2019. https://doi.org/10.1080/13685538.2019.1640194.
13. Park HJ, Park JK, Park K, Lee SW, Kim SW, Yang DY, et al. Prevalence of premature ejaculation in young and middle-aged men in Korea: A multicenter internet-based survey from the Korean Andrological Society. Asian J Androl. 2010;12(6):880–9. https://doi.org/10.1038/aja.2010.9.
14. Song WH, Yoo S, Oh S, Park J, Cho SY, Cho MC, et al. Ten-year interval changes in the prevalence of self-identified premature ejaculation and

premature ejaculation based on an estimated intravaginal ejaculation latency time of <3 minutes in the general population: The Korean Internet Sexuality Survey (KISS). J Sex Med. 2019;16(4):512–21. https://doi.org/10.1016/j.jsxm.2019.02.003.
15. Althof SE. Prevalence, characteristics and implications of premature ejaculation/rapid ejaculation. J Urol. 2006;175(3):842–8.
16. Serefoglu EC, Saitz TR. New insights on premature ejaculation: a review of definition, classification, prevalence and treatment. Asian J Androl. 2012;14(6):822–9. https://doi.org/10.1038/aja.2012.108.
17. Karabakan M, Bozkurt A, Hirik E, Celebi B, Akdemir S, Guzel O, et al. The prevalence of premature ejaculation in young Turkish men. Andrologia. 2016;48(9):895–9.
18. Shaeer O, Shaeer K, The Global Online Sexuality Survey (GOSS). Ejaculatory function, penile anatomy, and contraceptive usage among arabic-speaking internet users in the Middle East. J Sex Med. 2012;9(2):425–33.
19. Tang WS, Khoo EM. Prevalence and correlates of premature ejaculation in a primary care setting: a preliminary cross-sectional study. J Sex Med. 2011;8(7):2071–8.
20. McMahon CG, Lee G, Park JK, Adaikan PG. Premature ejaculation and erectile dysfunction prevalence and attitudes in the Asia-Pacific region. J Sex Med. 2012;9(2):454–65.
21. Corona G, Rastrelli G, Limoncin E, Sforza A, Jannini EA, Maggi M. Interplay between premature ejaculation and erectile dysfunction: a systematic review and meta-analysis. J Sex Med. 2015;12(12):2291–300. https://doi.org/10.1111/jsm.13041.
22. Xi Y, Colonnello E, Ma G, Limoncin E, Ciocca G, Zhang H, Jannini EA, Zhang Y. Validity of erectile function assessment questionnaires in premature ejaculation patients: a comparative study between the abridged forms of the international index of erectile function and proposal for optimal cutoff redefinition. J Sex Med. 2021;18(3):440–7.
23. Yusof F, Sidi H, Das S, Midin M, Kumar J, Hatta MH. Understanding the pathophysiology of premature ejaculation: bridging the link between pharmacological and psychological interventions. Curr Drug Targets. 2018;19(8):856–64.
24. Koon CS, Sidi H, Kumar J, Das S, Xi OW, Hatta MH, Alfonso C. The phosphodiesterase 5-inhibitors (PDE-5i) for erectile dysfunction (ED): a therapeutic challenge for psychiatrists. Curr Drug Targets. 2018;19:1366–77.

10

Hard bilateral syphilitic testes with vasculitis: A case report and literature review

Sat Prasad Nepal*, Takehiko Nakasato, Takashi Fukagai, Takeshi Shichijo, Jun Morita, Yoshiko Maeda, Kazuhiko Oshinomi, Yoshihiro Nakagami, Tsutomu Unoki, Tetsuo Noguchi, Tatsuki Inoue, Ryosuke Kato, Satoshi Amano, Moyuru Mizunuma, Masahiro Kurokawa, Yoshiki Tsunokawa, Sou Yasuda and Yoshio Ogawa

Abstract

Background: We report the case of a patient with syphilitic testicular gumma and vasculitis with adrenal failure due to chronic steroid use.

Case presentation: A 63-year-old male presented with hard right eye swelling and very firm bilateral testes on palpation, which he had for 2 years. Testicular tumor markers were negative; syphilis test was positive. Radiological examination suggested aortitis and bilateral testicular malignancy. The patient received ampicillin for the infection and prednisolone for vasculitis. Left orchidectomy was performed to confirm the presence of testicular tumor; histological examinations revealed granulomatous orchitis. The prednisolone doses were adjusted because of relapses and adverse effects of steroid use. Unfortunately, the patient died in the intensive care unit because of uncontrolled blood pressure and pneumonia.

Conclusions: This is a rare case of syphilis with testicular involvement and vasculitis. This report shows the importance of broadening the differential diagnoses of testicular firmness.

Keywords: Gumma, Testis, Syphilis, Vasculitis, Aortitis, Hard, Induration

Background

Syphilis involvement in the testis is extremely rare, and the literature has very few case reports. Testicular gummata are characterized by multiple swellings in the testis and granulomatous inflammation with a billiard ball-like hard consistency [1]. It is generally associated with patients with human immunodeficiency virus (HIV) infection. A literature search revealed this was the 24th recorded case of testicular syphilis but only the 2nd case of syphilitic vasculitis (aortitis) accompanying testicular gumma. Herein, we discuss a case of testicular gumma with vasculitis and review the current literature regarding the age at presentation, testicular characteristics, and other systemic findings of testicular syphilis.

Case presentation

In 2014, a 63-year-old patient initially presented at the medicine department with a cough and erythematous areas on the right ankle joint. The patient had a history of smoking (90 pack-years) and chronic obstructive pulmonary disease (COPD).

On examination, the bilateral testes were painless, very firm, smooth, and nonenlarged. There was bilateral decrease in breathing sounds. A painless right orbital mass—hard and immobile—was also noted, but it did not interfere with normal vision or eye movement. No other abnormal clinical signs were observed (Fig. 1).

Chest X-ray revealed bilateral pleural effusion. Thoracocentesis was normal. Testicular tumor marker levels

*Correspondence: satprasad1@gmail.com
Department of Urology, Showa University School of Medicine, 1-5-8 Hatanodai, Shinagawa-Ku, Tokyo 142-8555, Japan

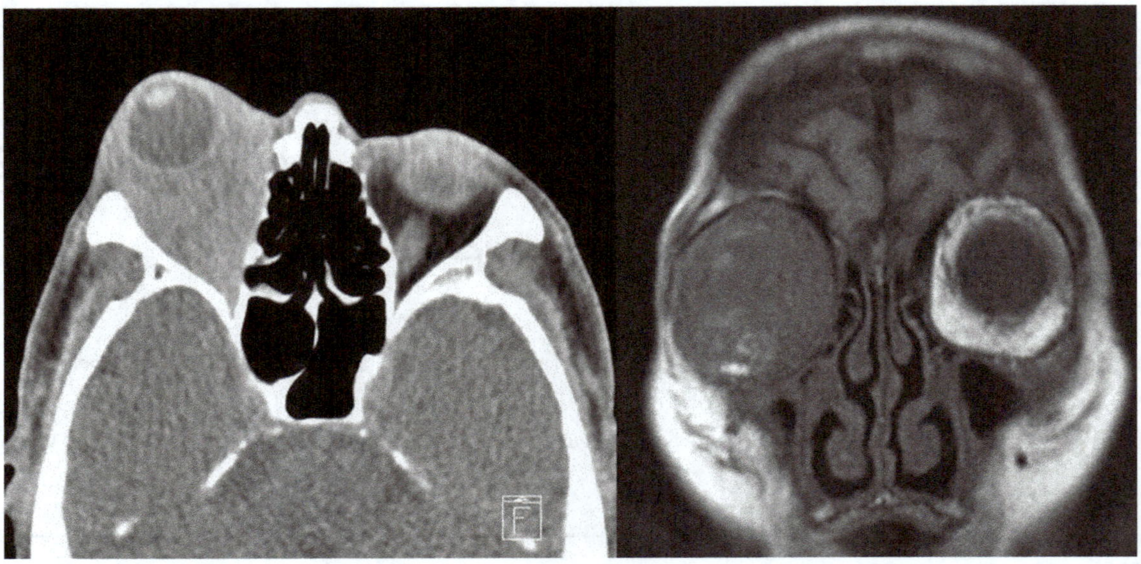

Fig. 1 **a** (left) Computed tomography examination of the right orbit showing a soft tissue shadow that occupies the roof of the right eye with no bone abnormality or damage. No abnormalities were noted in the brain parenchyma within the imaging range. **b** (right) Magnetic resonance imaging suggested an intraocular tumor probably because of an inflammatory pseudotumor

were not increased. Rapid plasma reagent, *Treponema pallidum* antibody, and absorbed fluorescent treponemal antibody quantitative tests were all positive. Lumbar puncture and magnetic resonance imaging (MRI) were performed, considering the possibility of neurosyphilis. Cerebrospinal fluid findings were normal.

Computed tomography examination from the aortic arch to the descending aorta revealed an edematous and thickened wall with swollen surroundings. Aortitis was suspected (Fig. 2). Left vertebral artery stenosis and left subclavian artery dilatation were also noted (Fig. 3).

Antineutrophil cytoplasmic antibodies tests were negative. Angiographies of the abdominal cavity, kidney, and superior and inferior mesenteric arteries were performed to assess vasculitis, all of which were negative. An MRI of the ankle was performed because of erythematous lesions in the lower limbs; this revealed inflammatory findings suggesting osteomyelitis. Skin biopsy indicated dermatopanniculitis.

Ultrasound revealed uniform echogenicity across the bilateral testes (right side: 20.3 × 40.8 mm; left side: 26.6 × 42.3 mm). However, the testicular condition was inconclusive (Fig. 4). Therefore, the patient underwent another MRI.

Testes MRI showed that the bilateral testes had higher signal than the muscle on T1 imaging and lower signal than that of a normal testis on T2. Thus, malignant lymphoma of the bilateral testes was considered (Fig. 5).

Left orchidectomy was performed, and the sample was sent for histological examinations. The testis and epididymis had a uniform yellowish-white tumor. The testis was hard in consistency (Fig. 6). Microscopic findings showed that seminiferous tubules were destroyed and surrounded by lymphocytes and plasma cells. CD68-positive epididymal cells were proliferated. No foreign body giant cells or necrotic foci were observed. There were few CD20 (L26)-positive B and CD3-positive T cells; no proliferation of atypical cells was noted. No pathogens were identified on Periodic acid–Schiff, Grocott`s mehtenamine silver and Gram, or Ziehl–Neelsen staining. Granulomatous orchitis was considered (Fig. 7; We used Olympus BX51 Microscope with an objective lens

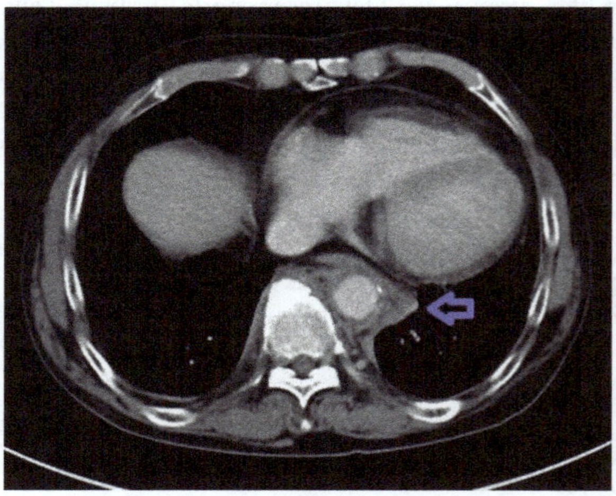

Fig. 2 Computed tomography examination of the abdomen showing thickened and edematous areas surrounding the aorta (blue arrow)

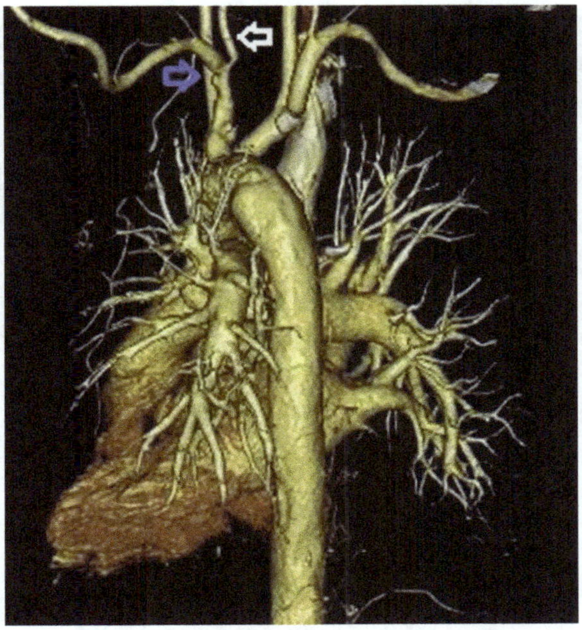

Fig. 3 Angiography showing stenosis of the left vertebral artery (white arrow) and left subclavian dilatation (blue arrow)

of × 10, Olympus DP73 Camera, and Olympus standard CellSens standard version 1.6 as acquisition software for the microscopy.). Because the histology of left testicle was nonmalignant, the right testicle was not removed.

Our patient was diagnosed with syphilitic gumma with vasculitis. He also had a 30-year-old history of sexual activity with a sex-service worker. Ampicillin (8 g/day) for 2 weeks was started for syphilis treatment. However, prednisolone (0.8 mg/kg/day, 35 mg) was introduced and continued because of a high inflammatory response, vasculitis, and pleural effusion. However, the tests for syphilis were positive even after the antibiotic therapy.

The patient refused treatment for the eye hardness; therefore, no biopsy was performed.

The steroid dose was frequently changed as the patient had relapses (i.e., shortness of breath, pleural effusion, and pericardial fluid accumulation) upon dose reduction and experienced steroid-induced adverse effects (i.e., surgery for avascular necrosis of femoral head, uncontrolled orthostatic hypotension with lower sodium and high potassium possibly due to steroid-induced adrenal insufficiency, and steroid-induced hypogammaglobulinemia).

He complained of numbness and tingling sensation in both upper limbs after 2 years of the diagnosis. An MRI of the cervical spine revealed C3–C4 cervical spinal canal stenosis with intervertebral disc swelling and spinal cord compression as well as similar narrowing of the spinal canal in C4–C7 (Fig. 8).

In 2020, the patient was admitted to the intensive care unit (ICU) owing to a deteriorating level of consciousness and uncontrolled blood pressure. He had pneumonia due to cytomegalovirus and *Pseudomonas aeruginosa* infections that led to acute respiratory distress syndrome. Unfortunately, the patient died on day 18 of ICU admission.

Discussion and conclusions

This report presents a rare case of tertiary syphilis with testicular gumma and syphilitic vasculitis. It could not be controlled with antibiotics and steroids and ultimately led to adrenal dysfunction and mortality. Only a few cases of testicular involvement in syphilis have been reported. Furthermore, testicular induration as the first presentation indicating syphilis is rare.

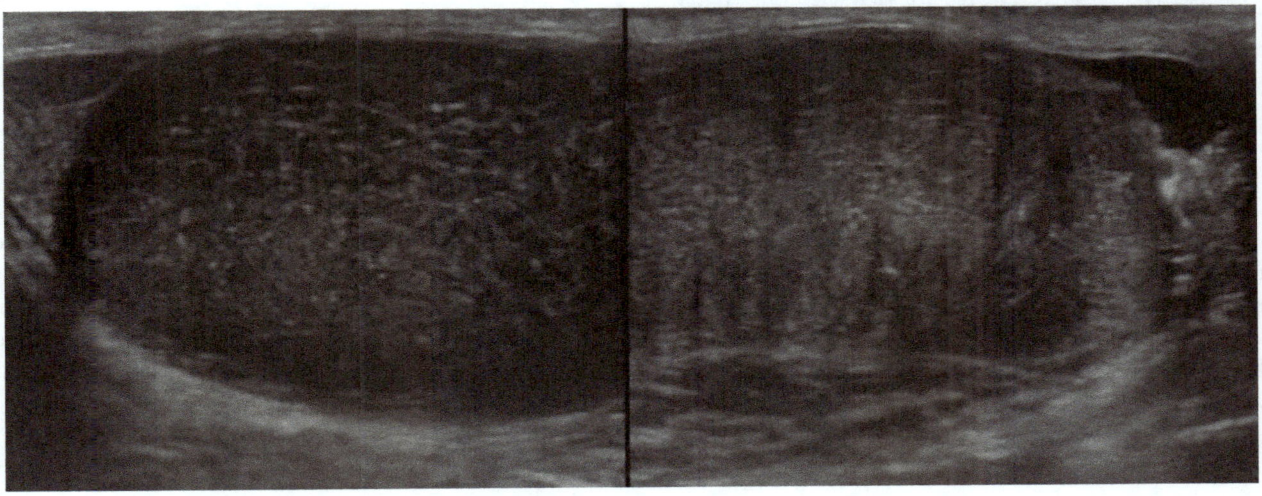

Fig. 4 Ultrasonography of bilateral testes showing similar echogenicity

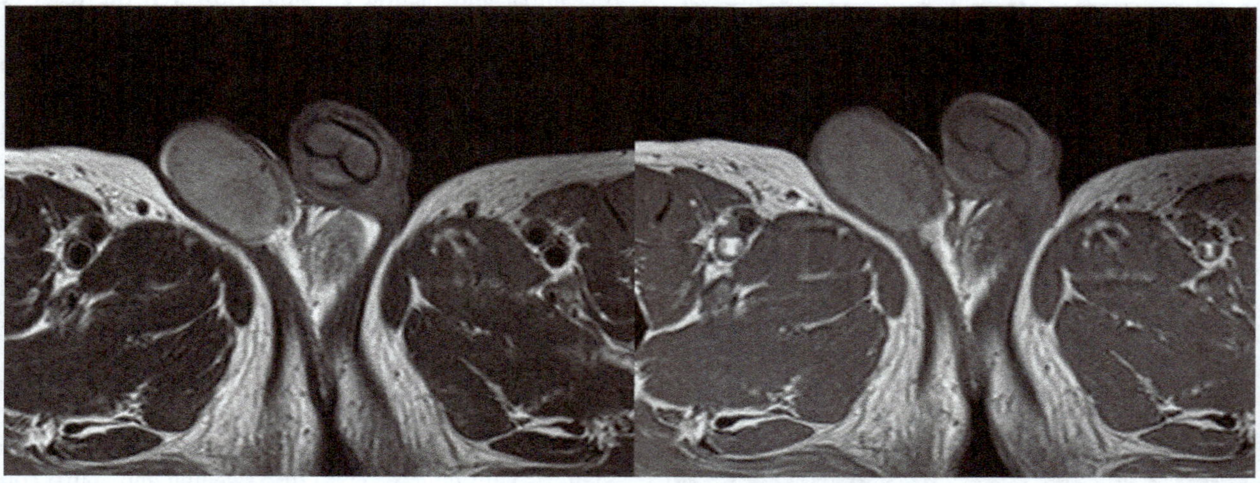

Fig. 5 Magnetic resonance imaging of the bilateral testes

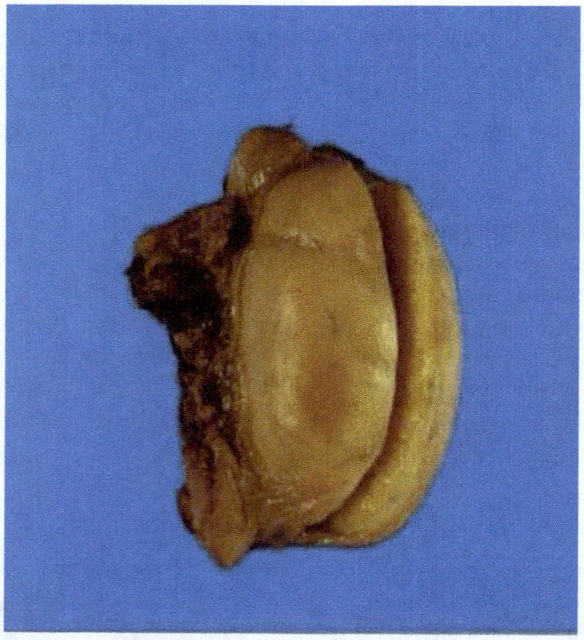

Fig. 6 Smooth yellowish left testis

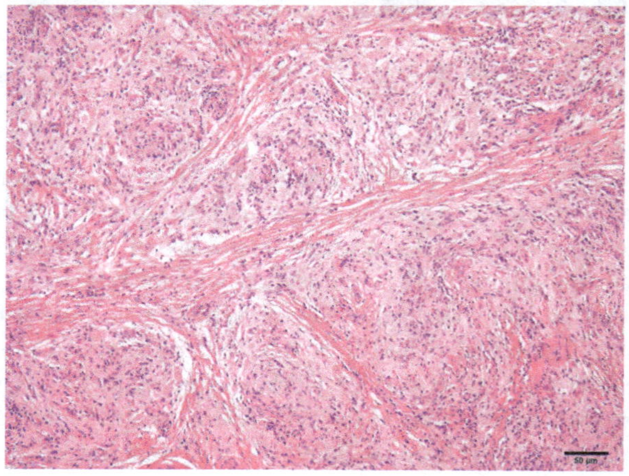

Fig. 7 Histology of the testicular gumma, showing epithelioid granulomas. (Horizontal and Vertical resolution at 72 dpi, Magnification × 10)

The indurated right eye may be due to syphilis. However, the reason for the hardened eye mass remains unknown because the patient denied undergoing a biopsy. Ocular syphilis can occur in any stage of syphilis and can infect any part of the eye, with panuveitis being the most common finding. Patients generally present with loss of vision, eye pain, floaters, and photophobia [2]. Orbital involvement is rare and characterized by gumma within the orbit, extraocular muscle, or lacrimal gland and the presence of periostitis [2–4].

The literature review revealed that the mean age of patients with testicular syphilis at disease presentation is 42 years and five patients had HIV infection (Table 1). In total, 14 patients (14/18, 77.7%; we were unable to collect the data of six patients mentioned in the study by Archimbaud et al. [5]) presented with enlarged testis or scrotal swelling. Six patients (6/18, 33.3%) presented with a firm or hard testicle accompanied by testicular

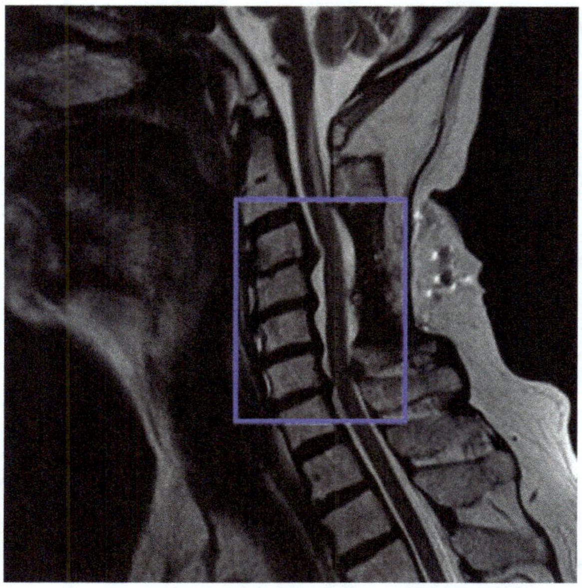

Fig. 8 Magnetic resonance imaging of the cervical spine showing C3–C4 cervical spinal canal stenosis due to cervical spondylosis (inside the blue box)

swelling. Our patient was unique in presenting with only hard bilateral testes.

The incidence of syphilis is currently increasing in developed countries. More than half of patients are males are owing to men having sex with men, and 42% of such patients were also HIV-positive [6]. The number of patients with syphilis is increasing by 1100 per year in Japan [7]; however, it is mainly because of heterosexual transmission rather than homosexual transmission [8]. It can also be caused by a direct *T. pallidum* (subspecies *pallidum*) infection and then is transmitted via blood products, either transplacentally or sexually.

Syphilis has three stages: primary (characterized by painless chancre occurring 2–6 weeks after infection), secondary (characterized by condylomata lata 1–2 months after primary syphilis), and tertiary (occurring 2–50 years after the initial infection, characterized by gummatous disease, meningovascular disease, tabes dorsalis, cardiovascular, ocular, and otic syphilis) [6].

Serologic testing is currently the standard approach for diagnosis; however, it lacks sensitivity in detecting early syphilis, congenital syphilis, neurosyphilis, tertiary syphilis, and HIV or Hepatitis C coinfection [9]. Hence, several other approaches such as immunohistochemistry (IHC), polymerase chain reaction (PCR), culture, morphological observation, and seroassay are considered for the detection of clinically undetected syphilis [10]. In a previous study, IHC had 49–92% sensitivity and excellent specificity for the diagnosis of secondary syphilis [9]. It can be used as a tool for further investigation when serological assays fail to identify the organism. However, there is a possibility of cross reaction with *Borrelia burgdorferi* and intestinal spirochetes [10]. PCR has a sensitivity of 89.1% in chancre specimens from patients with primary syphilis [10, 11]. In fact, the United States Centers for Disease Control and Prevention suggests that PCR is valuable for chancre samples [11]

Syphilitic gummata can mimic testicular tumors, which are usually diagnosed after surgery. Its differential diagnoses such as testicular neoplasms, mumps orchitis, tubercular epididymitis, and gonococcal epididymitis should be considered [1]. Gummata are usually multiple and regressive. It is clinically diagnosed with syphilis serology and treatment response [1]. On biopsy, obliterative endarteritis with palisading lymphocytes and plasma cells is visible. Over time, fibrous scarring causes tubular atrophy and sterility [1].

Ultrasonography shows lesions to be cystic with increased peripheral vascularity [12]. On contrast-enhanced ultrasonography, lesions show rapid wash-in and early washout [13]. Moreover, orchidectomy is generally performed for testicular syphilitic masses because of the concerns regarding missing out on the testicular tumor, thus requiring conservative management [13–15].

Penicillin G is the antibiotic of choice for syphilis. However, ampicillin treatment results in a higher cerebrospinal fluid concentration in the brain than penicillin G treatment. It was used in our patient to avoid neurosyphilis, although the investigations for this were negative [8]. Although intramuscular benzathine penicillin G is the first-line antibiotic recommended by the World Health Organization, it is unavailable in Japan and carries a risk of anaphylaxis [16]. Unfortunately, the syphilis tests were not negative in our patient even after the antibiotic therapy. Thus, therapy was inadequate due to severe inflammation.

The present case highlights the importance of broadening the differential diagnoses of testicular hardening or indurations. Patients with syphilitic gummata present only with hardness; this needs to be considered for timely treatment of and complication prevention in patients with similar presentations.

Table 1 Relevant literature on testicular involvement in syphilis

Case number	Authors	Age (years)	Testicular findings	Systemic findings
1	Lees et al. 1937 [15]	27	Bilateral (first right scrotal swelling, then left scrotal swelling) Congenital syphilis	NA
2	London et al. 1947 [17]	33	Hardening with painful swelling of testes	NA
3	Al-Egaily et al. 1977 [1]	37	Bilateral firm and enlarged testis with painless penile sores	NA
4–9	Archimbaud et al. 1984 [5]		Six cases	NA
10	Onishi et al. 1987 [18]	72	Right scrotal swelling with tenderness	Aortic aneurysm Aortitis
11	Terao et al. 1993 [19]	44	Enlarged firm right testis	NA
12	Nakano et al. 1999 [20]	75	Painless left scrotal swelling	NA
13	Varma et al. 2009 [21]	39	Right testis painful and firm lump	HIV
14	Silva et al. 2010 [22]	32	Bilateral testicular swelling	NA
15	Nakano et al. 2011 [8]	47	Painful right testicular swelling	NA
16	Sekita et al. 2012 [23]	40	Left scrotal swelling Left testis	NA
17	Teo et al. 2012 [14]	47	Right testis with firm, non-tender swelling Non-ulcerated indurated subprepuce Conservative treatment with doxycycline	NA
18	Liang et al. 2013 [24]	37	Left testicle and left kidney Painless swelling Doxycycline coz of penicillin allergy post-operation	HIV
19	Yogo et al. 2014 [25]	28	Right testis pain and swelling Jarisch–Herxheimer reaction in the testis following Penicillin G infusion	HIV with Bilateral Retinal detachment
20	Morlacco et al. 2015 [26]	31	Right testis pain and swelling	NA
21	Chu et al. 2016 [27]	33	Right testis hardening and swelling Non-granulomatous type	HIV
22	Tagliati et al. 2020 [13]	39	Testicular discomfort Multiple bilateral subcentimetric hypoechoic lesions	NA
23	Agrawal et al. 2020 [28]	40	Left scrotal abscess due to epididymo-orchitis Ulcerated enlarged left testis with indurated base	HIV
24	Our case	63	Bilateral testes induration	Aortitis Left subclavian artery aneurysm

HIV human immunodeficiency virus, *NA* not applicable

Abbreviations

COPD: Chronic obstructive pulmonary disease; HIV: Human immunodeficiency virus; ICU: Intensive care unit; MRI: Magnetic resonance imaging.

Acknowledgements

The authors would like to thank Dr. Toshiko Yamochi for interpreting histology findings and Enago (www.enago.jp) for the English language review.

Authors' contributions

SPN, TN1, TF, TS, JM, YM, and YO conceived the case report. KO, YN, TU, TN2, TI, RK, SA, MM, MK, YT, and SY were involved in the design and substantively revised the case report. TN1, TS, JM, YM, KO, YN, TU and TN2 were involved in the patient's medical check-up. TN1, YN, TN2, TI, RK, SA, MM, MK, YT, and SY were involved in the follow-up. SPN drafted the manuscript. All authors read and approved the final manuscript.

Competing interests

The authors declare that they have no competing interests.

References

1. Al-Egaily S. Gumma of the testis and penis. Br J Vener Dis. 1977;53:257–9. https://doi.org/10.1136/sti.53.4.257.
2. Dutta Majumder P, Chen EJ, Shah J, Ching Wen Ho D, Biswas J, See Yin L, et al. Ocular syphilis: an update. Ocul Immunol Inflamm. 2019; 27:117–125. https://doi.org/10.1080/09273948.2017.1371765.
3. Kemp JE. Syphilis of the orbit. Arch Dermatol. 1923;8:165. https://doi.org/10.1001/archderm.1923.02360140002001.
4. Sniderman HR. Late Syphilis with rare orbital gumma. Arch Derm Syphilol. 1940;42:559–65. https://doi.org/10.1001/archderm.1940.01490160019003.
5. Archimbaud A, Bonvalet D, Levy-Klotz B, Vallet C, Civatte J, et al. Syphilitic orchiepididymitis. Apropos of a pseudotumoral case. Ann Dermatol Venereol. 1984;111:169–71.
6. Ghanem KG, Ram S, Rice PA. The modern epidemic of syphilis. N Engl J Med. 2020;382:845–54. https://doi.org/10.1056/NEJMra1901593.
7. Syphilis, Japan. Tokyo: National Institute of Infectious Diseases. https://www.niid.go.jp/niid/en/basic-science/865-iasr/9542-479te.html. Accessed 19 Apr 2020.

8. Takahashi T, Arima Y, Yamagishi T, Nishiki S, Kanai M, Ishikane M, et al. Rapid increase in reports of syphilis associated with men who have sex with women and women who have sex with men, Japan, 2012 to 2016. Sex Transm Dis. 2018;45:139–43. https://doi.org/10.1097/OLQ.00000 00000000768.
9. Müller H, Eisendle K, Bräuninger W, Kutzner H, Cerroni L, Zelger B. Comparative analysis of immunohistochemistry, polymerase chain reaction and focus-floating microscopy for the detection of *Treponema pallidum* in mucocutaneous lesions of primary, secondary and tertiary syphilis. Br J Dermatol. 2011;165:50–60. https://doi.org/10.1111/j.1365-2133.2011. 10314.x.
10. Luo Y, Xie Y, Xiao Y. Laboratory diagnostic tools for syphilis: current status and future prospects. Front Cell Infect Microbiol. 2021;10: 574806. https:// doi.org/10.3389/fcimb.2020.574806.
11. Gayet-Ageron A, Sednaoui P, Lautenschlager S, Ferry T, Toutous-Trellu L, Cavassini M, et al. Use of *Treponema pallidum* PCR in testing of ulcers for diagnosis of primary syphilis. Emerg Infect Dis. 2015;21:127–9. https://doi. org/10.3201/eid2101.140790.
12. Mackenzie H, Mahmalji W, Raza A. The gumma and the gonad: syphilitic orchitis, a rare presentation of testicular swelling. Int J STD AIDS. 2011;22:531–3. https://doi.org/10.1258/ijsa.2009.009442.
13. Tagliati C, Macchini M, Argalia G, Giuseppetti GM, Giovagnoni A. Contrast-enhanced ultrasound evaluation of testicular syphilis: a case report. Med Ultrason. 2020;22:356–63. https://doi.org/10.11152/mu-2234.
14. Teo SY, Morris G, Fairley I. The great mimic: syphilis mimicking testicular tumour. Conservative management using antibiotics alone with testicular sparing. Int J STD AIDS. 2013; 24:415–8. https://doi.org/10.1177/09564 62412472833
15. Lees R. Calculus in the epididymis following bilateral syphilitic orchitis; a case report. Br J Vener Dis. 1957;33(4):258. https://doi.org/10.1136/sti.33.4. 258.
16. Tanizaki R, Nishijima T, Aoki T, Teruya K, Kikuchi Y, Oka S, et al. High-dose oral amoxicillin plus probenecid is highly effective for syphilis in patients with HIV infection. Clin Infect Dis. 2015;61:177–83. https://doi.org/10. 1093/cid/civ270.
17. London MZ. Bilateral calcified testicular gumma. J Urol. 1947;57:564–6. https://doi.org/10.1016/s0022-5347(17)69673-3.
18. Onishi N, Wakabayashi A, Sugiyama T, Mitsubayashi S, Kurita T. A case of syphilitic orchitis with aortic aneurysm. Hinyokika Kiyo. 1987;33:1496–9.
19. Terao T, Kura N, Ohashi H, Mizuo T, Kameda N. Syphilitic orchitis: report of a case. Hinyokika Kiyo. 1993;39:973–6.
20. Nakano Y, Chokyu H, Inaba Y, Harada M, Gotoh A, Maeda S. Syphilitic orchitis: a case report Hinyokika kiyo. Acta Urol Japon. 1999;45:289–91.
21. Varma R, Baithun S, Alexander S, Goh BT. Acute syphilitic interstitial orchitis mimicking testicular malignancy in an HIV-1 infected man diagnosed by *Treponema pallidum* polymerase chain reaction. Int J STD AIDS. 2009;20:65–6. https://doi.org/10.1258/ijsa.2008.008253.
22. de Silva A, Lee JD, Macdonald IW, Shekhar C. An unusual testicular lump. Int J STD AIDS. 2010;21:526–7. https://doi.org/10.1258/ijsa.2010.010051.
23. Sekita N, Nishikawa R, Fujimura M, Sugano I, Mikami K. Syphilitic orchitis: a case report. Hinyokika kiyo Acta Urologica Japonica. 2012;58:53–5.
24. Liang R, Chaudhry S. Testicular and kidney masses in a HIV-infected man. Int J STD AIDS. 2013;24:671–3. https://doi.org/10.1177/0956462413 482426.
25. Yogo N, Nichol AC, Campbell TB, Erlandson KM. Syphilis presenting as retinal detachment and orchitis in a young man with HIV. Sex Transm Dis. 2014;41:114–6. https://doi.org/10.1097/OLQ.0000000000000078.
26. Morlacco A, De Gobbi A, Dal Moro F, Zattoni F. Syphilis or cancer? A urological challenge. Urologia. 2015;82:245–6. https://doi.org/10.5301/ uro.5000128.
27. Chu CY, Chen WY, Yeh SD, Yeh HM, Fang CL. Syphilitic orchitis mimicking a testicular tumor in a clinically occult HIV-infected young man: a case report with emphasis on a challenging pathological diagnosis. Diagn Pathol. 2016;11:4. https://doi.org/10.1186/s13000-016-0454-x.
28. Agrawal V, Ranjan R. Scrotal abscess consequent on syphilitic epididymo-orchitis. Trop Doct. 2019;49:45–7. https://doi.org/10.1177/0049475518 809240.

11

The impact of lower urinary tract symptoms on the quality of life during pregnancy: A cross-sectional study from Palestine

Qais T. Ahmad[1], Jaffar H. Saffarini[1], Ahmad M. Samara[1], Dima S. Jabri[1], Zaina H. Safarini[1], Yousra M. Banijaber[1], Ahmad Jaradat[1,2], Faris Abushamma[1,2] and Sa'ed H. Zyoud[3,4,5*]

Abstract

Background: Lower urinary tract symptoms (LUTS) are prevalent among pregnant women. Several articles show the impact of LUTS on pregnant women's quality of life (QoL). This study was designed to examine the impact of non-pathological LUTS on QoL among pregnant Palestinian women.

Methods: A cross-sectional, hospital-based study was conducted on women who were pregnant and receiving regular antenatal care at the obstetrics and gynecology clinic in Rafidia Hospital, Palestine. This self-administered questionnaire included the Urinary Distress Inventory – short-form (UDI-6), the Incontinence Impact Questionnaire – short-form (IIQ-7), the European Quality of Life scale – 5 dimensions (EQ-5D), and the European Quality of Life – visual analogue scale (EQ-VAS). A convenience sampling method was used. In addition to this, multiple linear regression analyses were performed aiming to identify variables that have a significant relationship with QoL (i.e. socio-demographic variables, UDI-6 score, and IIQ-7 score).

Results: This study included a total of 306 pregnant women. Participants had a mean age of 26.9 years (SD, 3.6). The subjects scored an average of 31.2 ± 19.2 out of 100 points for the UDI-6 scale and an average of 31.9 ± 24.9 out of 100 points for the IIQ-7 scale. On the other hand, the subjects' average EQ-5D and EQ-VAS scores were 0.76 ± 0.17 and 67.96 ± 19.28 respectively. The subjects' responses on UDI-6 significantly correlated with their responses on both the EQ-5D and EQ-VAS scales ($r = -0.338$, $p < 0.001$ and $r = -0.206$, $p < 0.001$, respectively). Likewise, their responses on IIQ-7 also significantly correlated with their responses on both the EQ-5D and EQ-VAS scales ($r = -0.389$, $p < 0.001$ and $r = -0.329$, $p < 0.001$, respectively). Regression analysis found that the UDI-6 score ($p = 0.001$) and IIQ-7 score ($p < 0.001$), were significantly and negatively associated with EQ-5D index scores.

Conclusions: Our study shows a remarkable correlation between LUTS and QoL among pregnant women. Further longitudinal studies are required to assess the status of LUTS in the pre-pregnancy stage to ascertain a more accurate assessment of LUTS or LUTS related intervention and its impact on QoL during pregnancy.

Keywords: Lower urinary tract symptoms, Quality of life, Pregnancy, Palestine

Background

Pregnancy is a physiological process that entails several multisystem changes [1]. Pathological conditions may appear during pregnancy such as Urinary tract infections (UTIs), pre-eclampsia, and gestational diabetes [2]. Few reports have been conducted to date to assess the impact of lower urinary tract symptoms (LUTS) during pregnancy [3–5]. LUTS can have negative effects on the

*Correspondence: saedzyoud@yahoo.com; saedzyoud@najah.edu
[3] Department of Clinical and Community Pharmacy, Department of Pharmacy, College of Medicine and Health Sciences, An-Najah National University, Nablus 44839, Palestine
Full list of author information is available at the end of the article

social, physical, and emotional well-being of pregnant women [6]. Pregnancy-related LUTS, despite not being a pathological condition by definition, account for a significant amount of urinary distress and can affect quality of life (QoL) during pregnancy [7]. Moreover, the prevalence of urinary symptoms and distress during pregnancy could be under-reported due to the intimate nature of these symptoms [8].

QoL during pregnancy, with its effect on women's physical and mental health, is an important topic that can be directly affected by the presence of LUTS [9–11]. Several reports have been published in order to identify and manage these symptoms early in pregnancy, such as antenatal urinary incontinence screening, health education regarding risk factors for urinary incontinence, and highlighting the importance of early recognition and management [7].

In Palestine, there has been a growing interest in studying QoL indices in different populations and how this may be impacted by different variables and factors [12–19]. However, the impact of LUTS on the QoL among pregnant women has not been examined before. Therefore, this study aimed to examine the impact of non-pathological LUTS on the overall QoL during pregnancy, and to identify factors that might directly affect the QoL. The merit of this study shadows the growing trend to integrate LUTS management into routine pregnancy-care, and planning personalised care for pregnant women in relation to these symptoms based on their unique risks and needs. Our results provide key data from the clinical setting demonstrating the extent to which LUTS affects pregnant women's physical and psychological well-being. This in turn allows for better planning and establishment of management protocols for the problem in order to improve pregnancy and health outcomes in general. Finally, the current study will provide a reference point for health officials in order to assess the efficiency of any future interventions to address this problem.

Methods

Study design

This was a cross-sectional study that assessed the impact of LUTS on QoL during pregnancy. It used questionnaire-based interviews to collect data from the study subjects.

Study setting and study population

The survey took place at the obstetrics and gynecology clinic in Rafidia Hospital. The target population was pregnant women aged between 18 and 40 years. Data was collected between September 2019 and February 2020. The appointments were undertaken between 8 AM and 1 PM which are the official clinic hours allocated to conducting follow-up appointments for pregnant women in the studied clinic.

Sample size and sampling method

During the study period, the approximate number of pregnant women visiting the obstetrics and gynecology clinic at Rafidia Hospital was 1100. To determine the sample size required for analysis this number was used as a reference. Using the Raosoft sample size calculator, a sample size of 285 was determined by setting the response distribution at 0.50, the error margin at 5%, and the confidence interval at 95%. The target sample size was increased to 306 participants in order to decrease erroneous outcomes and improve research reliability. The convenience sampling technique was used for participants' selection.

Inclusion and exclusion criteria

For inclusion in the study, participants were required to be female, pregnant, able to speak Arabic, aged between 18 and 40 years, and have no history of a psychiatric illness. They were also required to be visiting the obstetrics and gynecology clinic in Rafidia Hospital for a pregnancy-related reason. Patients who had an established diagnosis of a urogenital condition or history of urological surgery were excluded.

Data collection tool

For data collection, a four-section, Arabic-language questionnaire was used. Section one asked for the participants' demographics. The structured questionnaire used in this study was based on previously published studies [20–23]. The Urinary Distress Inventory – short version (UDI-6) and the Incontinence Impact Questionnaire - Short Form (IIQ-7), were included in sections two and three respectively, to assess lower urinary tract symptoms including incontinence [20–22]. In the final section, we included the European Quality of Life scale 5 dimensions (EQ-5D) and the European Quality of Life visual analogue scale (EQ-VAS) [23, 24]. Data for this research was obtained through self-administered questionnaires. Physicians were available at all times to answer questions and explain any queries.

Section one asked the participants to fill in their age, weight, height, residency type, smoking status, employment status, education level, income, regular physical exercise, gestational trimester, parity (number of children), presence of psychiatric illness, medical disorders, long-term medication use, and previous surgeries. These factors were selected from those identified in previous studies that may affect QoL during pregnancy [25, 26].

Participants were put into one of five age groups: ≤ 20, 21–25 years, 26–30 years, 31–34 years, or ≥ 35 years [27]. The body mass index (BMI) for pregnancy was measured as pre-pregnancy weight in kilograms divided by height in meters squared, on the basis of self-reported weight and height. Based on their calculated body mass index (BMI), participants were classified into one of four groups: obese group (BMI $\geq 30\,kg/m^2$), overweight group (BMI = 25–29.9 kg/m^2), normal-weight group (BMI = 18.5–25 kg/m^2), or the underweight group (BMI $< 18.5\,kg/m^2$) [28].

In section two, we included the UDI-6 – short version. Similar to its full version, UDI-6 was designed to assess the severity of urinary distress symptoms based on the level of discomfort experienced during the past month. UDI-6 contains six questions that cover three areas: irritative symptoms (items one and two), stress symptoms (items three and four), and obstructive or discomfort symptoms (items five and six). Participants answer each section by choosing one of four options: 'greatly', 'moderately', 'a little bit', and 'not at all'. Each answer received a number of points between zero and three, with 'greatly' receiving three points and 'not at all' receiving zero points. Therefore, the highest possible UDI score was 18. The internal consistency of UDI, as previously tested by Cronbach's alpha test coefficient, was 0.720. Permission to include the Arabic version of this tool in our study was granted by the developer [21].

In section three, we included IIQ-7 – short version. IIQ-7 is a tool designed to gauge the impact of urinary incontinence on life quality in women. As in its full version, IIQ-7 focuses on four areas: physical activity (items one and two), travel (items three and four), social relations (item five), and emotional wellbeing (items six and seven). The participant rated the severity of symptoms on a zero-to-three scale, with zero as the least severe, and three as the most severe [22]. Therefore, the highest possible IIQ-7 score was 21. The internal consistency of this tool was previously tested and the reported Cronbach's alpha coefficient was 0.894. We obtained approval to include the Arabic version of this tool in our study from its developer.

All scores for UDI-6 and IIQ-7 were converted to a scale of 0–100 to allow comparison across measures [29]. UDI-6 and IIQ-7 proved to be valid and reliable questionnaires for evaluating the subjective phases of urinary incontinence severity. They were helpful in characterising the severity of incontinence, accessing treatment effectiveness, and making treatment decisions [30, 31].

In section four, we included the EQ-5D and the EQ-VAS scales to evaluate the health status and QoL of our subjects. EQ-5D is a standardized tool used to assess health outcomes. It studies five separate aspects of health: anxiety/depression, pain/discomfort, self-care, mobility, and usual activities. The subject rates each section on a 5-level scale (no problems, slight problems, moderate problems, severe problems and extreme problems). There are 3125 possible health states, obtained by using one number from each section, ranging from 11,111 (full health) to 55,555 (worst health). In the current study, we included the Arabic version [12, 15–19, 23] of EQ-5D in accordance with its developers' guidelines after receiving their approval to use it (ID: 35675). The EQ-5D score was calculated according to the United States General Population Score Algorithm (i.e. EQ-5D-5L Crosswalk Index Value Calculator) for measuring the index value by the value set (weights) [32]. The possible values of this algorithm ranged from − 0.109 to 1, with values below 0 representing states considered to be worse than death. The internal consistency for this tool was acceptable (Cronbach's alpha of 0.808). EQ-VAS, on the other hand, measures the subject's perspective of their life quality using a scale of 0–100 points [23, 24].

Statistical analysis

We used IBM SPSS, version 21 for data analysis. We presented the data as frequencies and percentages for participants' characteristics, and as means and standard deviations for their questionnaire scores. Participants' scores on EQ-5D and EQ-VAS scales were presented as medians and interquartile ranges. We tested the variables' normality using the Kolmogorov-Smirnov test. Mann-Whitney and Kruskal-Wallis tests were implemented to test the contrast between different categories based on the participants' characteristics. Possible correlations between all scales were evaluated by Pearson correlation coefficients. The significance was assumed at p-value < 0.05. We also carried out multiple linear regressions to predict the variables that had a significant relationship with QoL (EQ-5D and EQ-VAS scores as dependent variables). In our regression model, all variables with $p < 0.05$ in univariate analysis were used. Multicollinearity between the selected independent variables was tested with a variance inflation factor (VIF). Any VIF values of < 3 were considered to be appropriate due to a lack of collinearity.

Results

Demographic and clinical characteristics

A total of 306 participants took part in this study. Participants had a mean age of 26.9 years (SD, 3.6). The age and BMI categories which included the highest number of subjects were 21–30 years and normal BMI range, (70.2, and 46.1%, respectively). The majority of participants were educated to a university-level (71.2%). Most subjects were housewives (77.8%), and lived in a moderate-income household (48%). Over one-third of our subjects (41.2%) were pregnant in their third trimester. Only 8.2% had an established diagnosis of a chronic illness, and 10.1% practiced physical exercise regularly. Tables 1 and 2 summarise all demographic and clinical characteristics of the subjects.

QoL assessment findings (EQ-5D and EQ-VAS scores)

The participants' mean EQ-5D and EQ-VAS scores were 0.76 ± 0.17 and 67.96 ± 19.28, respectively. Table 1 shows the association between the characteristics of the participants and the scores achieved on the EQ-5D scale, whereas Table 2 presents the relationship between their characteristics and scores on the EQ-VAS scale. The participants' level of education significantly affected their scores on both EQ-5D and EQ-VAS scales (p-values were 0.005 and 0.004, respectively), whereas their level of income and history of previous chronic disease significantly correlated only with their EQ-VAS scores (p-values were < 0.001 and 0.008, respectively).

Urogenital symptoms' correlation with the QoL in pregnant women

Regarding urinary distress observations, the subjects scored an average of 5.6 ± 3.4 out of 18 (31.2 ± 19.2 out of 100) points for the UDI-6 scale, and an average of 6.7 ± 5.2 out of 21 (31.9 ± 24.9 out of 100) points for the IIQ-7 scale. Table 3 presents the correlations between urogenital symptom scales and QoL scales in pregnant women. The participants' responses on UDI significantly correlated with their responses on both the EQ-5D and EQ-VAS scales ($r = -0.338$, $p < 0.001$ and $r = -0.206$, p-value< 0.001, respectively). Likewise, their responses on IIQ-7 also significantly correlated with their responses on both the EQ-5D and EQ-VAS scales ($r = -0.389$, $p < 0.001$ and $r = -0.329$, $p < 0.001$, respectively). As expected, the participants' responses on the EQ-5D scale and EQ-VAS scale also showed significant correlation ($r = 0.329$, $p < 0.001$).

Results of multiple linear regression analysis

A multiple linear regression analysis was constructed according to BMI, educational level, UDI-6 score, and IIQ-7 score. Multiple linear regression models that were estimated to explore associations with the EQ-5D index score found that the UDI-6 score ($p = 0.001$) and the IIQ-7 score ($p < 0.001$) significantly and negatively correlated with the EQ-5D index score. The factors significantly associated with the EQ-5D index score based on multiple linear regression findings are illustrated in Table 4. There was no evidence of multicollinearity between independent variables (VIF ranged from 1.037–1.261).

The multiple linear regression analysis was performed by using the EQ-VAS score as a dependent variable after controlling for BMI, education level, income, presence of chronic disease, drug history, UDI-6 score, and IIQ-7 score (Table 5). This demonstrated that income (p value$= 0.036$) was significantly and positively associated with EQ-VAS scores, whilst IIQ-7 scores ($p < 0.001$) significantly and negatively correlated with EQ-VAS scores.

The factors significantly associated with the EQ-VAS score based on multiple linear regression findings are illustrated in Table 5. There was no evidence of multicollinearity between independent variables (VIF ranged from 1.089–2.962).

Discussion

There is scanty data to describe the prevalence of LUTS during pregnancy and its negative effect on QoL, which we believe is prevalent in Palestine, and may negatively affect the physical and mental health of pregnant women. We used two assessment tools for urinary symptoms (UDI-6 and IIQ-7) and two life quality assessment tools (EQ-5D and EQ-VAS) in order to explore this problem. In addition to this, factors that may affect QoL have also been studied. It was appropriate to use a generalised questionnaire to determine the subject's health-related quality of life (HRQoL) values [33–36], given that most pregnant women do not have a fatal illness [37]. As one of the most common means for assessing the overall health of the body, EQ-5D is a powerful generic tool, particularly in regards to evaluating symptoms of pain and anxiety/depression [38]. In addition, IIQ-7 is a seven-item questionnaire designed for the assessment of various QoL impairment areas [39]. The areas include social activities, moving far from home, mental wellbeing, household chores, entertainment activities, feelings of frustration, and physical recreation.

The mean EQ-5D in our study was 0.76 ± 0.17, whereas the mean EQ-VAS score was 67.96 ± 19.28. There was also a strong correlation between urinary distress symptoms assessment scores (UDI and IIQ-7) and QoL assessment scores (EQ-5D and EQ-VAS). Therefore our study confirms the hypothesis that LUTS during pregnancy has a detrimental effect on QoL, suggesting a negative impact on physical and mental health during pregnancy.

The participants' scores on QoL assessment scales showed significant correlations with some demographic variables such as BMI, education level, income level, history of other chronic illnesses, and use of chronic medication. This is supported by the Singaporean Integrated Women's Health Program findings which showed a notable association of BMI, parity, and education level with urinary distress symptoms and a higher likelihood of seeking medical care due to these symptoms [40].

Table 1 Association between the characteristics of the participants and the EQ-5D scores they achieved

Characteristic	No. (%); Total = 306	EQ-5D score Median [Q1-Q3]	*P*-value*
Age group (years)			
≤ 20	22 (7.2)	0.79 [0.68–0.82]	0.323 [a]
21–25	102 (33.3)	0.79 [0.67–0.86]	
26–30	113 (36.9)	0.79 [0.65–0.88]	
31–35	39 (12.7)	0.74 [0.60–0.82]	
> 35	30 (9.8)	0.80 [0.67–0.86]	
BMI group			
Healthy weight	141 (46.1)	0.81 [0.69–0.88]	**0.021** [a]
Overweight	118 (38.6)	0.77 [0.65–0.83]	
Obese	47 (15.4)	0.74 [0.60–0.83]	
Education level			
Elementary school	4 (1.3)	0.76 [0.63–0.81]	**0.005** [a]
Middle school	18 (5.9)	0.79 [0.71–0.84]	
High school	66 (21.6)	0.81 [0.71–1.00]	
University	218 (71.2)	0.77 [0.64–0.83]	
Employment status			
House-wife	238 (77.8)	0.70 [0.53–0.85]	0.133 [a]
Governmental employee	31 (10.1)	0.65 [0.50–0.80]	
Private sector	37 (12.1)	0.70 [0.57–0.82]	
Income			
Low (< 2000 NIS)	123 (40.2)	0.79 [0.64–0.86]	0.577 [a]
Moderate (2000–4999 NIS)	147 (48)	0.79 [0.68–0.84]	
High (≥5000 NIS)	36 (11.8)	0.80 [0.66–0.88]	
Gestational trimester			
First trimester	68 (22.2)	0.80 [0.70–0.87]	0.055 [a]
Second trimester	112 (36.6)	0.80 [0.68–0.87]	
Third trimester	126 (41.2)	0.75 [0.63–0.83]	
No. of children			
0	60 (19.6)	0.79 [0.67–0.82]	0.869 [a]
1	92 (30.1)	0.79 [0.67–0.86]	
2	64 (20.9)	0.80 [0.63–0.96]	
3	44 (14.4)	0.77 [0.65–0.84]	
≥ 4	46 (15.0)	0.78 [0.68–0.86]	
Presence of chronic diseases			
No	281 (91.8)	0.79 [0.68–0.86]	0.154 [b]
Yes	25 (8.2)	0.74 [0.63–0.83]	
Drug history			
No	287 (93.8)	0.79 [0.68–0.86]	
Yes	19 (6.2)	0.74[0.66–0.83]	
			0.361 [b]
Regular exercise			
No	275 (89.9)	0.79 [0.68–0.86]	0.401 [b]
Yes	31 (10.1)	0.80 [0.63–0.83]	

Abbreviations: *BMI* body mass index, *EQ-5D* European Quality of Life scale 5 dimensions, *NIS* New Israeli Shekel (1 New Israeli Shekel = 0.29 US Dollar)

* All significant *p*-values are displayed in bold

[a] Calculated by Kruskal–Wallis test

[b] Calculated by Mann–Whitney U test

Table 2 Association between the characteristics of the participants and the EQ-VAS scores they achieved

Characteristic	No. (%); Total = 306	EQ-VAS score Median [Q1-Q3]	*P*-value*
Age group (years)			
≤20	22 (7.2)	82.00 [68.00–90.00]	0.260 [a]
21–25	102 (33.3)	70.00 [50.00–80.00]	
26–30	113 (36.9)	70.00 [60.00–85.00]	
31–35	39 (12.7)	60.00 [45.00–80.00]	
>35	30 (9.8)	72.50 [63.75–86.25]	
BMI group			
Healthy weight	141 (46.1)	70.00 [57.50–90.00]	**0.031** [a]
Overweight	118 (38.6)	70.00 [55.00–80.00]	
Obese	47 (15.4)	65.00 [50.00–80.00]	
Education level			
Elementary school	4 (1.3)	37.50 [27.50–40.00]	**0.004** [a]
Middle school	18 (5.9)	55.00 [48.50–80.00]	
High school	66 (21.6)	70.00 [50.00–81.25]	
University	218 (71.2)	70.00 [60.00–85.00]	
Employment status			
House-wife	238 (77.8)	70.00 [53.75–85.00]	0.279 [a]
Governmental employee	31 (10.1)	65.00 [50.00–80.00]	
Private sector	37 (12.1)	70.00 [57.50–82.50]	
Income			
Low (<2000 NIS)	123 (40.2)	65.00 [50.00–80.00]	**<0.001** [a]
Moderate (2000–4999 NIS)	147 (48)	70.00 [55.00–80.00]	
High (≥5000 NIS)	36 (11.8)	80.00 [70.00–90.00]	
Gestational trimester			
First trimester	68 (22.2)	70.00 [60.00–80.00]	0.152 [a]
Second trimester	112 (36.6)	70.00 [60.00–85.00]	
Third trimester	126 (41.2)	70.00 [50.00–80.00]	
No. of children			
0	60 (19.6)	75.00 [60.00–90.00]	0.136 [a]
1	92 (30.1)	70.00 [60.00–85.00]	
2	64 (20.9)	70.00 [55.00–80.00]	
3	44 (14.4)	70.00 [50.00–80.00]	
≥4	46 (15.0)	62.00 [50.00–80.00]	
Presence of chronic diseases			
No	281 (91.8)	70.00 [57.50–85.00]	**0.008** [b]
Yes	25 (8.2)	60.00 [40.00–70.00]	
Drug history			
No	287 (93.8)	70.00 [55.00–85.00]	**0.033** [b]
Yes	19 (6.2)	60.00 [40.00–70.00]	
Regular exercise			
No	275 (89.9)	70.00 [50.00–80.00]	0.532 [b]
Yes	31 (10.1)	80.00 [70.00–90.00]	

Abbreviations: *BMI* body mass index, *EQ-VAS* European Quality of Life visual analogue scale, *NIS* New Israeli Shekel (1 New Israeli Shekel = 0.29 US Dollar)

* All significant *p*-values are displayed in bold

** We merged underweight and healthy weight groups as the former contained only 7 subjects

[a] Calculated by Kruskal–Wallis test

[b] Calculated by Mann–Whitney U test

Table 3 Correlation of urinary distress scales and quality of life scales among pregnant women

Scales	EQ-5D *P*-value	Correlation	EQ-VAS *P*-value	Correlation
UDI	< 0.001	− 0.338	< 0.001	− 0.206
IIQ-7	< 0.001	− 0.398	< 0.001	− 0.348
EQ-5D	-	-	< 0.001	0.329
EQ-VAS	< 0.001	0.329	-	-

Abbreviations: *EQ-VAS* European Quality of Life visual analogue scale, *EQ-5D* European Quality of Life scale 5 dimensions, *UDI* urinary distress inventory, *IIQ-7* incontinence impact questionnaire - short form

Participants with higher socioeconomic status had a better QoL score, which is consistent with findings from other studies that revealed a significant association between socioeconomic status and urinary incontinence. Furthermore, this cohort of patients is more likely to seek medical advice and treatment in earlier stages [41]. LUTS is a newly evolving concept in urology, as well as a broad term that can be applied to many urological abnormalities, such as lower urinary tract infections, idiopathic overactive bladder symptoms, etc. In general, higher-income and educated females are more likely to lead a healthy lifestyle in regards to eating healthily and undertaking regular exercise, as well as being less exposed to anxiety and other mental health issues. All of these elements reduce the risk of developing LUTS symptoms [41, 42]. This is also applicable to pregnant females, particularly as patients with a higher income have easier access to primary healthcare, allowing prompt treatment of LUTS and any underlying pathology. This observation should be taken into consideration if a screening program for LUTS were to be initiated, as prioritising lower-educated and lower-income females would likely identify a higher proportion of patients requiring treatment. Omitting higher-income and educated females from such a screening program would likely be a cost-effective approach.

Table 4 Multiple linear regression analysis of the association of variables with EQ-5D scores

Model		Unstandardized Coefficients		Standardized Coefficients	t	*p*-value*	95.0% Confidence Interval for B		Collinearity Statistics
		B	Std. Error	Beta			Lower Bound	Upper Bound	VIF
1	**(Constant)**	1.045	0.058		17.962	0.000	0.931	1.160	
	BMI	−0.013	0.013	−0.052	− 0.966	0.335	− 0.038	0.013	1.108
	Education level	−0.037	0.014	−0.040	−.992	0.052	−0.064	0.010	1.037
	UDI-6 score	−0.002	0.001	−0.191	−3.334	**0.001**	−0.004	−0.001	1.261
	IIQ-7 score	−0.002	0.000	−0.330	−5.927	**0.000**	−0.003	−0.002	1.196

BMI body mass index, *VIF* variance inflation factor, *EQ-5D* European quality of life scale 5 dimensions, *UDI* urinary distress inventory, *IIQ* incontinence impact questionnaire

* All significant p-values are displayed in bold

Table 5 Multiple linear regression analysis of the association between factors and EQ-VAS score

Model		Unstandardized Coefficients		Standardized Coefficients	t	*p*-value*	95.0% Confidence Interval for B		
		B	Std. Error	Beta			Lower Bound	Upper Bound	VIF
1	**(Constant)**	69.385	8.852		7.839	0.000	51.965	86.804	
	BMI	−0.669	1.508	−0.025	− 0.444	0.657	−3.637	2.298	1.140
	Education level	2.665	1.674	0.091	1.592	0.113	−0.630	5.960	1.162
	Income	3.373	1.604	0.116	2.102	**0.036**	0.215	6.530	1.089
	Presence of chronic diseases	−7.004	7.401	−0.100	−0.946	0.345	−21.569	7.562	2.962
	Drug history	1.251	8.509	0.016	0.147	0.883	−15.494	17.997	2.065
	UDI-6 score	−0.110	0.080	−0.082	−1.371	0.171	−0.269	0.048	1.285
	IIQ-7 score	−0.217	0.045	−0.280	−4.821	**0.000**	−0.306	−0.129	1.209

BMI body mass index, *EQ-VAS* European Quality of Life visual analogue scale, *UDI* urinary distress inventory, *IIQ* incontinence impact questionnaire, *VIF* variance inflation factor

* All significant *p*-values are displayed in bold

We also uncovered a significant correlation between the severity of the urinary distress symptoms (using both UDI-6 and IIQ-7 scales) and the subject's QoL. This emphasises the bothersome nature of these symptoms. This observation is in concordance with an increasing understanding of the fundamental effect of urinary incontinence symptoms on quality of life, and the importance of surveying and managing these symptoms as early as possible [43]. Proper and timely intervention for these problems should be of particular importance, as due to the intimate nature of urinary distress symptoms, affected women often delay seeking medical help.

Limitations and strengths

One of the limitations of this study was the cross-section design, which prevented us from interpreting the causality of significant associations in our results. Another limitation of this study is that it took place in one hospital, which may limit the generalisability of our data to all pregnant women in Palestine. However, this study had strengths as well, such as using two urinary distress assessment tools and two QoL tools that have proven validity, which attest to the accuracy of our assessment. The most fundamental limitation lies in the fact that we wanted to exclude any established diagnosis of lower urinary tract abnormalities, therefore our exclusion criteria mandates omission of subjects with any previously established diagnosis of urinary tract abnormalities or previous urological surgeries. Nevertheless, we do believe that a small percentage of pregnant females could have had overactive bladder symptoms prior to pregnancy which became more prominent or distressing during pregnancy. We did not go back and try to review all symptoms prior to pregnancy, as our goal was to assess the prevalence of LUTS during pregnancy and its impact on QoL. An additional question that was not addressed in this study was whether the effect on bladder function alters during different trimesters. Whilst we have the data available and could have undertaken sub-analysis, we felt the sample size too small to present viable conclusions. Therefore, we preferred to analyse the data as a whole, rather than sub-classifying it. Furthermore, the absence of control groups (i.e. pregnant versus non-pregnant) limits the interpretation of the disease burden on HRQoL.

Moreover, this was the first study to examine urinary distress symptoms' impact on the QoL during pregnancy in Palestine. As our study focus was towards pregnancy-associated, non–pathological LUTS, all of our participants had received a first-trimester negative urine test, and were screened for fever symptoms and dysuria at the time of the questionnaire. Patients with pre-existing urogenital conditions and a history of urological surgery were also excluded, as mentioned previously. Understanding of Pregnancy-associated LUTS/ Pregnancy non-pathological LUTS/ LUTS during pregnancy is an evolving concept in the literature [44] and we took the first step in the Middle East to evaluate its presence, risk factors, and impact on QoL.

Conclusions

There is a remarkable correlation between the severity of urinary distress symptoms and the QoL among pregnant women. Identification and characterisation of HRQoL-related factors in pregnant women with LUTS can potentially accelerate the development of diagnostic, preventive, and therapeutic strategies for the improvement of HRQoL in this population. Alerting healthcare providers to the presence of LUTS among pregnant women is recommended. Focusing on the prevention of risk factors for LUTS is necessary in order to minimise its detrimental effect on QoL. Further longitudinal studies are required to assess the status of LUTS in the pre-pregnancy stage and ascertain a more accurate assessment of LUTS and LUTS related intervention and its impact on QoL during pregnancy. Several strategies can be adapted to recognise and treat this problem from an early stage, such as community-based counselling for pregnant females and regular assessment of LUTS during different stages of pregnancy. Therefore, healthcare providers should consider the psychological effects of LUTS on pregnant women in order to raise and deal with possible evolving mental health issues through different trimesters.

Abbreviations

UTIs: Urinary tract infections; LUTS: Lower urinary tract symptoms; QoL: Quality of life; HRQoL: Health-related quality of life; NNU: An-Najah National University; NIS: New Israeli Shekel; UI: Urinary incontinence; EQ-5D: European Quality of Life scale 5 dimensions; UDI: Urinary distress inventory; IIQ: Incontinence impact questionnaire; EQ-VAS: European Quality of Life visual analogue scale; OBGYN: Obstetrics and gynecology; IRB: Institutional Review Board; VIF: Variance inflation factor.

Acknowledgements

The authors thank Samantha Kearley from the Bristol Urological Institute, UK for English editing of the manuscript.

Authors' contributions

JS and QA collected and analyzed the data, performed literature review and contributed to manuscript drafting. AS conducted data analysis and literature review and partially interpreted the data and drafted the manuscript. DJ, YB and ZS performed data collection and literature review. AJ and FA participated in the conception and design of the study and data interpretation, and revised the manuscript critically for strengthening intellectual contents. SZ played a key role in conceptualization, designing, coordination, supervision of this study and took the responsibility of the integrity of the data and the accuracy of the analysis; he also conducted a critical review of results' interpretation, revised the manuscript critically for strengthening intellectual contents, and took part in the final writing. All authors read the final manuscript and approve of it.

Competing interests

All authors declare there are no competing interests.

Author details

[1] Department of Medicine, College of Medicine and Health Sciences, An-Najah National University, Nablus 44839, Palestine. [2] Department of Urology, An-Najah National University Hospital, Nablus 44839, Palestine. [3] Department of Clinical and Community Pharmacy, Department of Pharmacy, College of Medicine and Health Sciences, An-Najah National University, Nablus 44839, Palestine. [4] Poison Control and Drug Information Center (PCDIC), College of Medicine and Health Sciences, An-Najah National University, Nablus 44839, Palestine. [5] Clinical Research Center, An-Najah National University Hospital, Nablus 44839, Palestine.

References

1. Soma-Pillay P, Nelson-Piercy C, Tolppanen H, Mebazaa A. Physiological changes in pregnancy. Cardiovasc J Afr. 2016;27(2):89–94.
2. Narayan B, Nelson-Piercy C. Medical problems in pregnancy. Clin Med (Lond). 2017;17(3):251–7.
3. Balik G, Güven ES, Tekin YB, Şentürk Ş, Kağitci M, Üstüner I, Mete Ural Ü, Şahin FK. Lower urinary tract symptoms and urinary incontinence during pregnancy. Low Urin Tract Symptoms. 2016;8(2):120–4.
4. Martins G, Soler ZA, Cordeiro JA, Amaro JL, Moore KN. Prevalence and risk factors for urinary incontinence in healthy pregnant Brazilian women. Int Urogynecol J. 2010;21(10):1271–7.
5. Liang CC, Chang SD, Lin SJ, Lin YJ. Lower urinary tract symptoms in primiparous women before and during pregnancy. Arch Gynecol Obstet. 2012;285(5):1205–10.
6. van der Vaart CH, de Leeuw JR, Roovers JP, Heintz AP. Measuring health-related quality of life in women with urogenital dysfunction: the urogenital distress inventory and incontinence impact questionnaire revisited. Neurourol Urodyn. 2003;22(2):97–104.
7. Mohd Yusoff D, Awang S, Kueh YC. Urinary incontinence among pregnant women attending an antenatal clinic at a tertiary teaching hospital in North-East Malaysia. J Taibah Univ Sci. 2018;14(1):39–46.
8. Narchi NZ. Prenatal care by nurses in the east zone of the city of Sao Paulo - Brazil. Rev Esc Enferm USP. 2010;44(2):266–73.
9. Herath INS, Balasuriya A, Sivayogan S. Physical and psychological morbidities among selected antenatal females in Kegalle district of Sri Lanka: a cross sectional study. J Obstet Gynaecol. 2017;37(7):849–54.
10. van Brummen HJ, Bruinse HW, van der Bom JG, Heintz AP, van der Vaart CH. How do the prevalences of urogenital symptoms change during pregnancy? Neurourol Urodyn. 2006;25(2):135–9.
11. Mallah F, Montazeri A, Ghanbari Z, Tavoli A, Haghollahi F, Aziminekoo E. Effect of urinary incontinence on quality of life among Iranian women. J Family Reprod Health. 2014;8(1):13–9.
12. Barham A, Ibraheem R, Zyoud SH. Cardiac self-efficacy and quality of life in patients with coronary heart disease: a cross-sectional study from Palestine. BMC Cardiovasc Disord. 2019;19(1):290.
13. Khatib ST, Hemadneh MK, Hasan SA, Khazneh E, Zyoud SH. Quality of life in hemodialysis diabetic patients: a multicenter cross-sectional study from Palestine. BMC Nephrol. 2018;19(1):49.
14. Alami YZ, Ghanim BT, Zyoud SH. Epworth sleepiness scale in medical residents: quality of sleep and its relationship to quality of life. J Occup Med Toxicol. 2018;13:21.
15. Abu Farha NH, Khatib MT, Salameh H, Zyoud SH. Cancer-related post-treatment pain and its impact on health-related quality of life in breast cancer patients: a cross sectional study in Palestine. Asia Pac Fam Med. 2017;16:7.
16. Zyoud SH, Daraghmeh DN, Mezyed DO, Khdeir RL, Sawafta MN, Ayaseh NA, Tabeeb GH, Sweileh WM, Awang R, Al-Jabi SW. Factors affecting quality of life in patients on haemodialysis: a cross-sectional study from Palestine. BMC Nephrol. 2016;17(1):44.
17. Al-Jabi SW, Zyoud SH, Sweileh WM, Wildali AH, Saleem HM, Aysa HA, Badwan MA, Awang R. Relationship of treatment satisfaction to health-related quality of life: findings from a cross-sectional survey among hypertensive patients in Palestine. Health Expect. 2015;18(6):3336–48.
18. Zyoud SH, Al-Jabi SW, Sweileh WM, Wildali AH, Saleem HM, Aysa HA, Badwan MA, Awang R, Morisky DE. Health-related quality of life associated with treatment adherence in patients with hypertension: a cross-sectional study. Int J Cardiol. 2013;168(3):2981–3.
19. Zyoud SH, Al-Jabi SW, Sweileh WM, Arandi DA, Dabeek SA, Esawi HH, Atyeh RH, Abu-Ali HA, Sleet YI, Abd-Alfatah BM, et al. Relationship of treatment satisfaction to health-related quality of life among Palestinian patients with type 2 diabetes mellitus: findings from a cross-sectional study. J Clin Transl Endocrinol. 2015;2(2):66–71.
20. Uebersax JS, Wyman JF, Shumaker SA, McClish DK, Fantl JA. Short forms to assess life quality and symptom distress for urinary incontinence in women: the incontinence impact questionnaire and the urogenital distress inventory. Continence program for women research group. Neurourol Urodyn. 1995;14(2):131–9.
21. Altaweel W, Seyam R, Mokhtar A, Kumar P, Hanash K. Arabic validation of the short form of urogenital distress inventory (UDI-6) questionnaire. Neurourol Urodyn. 2009;28(4):330–4.
22. Ghroubi S, El Fani N, Elarem S, Alila S, Ben Ayed H, Borgi O, Chmak J, Elleuch MH. Arabic (Tunisian) translation and validation of the urogenital distress inventory short form (UDI-6) and incontinence impact questionnaire short form (IIQ-7). Arab J Urol. 2020;18(1):27–33.
23. Horowitz E, Abadi-Korek I, Shani M, Shemer J. EQ-5D as a generic measure of health-related quality of life in Israel: reliability, validity and responsiveness. Isr Med Assoc J. 2010;12(12):715–20.
24. EuroQol Research Foundation. EQ-5D-5L User Guide. 2019. https://euroqol.org/publications/user-guides. Accessed 15 May 2020.
25. RezaeiNiaraki M, Roosta S, Alimoradi Z, Allen KA, Pakpour AH. The association between social capital and quality of life among a sample of Iranian pregnant women. BMC Public Health. 2019;19(1):1497.
26. Lagadec N, Steinecker M, Kapassi A, Magnier AM, Chastang J, Robert S, Gaouaou N, Ibanez G. Factors influencing the quality of life of pregnant women: a systematic review. BMC Pregnancy Childbirth. 2018;18(1):455.
27. Alzboon G, Vural G. Factors influencing the quality of life of healthy pregnant women in North Jordan. Medicina (Kaunas). 2019;55(6):278.
28. Klatsky AL, Zhang J, Udaltsova N, Li Y, Tran HN. Body mass index and mortality in a very large cohort: is it really healthier to be overweight? Perm J. 2017;21:16–142.
29. Utomo E, Korfage IJ, Wildhagen MF, Steensma AB, Bangma CH, Blok BF. Validation of the urogenital distress inventory (UDI-6) and incontinence impact questionnaire (IIQ-7) in a Dutch population. Neurourol Urodyn. 2015;34(1):24–31.
30. Nusee Z, Rusly A, Jamalludin AR, Abdulwahab DF, Ismail R. Translation and validation of Bahasa Malaysia version of urogenital distress inventory (UDI-6) and incontinence impact quality of life questionnaires (IIQ-7) a Cross Sectional Study. Malays J Med Sci. 2016;23(3):57–63.
31. Lasserre A, Pelat C, Gueroult V, Hanslik T, Chartier-Kastler E, Blanchon T, Ciofu C, Montefiore ED, Alvarez FP, Bloch J. Urinary incontinence in French women: prevalence, risk factors, and impact on quality of life. Eur Urol. 2009;56(1):177–83.
32. Visser E, de Bock GH, Kollen BJ, Meijerink M, Berger MY, Dekker JH. Systematic screening for urinary incontinence in older women: who could benefit from it? Scand J Prim Health Care. 2012;30(1):21–8.
33. Heslin M, Chua KC, Trevillion K, Nath S, Howard LM, Byford S. Psychometric properties of the five-level EuroQoL-5 dimension and short Form-6 dimension measures of health-related quality of life in a population of pregnant women with depression. BJPsych Open. 2019;5(6):e88.
34. Morin M, Claris O, Dussart C, Frelat A, De Place A, Molinier L, Matillon Y, Ehlinger V, Vayssiere C. Quality of life during pregnancy: is there a link with breastfeeding at birth? Breastfeed Med. 2020;15(5):321–30.
35. Sut HK, Asci O, Topac N. Sleep quality and health-related quality of life in pregnancy. J Perinat Neonatal Nurs. 2016;34(4):302–9.
36. Morin M, Claris O, Dussart C, Frelat A, de Place A, Molinier L, Matillon Y, Elhinger V, Vayssiere C. Health-related quality of life during pregnancy: a repeated measures study of changes from the first trimester to birth. Acta Obstet Gynecol Scand. 2019;98(10):1282–91.
37. Ming WK, Wu H, Wu Y, Chen H, Meng T, Shen Y, Wang Z, Huang X, Sun W, Chow TS, et al. Health-related quality of life in pregnancy with uterine fibroid: a cross-sectional study in China. Health Qual Life Outcomes. 2019;17(1):89.
38. Sarkin AJ, Groessl EJ, Carlson JA, Tally SR, Kaplan RM, Sieber WJ, Ganiats TG. Development and validation of a mental health subscale from the quality of well-being self-administered. Qual Life Res. 2013;22(7):1685–96.
39. El-Azab AS, Mascha EJ. Arabic validation of the urogenital distress inventory and adapted incontinence impact questionnaires--short forms. Neurourol Urodyn. 2009;28(1):33–9.

40. Ng KL, Ng KWR, Thu WPP, Kramer MS, Logan S, Yong EL. Risk factors and prevalence of urinary incontinence in mid-life Singaporean women: the integrated Women's health program. Int Urogynecol J. 2020;31(9):1829–37.
41. Lee JA, Johns TS, Melamed ML, Tellechea L, Laudano M, Stern JM, Abraham NE. Associations between socioeconomic status and urge urinary incontinence: an analysis of NHANES 2005 to 2016. J Urol. 2020;203(2):379–84.
42. Biswas B, Bhattacharyya A, Dasgupta A, Karmakar A, Mallick N, Sembiah S. Urinary incontinence, its risk factors, and quality of life: a study among women aged 50 years and above in a rural health Facility of West Bengal. J Midlife Health. 2017;8(3):130–6.
43. Aoki Y, Brown HW, Brubaker L, Cornu JN, Daly JO, Cartwright R. Urinary incontinence in women. Nat Rev Dis Primers. 2017;3:17042.
44. Li Z, Xu T, Zhang L, Zhu L. Prevalence, potential risk factors, and symptomatic bother of lower urinary tract symptoms during and after pregnancy. Low Urin Tract Symptoms. 2019;11(4):217–23.

12

Circumferential dissection of deep fascia as ancillary technique in circumcision: Is it possible to correct phimosis increasing penis size?

Pagano Carmine[1], Faenza Mario[2*], Guastafierro Antonio[2], Manfellotto Vincenzo[2], Grella Elisa[2], Cosenza Angelo[3], Pieretti Gorizio[2] and Izzo Sara[2]

Abstract

Background: Phimosis is the inability to retract the preputium downward over the glans penis. Despite the various techniques of preputial plasty described in literature, the most performed surgical treatment is still the conventional circumcision.

Methods: In this paper we retrospectively reviewed data of a homogeneous population of 36 consecutive adult patients who underwent phimosis correction by circumcsion with dissection of the Deep Fascia. Patients were followed up by one independent plastic surgeon that measured penis length and circumference in nonerected state preoperatively and at 6 month time postoperatively.

Results: The Wilcoxon Signed Rank Test showed a significant ($p < 0.0001$) difference between the two groups both in terms of length and circumference.

Conclusions: In conclusion, the ancillary technique we described leads to an increase of penis size, is safe and easy to perform and does not increase significantly operative time nor complication rate to the conventional procedure.

Background

Phimosis is a clinical condition in which the prepuce cannot be retracted over the glans. In pediatric population it is common and can be considered physiologic, whereas in adult population is always considered pathologic and is related to many conditions such as diabetes, or recurrent balanitis or trauma [1, 2]. Phimosis had been classified by Kayaba et al. [3] in four grades according to the retractability of the prepuce.

The most performed surgical treatment of this clinical condition is circumcision but alternative surgical techniques with preputial preservation have been described [4–6].

The chronic inflammatory conditions that lead to phimosis in adults are often associated with a certain grade of fibrosis, from simple glanular adhesions to constricting bands affecting a larger portion of penile skin.

These fibrotic reactions could consequently lead to a reduction in penis size due to chronic and progressive constriction [12].

During the last 30 years augmentative surgery of penis has gradually increased its appeal to the point of being considered equivalent to the need of some women to ask for breast augmentation [18].

*Correspondence: dottmariofaenza@gmail.com
[2] Multidisciplinary Department of Medical Surgical and Dental Sciences - Plastic Surgery Unit, Università degli Studi della Campania "Luigi Vanvitelli", Caserta, Italy
Full list of author information is available at the end of the article

In this paper we described an ancillary procedure in circumcision that can lead to an augmentation both in terms of penile length and circumference.

Methods

We retrospectively reviewed data of a homogeneous population of 36 consecutive adult patients, aged between 19 and 45 years old, who underwent phimosis correction between November 2018 and March 2019. All patients were classified in terms of phimosis grade, symptoms and characteristics (Table 1). No patients reported history of previous surgery or scarring at prepuce level.

Written informed consent was obtained from all participants.

A two-step surgical procedure was performed under local anaesthesia obtained by peripheral block of the dorsal penile nerve with 2% Xylocaine.

The first step consisted in a conventional circumcision (Fig. 1).

In the second step the skin of the penis body was retracted to the base showing ventrally the presence of the areolar tissue and Buck's Fascia (Fig. 2).

Adherent bridles were identified and bluntly dissected (Fig. 3). With the ventral face of the penis exposed, a manual traction was performed causing a partial relaxation of the Buck's Fascia and determining the expansion both of the corpora cavernosa and the spongious body of the urethra (Fig. 4). At the end of the surgery, the entire cut edges were approximated with interrupted fine absorbable stitches.

Results

Patients were followed up by one independent plastic surgeon that measured the stretched penis length from radix to the apex of glans and circumference at midpoint of the penile shaft in nonerected state after 10 min of acclimatization at room temperature preoperatively and at 6 month time postoperatively.

In 8 patients out of 36 (22.22%) we registered a gain only in terms of length, whereas in 5 patients out of 36 we found an increment only in terms of circumference.

Only 1 patient out of 36 did not show any dimensional change (Table 2).

The Wilcoxon Signed Rank Test showed a significant ($p < 0.0001$) difference between the two groups both in terms of length and circumference. The mean of gain of

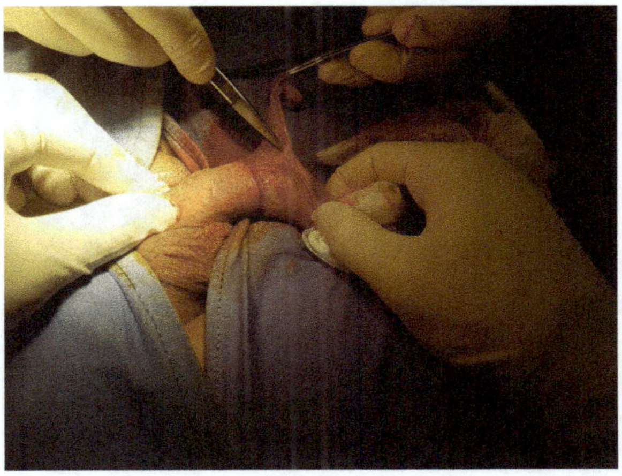

Fig. 1 Removal of the constricting fibrous band and consensual penile frenulectomy

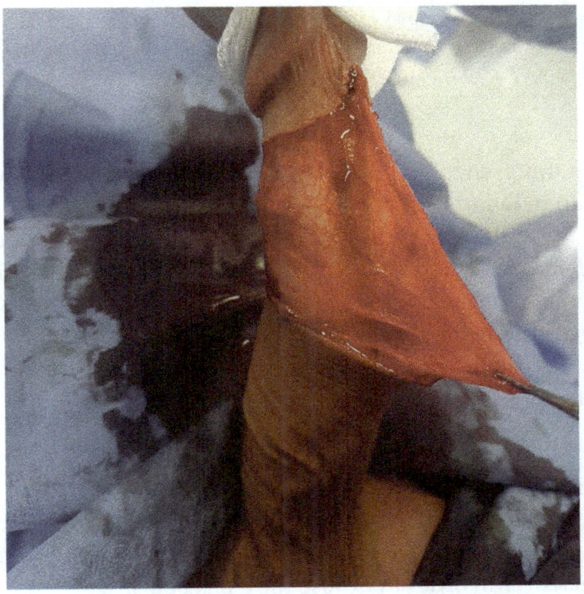

Fig. 2 Skin of the penis body was retracted to the base, showing ventrally the presence of the areolar tissue and deep fascia

Table 1 The deep fascia

Characteristics	Patients n = 36
Age (years old)	19–45 (average 23,7)
Kayaba's grade 1	6 (16.66%)
Kayaba's grade 2	19 (52.77%)
Kayaba's grade 3	11 (30.55%)
Smoking habit	11 (30.55%)
Diabetes	8 (22.22%)
History of recurrent balanoposthitis	6 (16.66%)
Painful erections	15 (41.66%)
Postoperative complications	
Huge edema	3 (8.33%)
Sensory impairments	10 (27.77%)

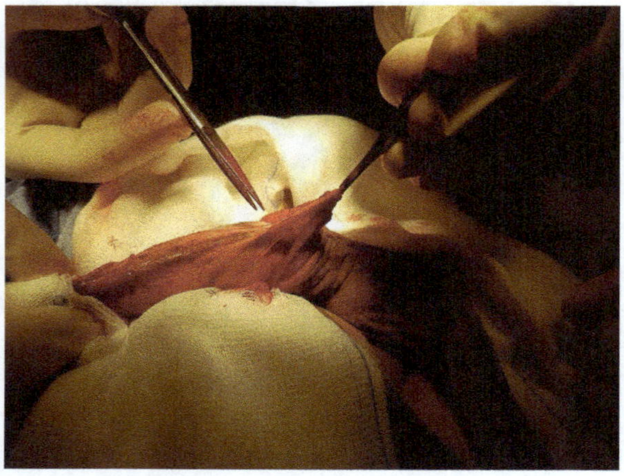

Fig. 3 Adherent bridles were identified and carefully dissected

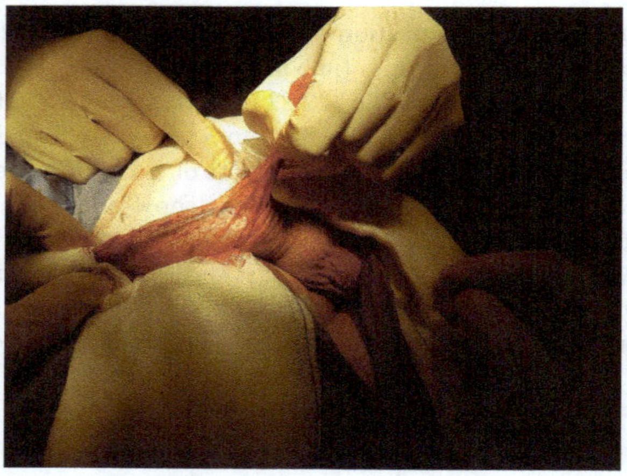

Fig. 4 With the ventral aspect of the penis exposed, a manual traction was performed, causing a partial relaxation of the deep fascia, determining the expansion of the corpora cavernosa and the spongeous body of the urethra

circumference was 0.95 + 0.71 cm, while the mean for gain in length was 0.7 + 0.56 cm.

The only complications registered were due to huge edema in 3 patients and sensory impairment in 10 patients occurred postoperatively and spontaneously regressed in 2 weeks time.

No recurrence of phimosis at 6 months follow-up have been registered.

Discussion

Phimosis is a clinical condition in which the foreskin, due to adherences or fibrotic preputial ring, cannot be pulled back over in order to expose the glans penis.

Phimosis can be classified into two groups: congenital and acquired.

The first type is usually seen in young children and could be considered physiological.

Acquired phimosis is mostly seen in adolescents and adults. Apart from discomfort during coitus in adult life, if the distal preputial ring is too narrow it can cause ballooning during voiding, making it difficult to maintain penile hygiene leading to chronic balanoposthitis.

This chronic condition leads to the development of adhesions between the glans and the inner leaf of the preputium and also the development of a fibrotic ring, severely narrowing the opening of the prepuce.

In 1996 Kayaba et al. [3] classified phimosis condition in four grades according to the level of preputial retractability.

Type I the preputial retractability is totally absent.

In Type II the preputial opening allows only exposure of the external urethral meatus.

In Type III the preputium can be partially retracted from the apex to the middle of the glans.

In Type IV the preputium can be retracted allowing the exposure to above the crown of the glans, because of adhesions between the inner leaf of the preputium and the corona.

Despite the various techniques of preputial plasty described in literature [4–6], the most performed surgical treatment is still the conventional circumcision.

This should be preferred if the preputium becomes scarred from previous attempts to release the glans or in the presence of balanitis xerotica obliterans.

Differing from reconstructive surgery, cosmetic surgery was developed by surgeons especially for people who felt the need to improve on nature, to improve the results of previous injuries or interventions by surgery.

Until 30 years ago, penis size either nonerected or erected was not mentioned in literature.

Cosmetic surgery for the penis cannot and should not be compared to rhinoplasty, breast augmentation, or breast reduction surgery, where obtained results are generally very acceptable.

Unfortunately, the expectations of patients of augmentation phalloplasty are far greater than the real results that can be obtained with the current surgical techniques.

When performed on a normal-looking penis which has an average size, a penile cosmetic procedure yields aesthetically less than the desired result. An increase of 2–4 cm should be considered a success.

The historical Kinsey report showed that only 5% of men have an erection of less than 9 cm and that 1% are very well endowed with an erection of longer than 20 cm [7].

A more recent study by Ponchietti et al. [8] of penile size in 3300 young Italian men showed these differences in a large sample: flaccid penile length: 5–13 cm

Table 2 Deep fascia the expansion

Patients	Circumference (cm)			Lenght (cm)		
	Pre-op	6 months Post-op	Gain	Pre-op	6 months Post-op	Gain
1	9.7	10.5	0.8	9.8	11	1.2
2	9	10.5	1.5	9.2	9.5	0.3
3	10.1	11.5	1.4	7.2	9.5	2.3
4	12	12	0	9.5	10.5	1
5	8.5	11.5	3	10.5	12.5	2
6	8.5	10	1.5	10.5	10.5	0
7	9.2	10.5	1.3	9.5	9.8	0.3
8	11.5	11.5	0	12.5	13	0.5
9	11	11	0	11.5	12	0.5
10	9	10.5	1.5	10	11	1
11	8.5	10	1.5	8.5	9.5	1
12	9.5	10.5	1	8.5	9	0.5
13	8	9.5	1.5	7	8	1
14	8.5	9.5	1	10	10.5	0.5
15	10	10.3	0.3	10	10	0
16	10.5	11.5	1	11	11.5	0.5
17	9	10.5	1.5	9.2	9.5	0.3
18	12	12	0	9.5	10.5	1
19	8.5	10	1.5	10.5	10.5	0
20	11	11	0	11.5	12	0.5
21	8.5	10	1.5	8.5	9.5	1
22	8.5	9.5	1	10	10.5	0.5
23	10	10.5	0.5	10	10	0
24	9	10.5	1.5	9.2	10	0.8
25	9	10.5	1.5	9	9.5	0.5
26	9.5	11	1.5	8	9.3	1.3
27	11	11	0	9.5	10.5	1
28	9.5	11.5	2	10.5	11	0.5
29	9	10	1	10.5	10.5	0
30	8.4	9.5	1.1	9.5	10	0.5
31	11.5	11.5	0	12	13	1
32	10	10	0	11	12	1
33	9	9.5	0.5	10	11	1
34	10	10	0	8.5	8.5	0
35	9.5	10.8	1.3	8.5	9	0.5
36	8.5	9	0.5	9	11	2

(average 9.0 cm), stretched penile size: 7.5–17.5 cm (average 12.5 cm), flaccid penile circumference: 8.5–11.5 cm (average 10 cm).

Another study by Wessels et al. [9] found that the average length of a flaccid penis was 8.8 cm, stretched length 12.4 cm and erect length 12.9 cm.

Khan et al. [10] asserted that men referred with penile disease had a marginally shorter penile length. In his study, men affected by penile disease, showed a flaccid length of 8.37 cm, a penopubic length of 9.97 cm and a stretched length of 13.70 cm.

In literature several surgical techniques have been described for penis augmentation, such as section of the suspensory ligament of the penis, lipectomy or liposuction of prepubic fat, inverted V-plasty of the radix of the penis and fat grafting of the penis [11].

Anyway is widely understood how a penis enlargement surgical or non surgical procedure is highly contraindicated in patients affected by uncorrected penile pathological conditions.

In 2011 Montag and Palmer [12] published a review about abnormalities of penile curvature and size, stating that these conditions can be related both to phimosis itself, because of the thickening of the Buck's fascia, and also to scar contraction after circumcision.

Many factors such as genetic predisposition, history of non-gonococcal urethritis, smoking habit, fibrotic lesions of the genital tract or previous urologic surgical procedures can lead to formation of asymptomatic fibrous cords at the level of penile fascia, with various degrees of contraction [13–15].

The suspensory apparatus of the penis is part of the deep fascia of the abdominal wall, it consists in the fundiform ligament, the suspensory ligament proper and the arcuate subpubic ligament.

The fundiform ligament is superficial and not adherent to the tunica albuginea, whilst the suspensory ligament proper bridges between the symphysis pubis and the Dartos and Buck's fascia of the corpora cavernosa, it splits to surround the penis and then unites and blends inferiorly with the Dartos' fascia forming the scrotal septum.

In our paper we described an ancillary technique in circumcision procedure in which we performed a release of the areolar tissue of the preputial skin, inducing a relaxation of the adherences of the Buck's fascia of penis.

In this way the corpora cavernosa are decompressed and, in our opinion, that is the reason why the circumference of the penis is significantly lengthened after the procedure.

The technique we described does not differ in its rationale from scar revision and nerve decompression procedures [16, 17].

For what concerns the gain in terms of penile length, the rationale should be related to the fact that Buck band is in continuity with the suspensory ligament of the penis, consequently its surgical release determines an elongation of the penis shaft.

After surgery the mean of gain of circumference observed was $0.95 + 0.71$ cm, while in terms of length was $0.7 + 0.56$ cm.

These data are comparable to the results obtained by other penis enlargement techniques, but to date there is no evidence of a contraction of the buck band in healthy patients, and therefore there is no evidence that this operation can lead to an increase in penis size even in healthy patients.

Further studies will be necessary to verify these premises in order to determine the real effectiveness of the technique also in penile cosmetic surgery.

Conclusions

In conclusion, the ancillary technique we described is safe and easy to perform and does not increase significantly operative time, since the degloving procedure takes just 15 min, nor complication rate to the conventional procedure.

For these reasons it could be done in every adult patient affected by phimosis, regardless of grade, who undergoes circumcision procedure.

Authors' contributions

CP: performing surgical procedures. MF: performing surgical procedures. AG: major contributor in writing the article. VM: collecting data. EG: data analysis. AC: data analysis. GP: design of the study. SI: design of the study. All authors have read and approved the manuscript

Competing interests

The authors declare that they have no competing interests.

Author details

[1] Clinica Nostra Signora di Lourdes, Somma, Italy. [2] Multidisciplinary Department of Medical Surgical and Dental Sciences - Plastic Surgery Unit, Università degli Studi della Campania "Luigi Vanvitelli", Caserta, Italy. [3] Department of Advanced Medical and Surgical Sciences - General Surgery Unit, Università degli Studi della Campania "Luigi Vanvitelli", Caserta, Italy.

References

1. Cold CJ, Taylor JR. The prepuce. BJU Int. 1999;83(Suppl 1):34–44.
2. Drivsholm T, De Fine ON, Nielsen AB, Siersma V. Symptoms, signs and complications in newly diagnosed type 2 diabetic patients, and their relationship to glycaemia, blood pressure and weight. Diabetologia. 2005;48:210–4.
3. Kayaba H, Tamura H, Kitajima S, Fujiwara Y, Kato T, Kato T. Analysis of shape and retractability of the prepuce in 603 Japanese boys. J Urol. 1996;156:1813–5.
4. Benson M, Hanna MK. Prepuce sparing: use of Z-plasty for treatment of phimosis and scarred foreskin. J Pediatr Urol. 2018;14:545e541–4.
5. Cuckow PM, Rix G, Mouriquand PD. Preputial plasty: a good alternative to circumcision. J Pediatr Surg. 1994;29:561–3.
6. Angotti R, Molinaro F, Ferrara F, Pellegrino C, Bindi E, Fusi G, Messina M. Preputialplasty: can be considered an alternative to circumcision? When, how, why? Experience of Italian centre. Gland Surg. 2018;7:228–33.
7. Kinsey AC, Pomeroy WB, Martin CE. Sexual behavior in the human male. Philadelphia: WB Saunders; 1948.
8. Ponchietti R, Mondaini N, Bonafe M, et al. Penile length and circumference: a study on 3,300 young Italian males. Eur Urol. 2001;39:183–6.
9. Wessels H, Lue TF, McAninch JW. Penile length in the flaccid and erect states: guidelines for penile augmentation. J Urol. 1996;156:995–7.
10. Khan S, Somani B, Lam W, Donat R. Establishing a reference range for penile length in Caucasian British men: a prospective study of 609 men. BJU Int. 2012;109:740–4.
11. Chapter 12. Int J Impot Res 15, S44–S45 (2003). https://doi.org/10.1038/sj.ijir.3901137
12. Montag S, Palmer LS. Abnormalities of penile curvature: chordee and penile torsion. Sci World J. 2011;11:1470–8.
13. Bjekic MD, Vlajinac HD, Sipetic SB, Marinkovic JM. Risk factors for Peyronie's disease: a case-control study. BJU Int. 2006;97:570–4.
14. Carrieri MP, Serraino D, Palmiotto F, Nucci G, Sasso F. A case-control study on risk factors for Peyronie's disease. J Clin Epidemiol. 1998;51:511–5.
15. Li CY, Agrawal V, Minhas S, Ralph DJ. The penile suspensory ligament: abnormalities and repair. BJU Int. 2007;99:117–20.
16. Rubino C, Faenza M, Di Pace B, Campitiello N, Brongo S, Zingone G. A new keystone flap "Plus" design: case series and analysis of follow-up. J Plast Reconstr Aesthet Surg. 2017;70(7):976–9.
17. Trignano E, Fallico N, Chen HC, Faenza M, Bolognini A, Armenti A, Santanelli Di Pompeo F, Rubino C, Campus GV. Evaluation of peripheral microcirculation improvement of foot after tarsal tunnel release in diabetic patients by transcutaneous oximetry. Microsurgery. 2016;36(1):37–41.

13

Prevalence of nocturia among community-dwelling adults: A population-based study in Malaysia

Hui-Yin Yow[1], John Jeh Lung Tiong[2], Chun-Wai Mai[3], Esther van der Werf[4], Zulkifli Md Zainuddin[5], Charng-Chee Toh[6], Kay-Seong Ngoo[7], Eng-Hong Goh[8], Ahmad Nazran Fadzli[9], Sze-Han Lok[1] and Teng-Aik Ong[9*]

Abstract

Background: Nocturia is widely prevalent condition with detrimental effects on quality of life and general health. In Malaysia, there is a lack of up-to-date prevalence study on nocturia. This study aimed to investigate the prevalence of nocturia and awareness pertaining to nocturia among Malaysian adults.

Methods: A cross-sectional population-based study was conducted among Malaysian adults aged ≥ 18 years old. The data was collected by mixed mode self-administered questionnaire from May 2019 to September 2019. Nocturia was defined as one or more voids at night.

Results: There were a total of 4616 respondents with 74.5% of response rate. The overall prevalence of nocturia among Malaysian adults was found to be 57.3%. In multivariate analysis, respondents aged 31–40 (1.91 [1.52–2.40]) or > 60 years old (2.03 [1.48–2.71]), and those who presented with hypertension (2.84 [2.28–3.53]), diabetes mellitus (1.78 [1.42–2.25]), renal disease (3.58 [1.93–6.63]) or overactive bladder (1.61 [1.10–2.35]) were associated with higher prevalence of nocturia. A significantly lower disease prevalence ($p < 0.05$) was noted among those aged 41–50 (0.73 [0.59–0.91]), male (0.78 [0.69–0.88]) and Chinese (0.47 [0.30–0.74]) or Indian (0.34 [0.21–0.54]) ethnicities. A total of 37.3% of respondents with nocturia reported that they faced sleeping difficulty about half the time or more after waking up in the middle of night. Those who had ≥ 2 voids per night experienced significantly higher mean bother score than those who had 1 void per night ($p < 0.001$). Approximately half (56.7%) of all respondents were not aware that night time urination is a medical condition. Only 25.2% of respondents with nocturia had sought medical attention for their nocturia.

Conclusions: The prevalence of nocturia among Malaysian adults is high and strongly influenced by age, sex, race and comorbidities. However, the general awareness pertaining to nocturia being a health issue remains low among Malaysians. The findings also highlighted the impact of nocturia on sleep and the need for nocturia education to better address this disease.

Keywords: Prevalence, Nocturia, Awareness, Malaysia, Survey

Background

Nocturia is defined as 'the complaint that the individual has to wake at night one or more times to void' by International Continence Society (ICS) [1]. Until recently, the definition has been revised as 'waking up to pass urine

*Correspondence: taong@um.edu.my
[9] Department of Surgery, Faculty of Medicine, University of Malaya, 50603 Kuala Lumpur, Malaysia
Full list of author information is available at the end of the article

during the main sleep period' [2]. Nocturia can affect all age groups although the disease prevalence does increase with age. Bosch and Weiss reviewed the nocturia prevalence studies in community based, predominantly populations in the western countries and some Asian countries (including China, Taiwan, Japan, Korea, Hong Kong and Singapore) [3]. They reported that prevalence of nocturia among younger populations (20–40 years old) with one or more voids per night varies from 11–44% whilst those with two or more voids per night has been reported to range between 2–18% [3]. Nevertheless, nocturia is more frequent among the older populations (>70 years old), with 69–93% having one or more voids per night while 28–62% reported two or more voids per night [3]. Similarly, a longitudinal study conducted by van Doorn and colleagues in the Dutch municipality Krimpen aan den IJssel showed that the prevalence of nocturia increases over time and with increasing age among men aged 50 to 78 years [4].

Several studies have demonstrated that nocturia has negative impact on quality of life and general health [5–8]. Increase in the number of voids per night has serious consequences on sleep, symptoms, morbidity from fatigue and falls and health-related quality of life [5–7]. Unfortunately, nocturia is often unreported, with the general lack of knowledge that nocturia is a treatable medical condition being cited as a crucial barrier to treatment seeking [9].

In Malaysia, there is lack of up-to-date prevalence studies on nocturia, only very limited studies are available as reference. A cross-sectional study had been carried out in Institute of Urology and Nephrology (IUN), Kuala Lumpur, Malaysia in 2007 and reported that the prevalence of nocturia was 29% among patients presented with lower urinary tract symptoms (LUTS) [10]. Similarly, Low and colleagues reported that high prevalence (19%) of LUTS was found among women in Northern Malaysia in 2006 and many of them did not seek treatment due to low disease awareness [11]. Most of these studies were at least 10 years ago, and thus the relevance remains questionable. Therefore, the aim of this present population-based study was to investigate the prevalence of nocturia and awareness pertaining to nocturia among community-dwelling adults in Malaysia.

Methods

A cross-sectional population-based study was conducted among community-dwelling Malaysian adults aged ≥ 18 years old across all states in Malaysia from May 2019 to September 2019 (Fig. 1). Convenience sampling was applied to obtain responses from any Malaysian adult aged ≥ 18 years old. The respondents were

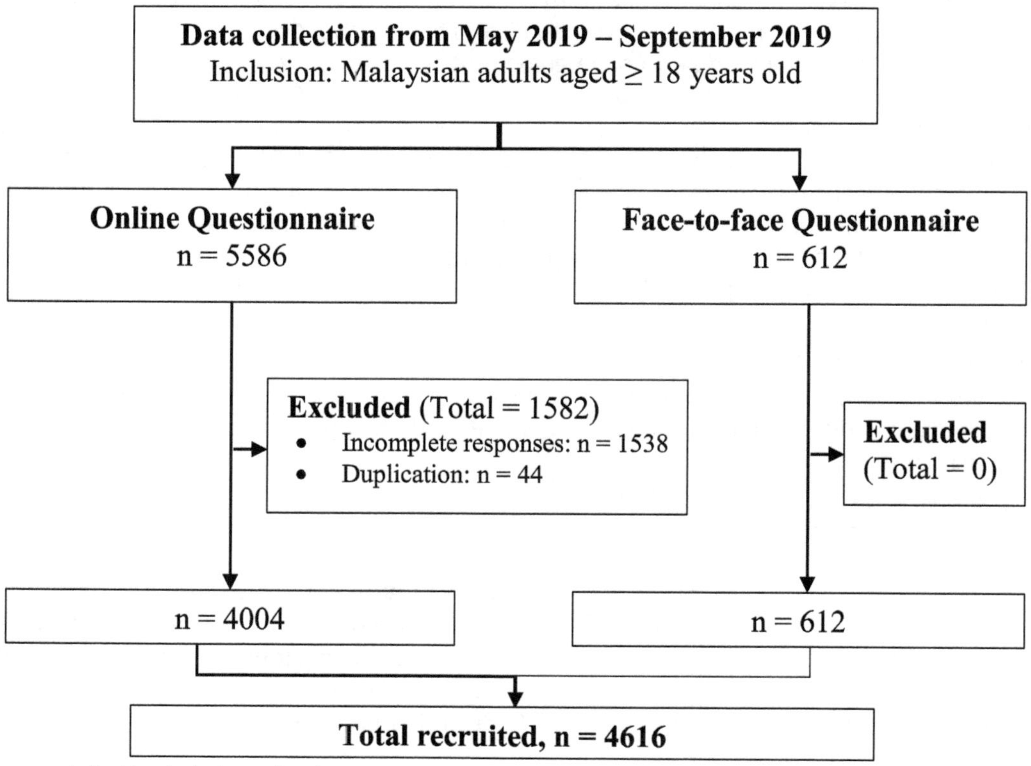

Fig. 1 Study protocol of subject inclusion and exclusion

approached based on the age population percentage reported by Department of Statistics Malaysia (https://www.dosm.gov.my). Individuals who were unable to read or understand English, Malay or Chinese, or with cognitive impairment or active mental illness, and all incomplete responses were excluded. A complete response was considered when the respondent answered all required questions until the last page of the survey, whereas for the questionnaire that was not done until the last page of survey was categorised as 'incomplete response'.

Questionnaire

The questionnaire consisted of three sections was developed for this study (Additional file 1). The first section of the research questionnaire consisted of items to extract the demographic data of the subjects. The second part was made up of three domains, namely present medical condition and disease pattern (2 items), night urination and sleeping issues (5 items) and treatment-seeking behaviour (2 items). Nocturia was defined as one or more voids at night based on the definition from ICS [1]. Those who had to wake up from sleep at night to urinate at least once were required to answer all items, while those without night urination were exempted from some questions pertaining to night urination and sleeping issues and treatment-seeking behaviour. The questionnaire was validated by a panel of experts on content validity and clarity. The English version of the questionnaire was checked by a native English speaker. The questionnaire was translated into Malay and Chinese languages based on ISPOR guideline with two forward-translation and two back-translation [12]. Three languages of questionnaire were pre-tested with a pilot study (n = 40, respectively) to confirm on the simplicity of language used and to assess the comprehension of the questions. Feedbacks were taken into consideration to incorporate into the final questionnaire. A second pilot study was conducted after the changes made to the questions, followed by a retest of the pilot study to assess internal consistency.

Data collection

Previous to the data collection, the researchers or the trained research assistants used a pre-trained structured protocol to introduce the instrument to the participants based on the inclusion criteria. In order to increase the response rate and outreach nationwide, data was collected by mixed mode, i.e. face-to-face and online modes. Face-to-face data collection was important to address the low level of technology literacy and/or limited access to the internet among certain segments of the population i.e. the elderly as well as the suburban and rural folks. It took place in public areas i.e. shopping malls, parks, restaurants, cafeteria and markets in rural and urban areas. The approached subjects spent approximately 5–10 min on the printed self-administered questionnaires. For the online mode, a third-party online platform was utilised to collect the responses. An information sheet about this research study along with a written consent form were attached to each copy of the questionnaire. All subjects signed the written informed consent form prior to answering the questionnaire.

Data analysis

Continuous variables were presented as mean and standard deviation; whilst categorical variables were presented as frequency and percentage. All data collected were tabulated and analysed using the Statistical Package for Social Sciences software, version 24.0. Pearson's chi-squared (χ^2) test was used to assess the significance in prevalence differences between dichotomous variables, such as sex, age group and employment status (or Fisher's exact test when the frequency of respondents was less than 5 for any category). For ordinal or continuous variables (e.g. age and degree of bother), the Mann–Whitney U test was used to determine the difference between two independent groups (or Kruskal Wallis test if there was more than two independent groups). Univariable analysis were performed for the respondents' characteristics in relation to prevalence of nocturia using logistic regression analysis. Variables with an association of $p < 0.05$ were selected for multivariable analysis using logistic regression analysis. Significance was defined as $p < 0.05$.

Results

The response rate was 74.5%, meaning that a total of 6198 respondents across the states in Malaysia participated in this study. There were 1538 of incomplete responses and 44 duplication of responses, which were excluded from the study. The demographic data of the study population was shown in Table 1. The comparison of demographic characteristics of study population with and without nocturia was shown in Table 2. Statistical analysis revealed that there was significant difference in prevalence between mean age, sex, race employment status and comorbidities ($p < 0.05$, respectively).

The overall prevalence of nocturia (at least one void per night) among Malaysian adults was 57.3% (Table 2), with 34.1%, 15.3% and 7.9% having an of an average of one void per night, two voids per night and three or more voids per night respectively. Figure 2 illustrated the increasing trend of prevalence with age in both sex and frequency of nocturnal voids was associated significantly with sex in different age groups. Younger (18–40 years old) and older women (> 60 years old) were more likely to have one void per night than men from the same age group ($p < 0.05$). Whereas middle-aged men (41–60 years

Table 1 Demographic characteristic of study population

Variable	Overall (n, %)	Mode of questionnaire		*p* value*
		Online (n, %)	Face-to-Face (n, %)	
Total respondents	4616 (100)	4004 (86.7)	612 (13.3)	
Mean age (years ± SD)	38.4 ± 14.58	38.0 ± 14.08	40.9 ± 17.31	0.025[φ]
18–30	1794 (38.9)	1573 (39.2)	221 (36.2)	
31–40	889 (19.3)	835 (20.9)	54 (8.8)	
41–50	760 (16.5)	692 (17.3)	68 (11.1)	
51–60	865 (18.7)	664 (16.6)	201 (32.9)	
> 60	307 (6.7)	240 (6.0)	67 (11.0)	
Sex				
Male	1982 (42.9)	1646 (41.1)	336 (54.9)	< 0.001[#]
Female	2634 (57.1)	2358 (58.9)	276 (45.1)	
Race				
Malay	1796 (38.9)	1222 (30.5)	574 (94.1)	< 0.001[#]
Chinese	2126 (46.1)	2115 (52.8)	11 (1.8)	
Indian	595 (12.9)	574 (14.4)	21 (3.4)	
Others	96 (2.1)	92 (2.3)	4 (0.7)	
Employment status				
Student	920 (19.9)	724 (18.1)	196 (32.0)	< 0.001[#]
Employed for wages	2659 (57.4)	2370 (59.2)	280 (45.8)	
Self-employed	394 (8.5)	319 (8.0)	75 (12.2)	
Unemployed	652 (14.1)	591 (14.7)	61 (10.0)	
Comorbidities				
Hypertension	638 (13.8)	502 (12.5)	136 (22.2)	< 0.001[#]
Diabetes mellitus	524 (11.4)	402 (10.0)	122 (19.9)	< 0.001[#]
Renal disease	90 (1.9)	39 (1.0)	51 (8.3)	< 0.001[#]
Heart failure	22 (0.5)	16 (0.4)	6 (1.0)	0.052[#]
Enlarged prostate	61 (1.3)	59 (1.5)	2 (0.3)	0.021[#]
Overactive bladder	141 (3.1)	121 (3.0)	20 (3.3)	0.742[#]
Prostate cancer	9 (0.2)	8 (0.2)	1 (0.2)	1.000[φ]
Bladder cancer	6 (0.1)	6 (0.1)	0 (0)	1.000[φ]
Snoring	781 (16.9)	714 (91.4)	67 (11)	< 0.001[#]
Prevalence of Nocturia	2646 (57.3)	2166 (54.1)	480 (78.4)	< 0.001[#]

*The statistical significance level was 0.05; [φ]Mann–Whitney U test; [#]Chi-square test; [φ]Fisher's Exact test; SD: standard deviation; n = 4616

old) were more likely to have two voids per night as compared to the middle-aged women ($p < 0.05$; Fig. 2).

The variables univariately associated with nocturia are presented in Table 3. Age group, sex, race, employments status and comorbidities such as hypertension, diabetes mellitus, renal disease and overactive bladder were significantly associated with the prevalence of nocturia. In the multivariate analysis, age group between 31 and 40 or > 60 years old, and those who were presented with comorbidities included hypertension, diabetes mellitus, renal disease or overactive bladder were associated with significantly higher prevalence of nocturia, whereas age group of 41–50, male and Chinese or Indian were associated with a decreased prevalence (Table 3). This study also revealed that the prevalence of nocturia was significantly increased with the drink consumption in the late evening, including large volume of water, tea and coffee (Fig. 3; $p < 0.001$) although evening drinking habit was only one of the few factors predisposing to nocturia since the prevalence of nocturia was also significantly high among those without any drink consumption in the late evening ($p < 0.001$).

From the sub analyses, the frequency of nocturnal voids among respondents with nocturia and among different age groups has been depicted in Fig. 4. Those who were more than 60 years old were more likely to experience more than one nocturnal void as compared to their younger counterparts (Fig. 4). The mean age

Table 2 Demographic characteristic of study population with and without nocturia

Variable	Nocturia (n, %)	No nocturia (n, %)	*p* value*
Total respondents	2646 (57.3)	1970 (42.7)	
Mean age (years ± SD)	39.14 ± 14.98	37.33 ± 13.96	< 0.001^φ
18–30	948 (35.8)	846 (43.0)	
31–40	591 (22.4)	298 (15.1)	
41–50	366 (13.8)	394 (20.0)	
51–60	508 (19.2)	357 (18.1)	
> 60	233 (8.8)	74 (3.8)	
Sex			
Male	1103 (41.7)	879 (44.6)	0.046^#
Female	1543 (58.3)	1091 (55.4)	
Race			
Malay	1239 (46.9)	557 (28.2)	< 0.001^#
Chinese	1087 (41.1)	1039 (52.8)	
Indian	253 (9.6)	342 (17.4)	
Others	65 (2.4)	31 (1.6)	
Employment status			
Student	490 (18.5)	430 (21.8)	0.019^#
Employed for wages	1555 (58.8)	1095 (55.6)	
Self-employed	216 (8.2)	178 (9.0)	
Unemployed	385 (14.5)	267 (13.6)	
Comorbidities			
Hypertension	500 (18.90)	138 (7.0)	< 0.001^#
Diabetes mellitus	369 (13.95)	155 (7.9)	< 0.001^#
Renal disease	77 (2.91)	13 (0.7)	< 0.001^#
Heart failure	17 (0.64)	5 (0.3)	0.058^#
Enlarged prostate	41 (1.55)	20 (1.0)	0.116^#
Overactive bladder	93 (3.51)	48 (2.4)	0.035^#
Prostate cancer	6 (0.23)	3 (0.2)	0.741^φ
Bladder cancer	4 (0.15)	2 (0.1)	1.000^φ
Snoring	471 (17.80)	310 (15.7)	0.064^#

*The statistical significance level was 0.05; ^φMann-Whitney U test; ^#Chi-square test; ^φFisher's Exact test; SD: standard deviation; n = 4616

for those with once, twice and three or more times of nocturnal voids was 35.51 ± 14.03, 43.41 ± 14.49 and 46.55 ± 14.97, respectively. The association was significant, which indicated that frequency of nocturnal void is higher in older age groups ($p < 0.001$).

The disease pattern of nocturia encountered by the respondents with nocturia has been summarised in Table 4. Post urination dribble was the only symptom that differed significantly in male respondents with nocturia compared to female ($p < 0.001$). Those with higher age (> 50 years old) were more likely to present with almost all the symptoms ($p < 0.05$).

In terms of impact of nocturia on sleep disturbance, 37.3% of respondents with nocturia reported that they faced sleeping difficulty about half the time or more after waking up in the middle of night, particularly among those with ≥ 2 voids per night (66.5%), aged > 50 (40.6%) and employed for wages (62.3%) (Table 5; $p < 0.001$). As consequences of sleep disturbance due to nocturia, they complaint of fatigue (60.9%), difficulty in concentrating (43.2%), bad mood (41.2%), lack of motivation to work (34.5%), forgetfulness (24.6%), depression (15.6%), lack of sex drive (4.61%) and erectile dysfunction (3.5%; only male respondents). On a scale of 1 to 10 for degree of bother, those who had two voids as well as ≥ 3 voids per night experienced significantly higher mean bother score (3.96 ± 2.41 and 3.91 ± 2.20, respectively) than those who had one void per night (3.29 ± 2.63) ($p < 0.001$).

Our study also found that the awareness on nocturia was poor among study population. Out of 4616 respondents, 56.7% of them were not aware that night time urination is a medical condition. Unfortunately, the majority (62.2%) of respondents with nocturia did not think that it is a medical condition. Only a minority (25.2%) of respondents with nocturia had sought medical attention for their nocturia (Fig. 5). There was a correlation between treatment-seeking behaviour with age, sex, employment status, frequency of nocturia, degree of sleep disturbance, bother score and nocturia disease awareness among respondents with nocturia ($p < 0.05$; Table 6). A total of 60.7% out of 4616 respondents had sought or would consider seeking medical attention for nocturia from urologist. There were 39.6% and 21.3% who opted for general practitioner and gynecologist, respectively. This was followed by 17.7% and 17.2% who had chosen pharmacist and nephrologist, respectively.

Discusssion

This study presented the first nation-wide report on prevalence of nocturia (at least one void at night) in a multiracial population of Malaysia. The overall prevalence of nocturia among Malaysian adults was high (57%), which was comparable with those reported from studies in Asian population, yet relatively higher compared to Western populations. Liew and colleagues reported that the prevalence of nocturia among Singaporean adults was 55% [13]. Meanwhile, the reported prevalence were 46% in the Dutch population [14], 31% in the US population [5] and 28.4% in the Turkish population [15]. In the present study, there was a significant higher prevalence among women. This finding is consistent with the report from previous studies [13, 14, 16, 17]. Nevertheless, information on the exact etiology pertaining to high prevalence of nocturia in women is lacking. Nocturia was found to be more common among younger women

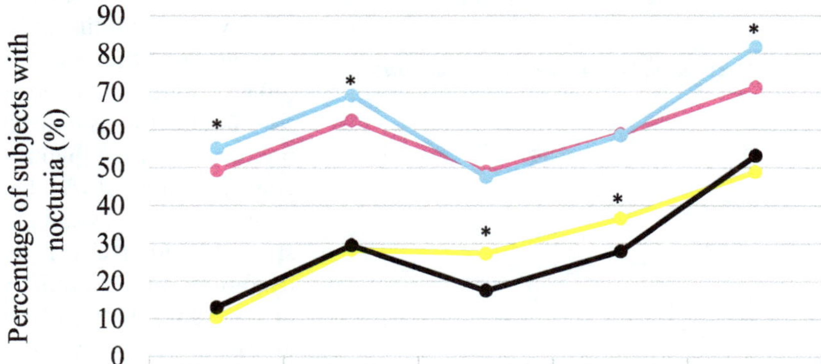

	18 - 30	31 -40	41 - 50	51 - 60	>60
Once or more (Male)	49.3	62.5	49	58.9	71.2
Twice or more (Male)	10.3	28.2	27.3	36.5	48.8
Once or more (Female)	55.2	69.1	47.6	58.5	81.8
Twice or more (Female)	13.1	29.6	17.6	28	53.3

Age group

Once or more (Male) Twice or more (Male)
Once or more (Female) Twice or more (Female)

Fig. 2 The prevalence of nocturia based on sex and frequency of nocturia. n = 4616. *According to the Chi-Square test, younger (18–40 years old) and older women (> 60 years old) were more commonly to have one void per night than men from the same age group ($p < 0.05$). Whereas middle-aged men (41–60 years old) were more likely to have two voids per night as compared to the middle-aged women ($p < 0.05$)

(18–40 years old). This is congruent with the finding from study in Finland [17].

In addition, the prevalence of nocturia was found to increase with age, which corroborated the findings of other studies [4, 5, 18]. This may be due to various pathophysiological mechanisms that related to ageing. In the elderly, nocturia can be resulted from decline in functional bladder capacity with high post void residual, deregulation of arginine vasopressin level, sleep disorders and comorbidities including diabetes mellitus and diabetes insipidus [19]. This also further explains the finding in current study that the frequency of nocturnal voids was higher among the elderly population than younger population. On the other hand, there was higher nocturia prevalence among those 31–40 years old than those between 41 and 50 years old. The underlying etiology for this finding is unknown, but it may be due to the alcoholic beverage consumption among this age group. Based on the previous National Health and Morbidity Survey 2011 in Malaysia, those 30–39 years old presented with highest prevalence of alcohol consumption than other age groups and the drinking pattern waned by older population [20]. Nevertheless, further investigation is required to reveal the exact etiology of this finding.

Previous studies have reported the differences in prevalence of nocturia among races in the US population. The prevalence of nocturia was reported to be higher among Black and Hispanic respondents compared to the White respondents [21, 22]. Consistently, similar observation was reported among the multi-ethnic groups in Malaysia. Malay respondents had a significant higher prevalence compared to other races as revealed by the univariate analysis, yet this prevalence was not significant in multivariate analysis. Chinese and Indian respondents on the other hand, had significantly lower prevalence compared to Malay in both univariate and multivariate analyses. However, Liew and colleagues reported that there was no significant difference between Malay, Chinese and Indian respondents in Singapore [13]. Kupelian and colleagues reported that socioeconomic status was accounted for the ethnic discrepancies in prevalence of nocturia [22]. Further investigation is required in order to identify the underlying etiology of ethnic discrepancies among Malaysians in term of prevalence of nocturia.

Nocturia is strongly associated with various risk factors and comorbidities, including cardiovascular diseases, diabetes, sleep disorders, somatic and mental health [6, 13, 18, 23, 24]. This supports the findings of this study which also showed the significant higher disease prevalence among respondents with comorbidities such as hypertension, diabetes mellitus, renal disease or overactive bladder. The pathophysiological changes

Table 3 Univariable and multivariable analysis for respondents' characteristic in relation to prevalence of nocturia

	Univariate Analysis*		Multivariate Analysis*,#	
	OR (95% CI)	*p* value	OR (95% CI)	*p* value
Age group				
18–30	0.741 (0.658–0.835)	< 0.001	1.161 (0.931–1.449)	0.185
31–40	1.513 (1.383–1.880)	< 0.001	1.909 (1.521–2.396)	< 0.001
41–50	0.642 (0.549–0.750)	< 0.001	0.733 (0.592–0.908)	0.005
51–60	1.073 (0.923–1.803)	0.358	Not included	–
> 60	2.473 (1.891–3.234)	< 0.001	2.027 (1.478–2.708)	< 0.001
Sex				
Male	0.887 (0.789–0.998)	0.046	0.779 (0.687–0.884)	< 0.001
Female	1.127 (1.002–1.268)	0.046	–	–
Race				
Malay	2.235 (1.974–2.531)	< 0.001	0.891 (0.569–1.396)	0.615
Chinese	0.625 (0.556–0.703)	< 0.001	0.471 (0.302–0.735)	0.001
Indian	0.503 (0.423–0.599)	< 0.001	0.336 (0.210–0.537)	< 0.001
Others	1.576 (1.023–2.427)	0.039	–	
Employment status				
Student	0.814 (0.704–0.941)	0.005	1.154 (0.911–1.463)	0.235
Employed for wages	1.139 (1.012–1.281)	0.031	1.141 (0.963–1.352)	0.129
Self-employed	0.895 (0.727–1.101)	0.294	Not included	–
Unemployed	1.086 (0.918–1.285)	0.336	Not included	–
Comorbidities				
Hypertension	3.093 (2.536–3.772)	< 0.001	2.837 (2.281–3.530)	< 0.001
Diabetes mellitus	1.898 (1.558–2.312)	< 0.001	1.783 (1.416–2.245)	< 0.001
Renal disease	4.512 (2.500–8.145)	< 0.001	3.579 (1.933–6.625)	< 0.001
Heart failure	2.541 (0.936–6.900)	0.067	Not included	–
Enlarged prostate	1.535 (0.896–2.627)	0.119	Not included	–
Overactive bladder	1.459 (1.024–2.077)	0.036	1.606 (1.097–2.352)	0.015
Prostate cancer	1.490 (0.372–5.966)	0.573	Not included	–
Bladder cancer	1.490 (0.273–8.142)	0.645	Not included	–
Snoring	1.160 (0.991–1.357)	0.064	Not included	–

*Based on logistic regression analysis, the statistical significance level was 0.05; #Variables with an association of $p < 0.05$ were selected for a multivariable analysis; OR: Odd ratio; CI Confidence interval; n = 4616

in hypertensive patients appear to be a significant risk factor for nocturia [25, 26]. A prolonged hyperglycemic state in diabetes mellitus patients on the other hand, may cause an alteration in urinary bladder activity, predisposing to diabetic cystopathy [27]. Diabetic cystopathy is primarily induced by paralysis of detrusor muscle and hyperglycemia-induced polyuria that can further lead to bladder hypertrophy in patients with diabetes mellitus [27]. Moreover, microvascular complications of diabetes, particularly diabetic nephropathy and neuropathy have been implicated in nocturia [28]. Diabetic nephropathy is associated with polyuria and an increase in mean void volume, whereas, diabetic neuropathy may lead to impaired bladder sensation, poor detrusor contractility and increased post void residual [28]. This explains the mechanistic link between diabetes mellitus and nocturia.

Several studies have reported that nocturia is associated with chronic kidney disease [13, 29, 30]. This may be attributed to the failure of kidneys to concentrate the urine as the renal function worsens, and ultimately leads to nocturnal polyuria and increased nocturnal urine volume in patients with chronic kidney disease [31]. Additionally, overactive bladder was also found to be one of the risk factors in this study. Indeed, nocturia is a common urinary symptom in overactive bladder patients [32]. However, in this study, there was no significant association between nocturia and benign prostatic hyperplasia, prostate cancer, bladder cancer and snoring, which had been reported in previous studies [22, 23, 33]. This could

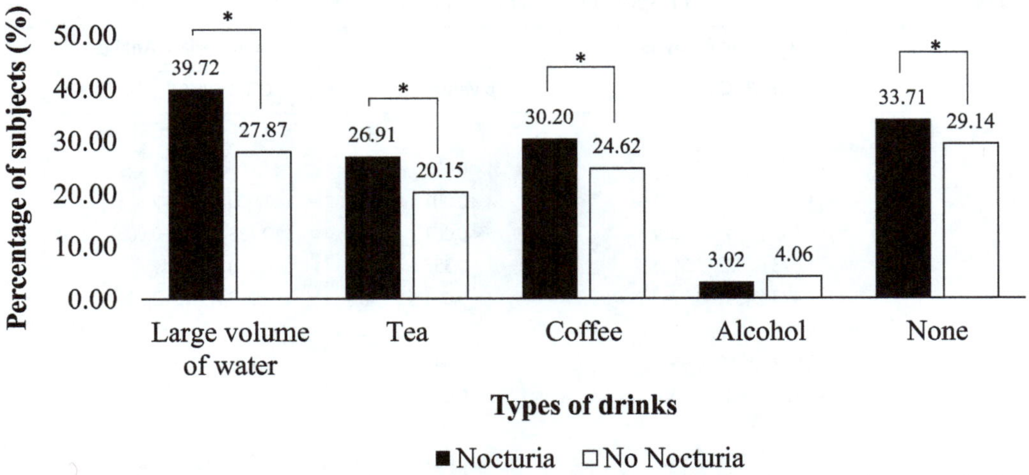

Fig. 3 Relationship between prevalence of nocturia and drinks consumption in the late evening. n = 4616. *According to the Chi-Square test, the prevalence of nocturia was significantly associated with the drink consumption in the late evening, including large volume of water, tea and coffee ($p < 0.001$). The prevalence of nocturia was significant among those without any drink consumption in the late evening ($p < 0.001$)

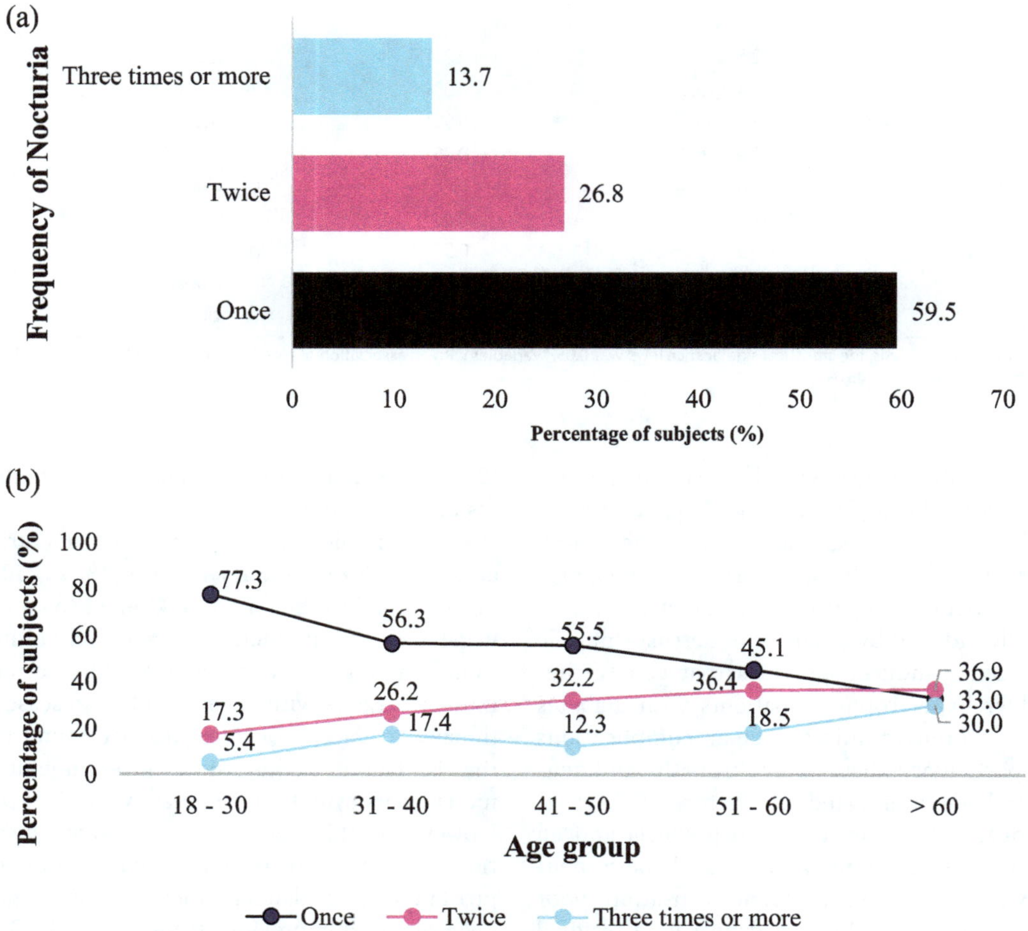

Fig. 4 Frequency of nocturia **a** among respondents with nocturia, **b** in different age groups. n = 2646

Table 4 Disease pattern of nocturia among study population based on sex and age

Symptom	Sex (n, %)		Age group (n, %)	
	Male	Female	18–50	>50
Total respondents	1103 (41.7)	1543 (58.3)	1905 (72.0)	741 (28.0)
Post urination dribble	172 (15.6)	139 (9.0)	237 (12.4)	74 (10.0)
	$p<0.001$*		$p=0.078$*	
Frequent urination during the day	276 (25.0)	274 (17.8)	438 (23.0)	212 (28.6)
	$p=0.644$*		$p=0.003$*	
Frequent urinary urgency	129 (11.7)	168 (10.9)	155 (8.1)	142 (19.2)
	$p=0.516$*		$p<0.001$*	
Urinary Incontinence	90 (8.2)	124 (8.0)	73 (3.8)	141 (19.0)
	$p=0.909$*		$p<0.001$*	
Slow urine flow	63 (5.7)	78 (5.1)	69 (3.6)	72 (9.7)
	$p=0.458$*		$p<0.001$*	
Feeling of incomplete bladder emptying after urination	143 (13.0)	165 (10.7)	166 (8.7)	142 (19.8)
	$p=0.072$*		$p<0.001$*	

*Based on Chi-square test, the statistical significance level was 0.05; n=2646

Table 5 The impact of nocturia on sleep disturbance and factors affecting the sleep disturbance

Variable	Degree of sleep disturbance (n, %)		*p* value*
	Less than half the time	About half the time or more	
Total respondents	1655 (62.7)	983 (37.3)	
Frequency of nocturia			
Once	1241 (75.0)	329 (33.5)	<0.001
Twice	273 (16.5)	433 (44.0)	
Three times or more	141 (8.5)	221 (22.5)	
Age			
18–30	730 (44.1)	215 (21.9)	<0.001
31–40	375 (22.6)	215 (21.9)	
41–50	210 (12.7)	154 (15.6)	
51–60	233 (14.1)	273 (27.8)	
>60	107 (6.5)	126 (12.8)	
Sex			
Male	681 (41.1)	417 (42.4)	0.521
Female	974 (58.9)	566 (57.6)	
Employment status			
Student	391 (23.6)	98 (10.0)	<0.001
Employed for wages	938 (56.7)	613 (62.3)	
Self-employed	116 (7.0)	98 (10.0)	
Unemployed	210 (12.7)	174 (17.7)	

*Based on Chi-square test, the statistical significance level was 0.05; n=2638

be due to the comorbidities determined by self-reporting of respondents in the present study, which might have led to underestimation of the prevalence of these comorbidities in Malaysia.

Excessive evening intake of fluid, caffeinated drinks or alcohol is known to be one of the causes of nocturnal polyuria [1]. In the current study, approximately one third of the respondents with nocturia have the habit of consuming large volume of water, tea or coffee in the late evening. This may suggest that limiting fluid or caffeinated drink intake in the late evening among Malaysian could be one of the modifiable lifestyle risk factors for nocturia. Shiri and colleagues reported that there was no significant association between coffee consumption and nocturia among 50 to 70 years old men in Finland, yet the risk of moderate or severe nocturia was twofold higher among men who drank 6 cups coffee or more per day than non-drinkers or those who consumed one cup per day for this age group [34]. Interestingly, the prevalence of nocturia was about one third of respondent despite any drink consumption. The actual prevalence of nocturia with underlying pathological causes in the population may be reflected by eliminating the potential confounding factor of drink consumption in the late evening.

LUTS can be classified according to voiding or obstructive symptoms (such as hesitancy, poor stream, straining, prolonged micturition, feeling of incomplete bladder emptying, post-micturition dribble) and storage or irritative symptoms (such as frequency, urgency, urge incontinence and nocturia). In the present study, the disease pattern of nocturia was not sex-specific, except for post-micturition dribble. This interpretation is supported by the fact that post-micturition dribble is more common in men [35]. Studies also showed that prevalence of LUTS was comparable between men and women [36, 37]. In addition, with advancing age, the prevalence and severity of LUTS increase regardless of sex [36]. This is supported

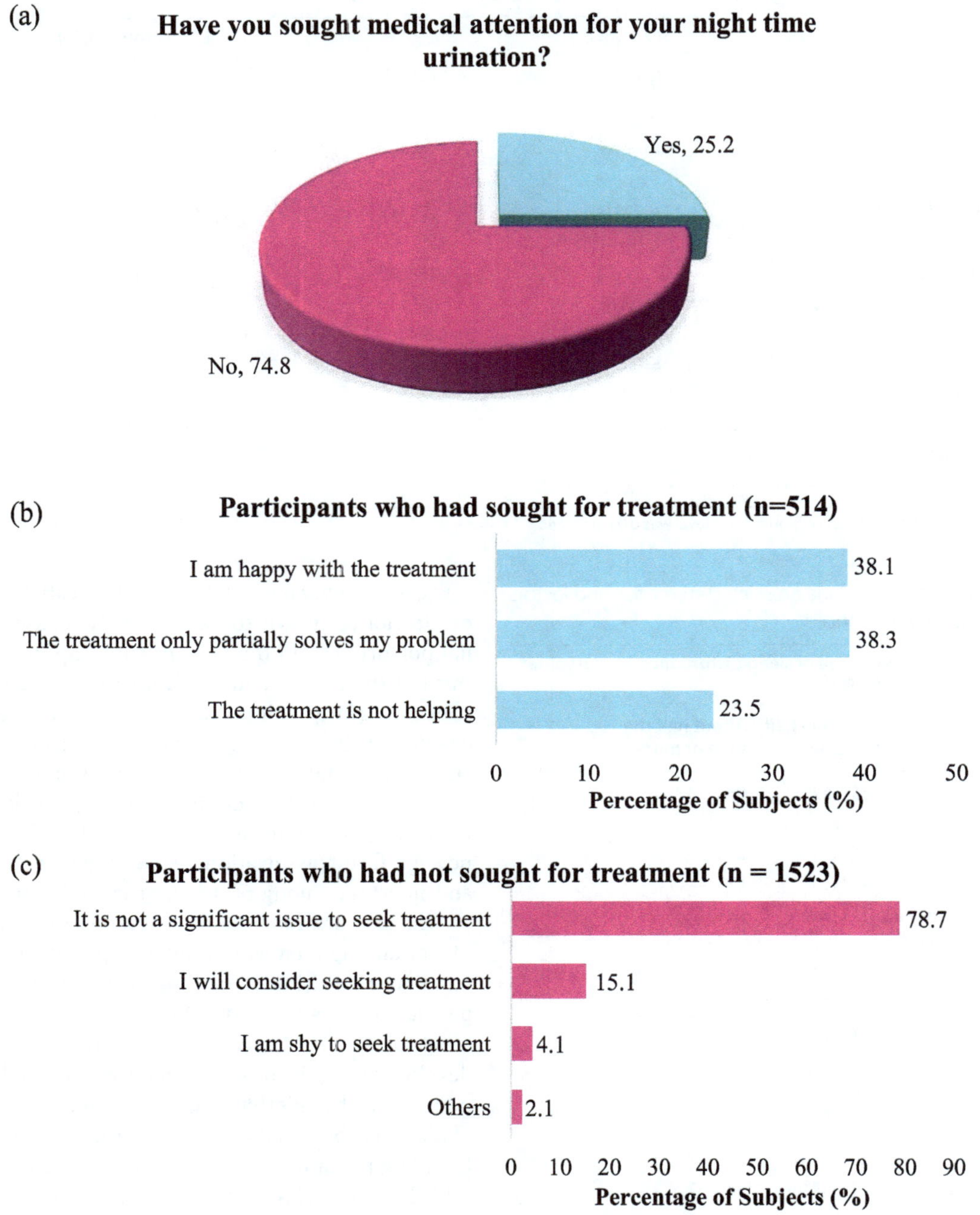

Fig. 5 Treatment seeking behaviour among participants with nocturia. n = 2037. **a** The overall treatment seeking behaviour among participants with nocturia. **b** The responses from those participants who had sought for treatment. **c** The responses from participants who had not sought for treatments

by the finding of this study where elderly respondents are more likely to exhibit almost all the LUTS compared to the younger population.

Nocturia has been regarded as not only 'bothersome', but also negatively affects sleep and quality of life [5–8]. This study also revealed that nocturia was regarded as moderately bothersome for Malaysians, particularly those with two or more nocturnal voids. This alluded to the clinical relevance of at least 2 voids being the threshold to patient-reported impaired health-related quality of life [38]. Furthermore, more than one-third of respondents in this study claimed to have disturbed sleep about half the time or more after nocturnal awakening. The sleep disturbance was proportionately increased with

Table 6 Characteristics comparison between respondents who had and did not seek treatment

Variable	Treatment seeking behaviour (%)		p value*
	Yes (n = 514)	No (n = 1523)	
Age (years ± SD)	44.43 ± 16.34	38.59 ± 14.67	< 0.001$^{\varphi}$
Sex			
Male	49.4	42.9	0.011$^{\#}$
Female	50.6	57.1	
Employment status			
Student	14.6	19.7	< 0.001$^{\#}$
Employed for wages	51.6	61.5	
Self-employed	10.7	7.3	
Unemployed	23.2	11.4	
Frequency of nocturia			
Once	47.3	62.1	< 0.001$^{\#}$
Twice	34.2	27.5	
Three times or more	18.5	10.4	
Degree of sleep disturbance			
Less than half the time	49.0	62.1	< 0.001$^{\#}$
About half the time or more	51.0	37.9	
Bother score (mean ± SD)	4.51 ± 2.55	3.19 ± 2.4	< 0.001$^{\varphi}$
Awareness of nocturia as a medical condition			
Yes	54.3	35.4	< 0.001$^{\#}$
No	45.7	64.6	

*The statistical significance level was 0.05; $^{\varphi}$Mann-Whitney U test; $^{\#}$Chi-square test; SD: standard deviation; n = 2037

the frequency of nocturnal voids and age. This finding is consistent with previous studies [5, 13, 14, 39]. As a result of sleep disturbance, nocturia has also been associated with excessive daytime sleepiness (7–18%), increased sick leaves (27–27%), insomnia (43%), psychiatric disorders (28–35%) and poorer health status (15–40%) [40, 41] In addition, people with nocturia have a lower productivity at work and decreased activity levels [6]. Consistently, the respondents with nocturia in this study also reported to experience fatigue, difficulty in concentrating, lacking of motivation to work, bad mood, forgetfulness and depression as consequences of disturbed sleep. Hence, it is obvious that nocturia should not be overlooked or underestimated due to its serious repercussions on sleep quality, work productivity and quality of life.

Treatment-seeking behaviour for LUTS is correlated with the symptom severity, degree of bother, costs and benefits of treatment [42, 43]. Consistently, this study found that those who had not sought treatment were presented with less than two nocturnal voids, less degree of sleep disturbance and lower bother score as compared to those who had sought treatment. To the best of our knowledge, this is the first study to report on the association between awareness of nocturia and treatment-seeking behaviour in Malaysia. Approximately two-thirds of respondents with nocturia in this study were not aware that nocturia is a medical condition and this was significantly associated with behaviour of not seeking medical attention. This finding suggests that poor awareness might be a factor affecting their treatment-seeking behaviour. In Taiwan, Chen and colleagues found that the lack of knowledge on nocturia appeared to be an important barrier to medical consultation among Taiwanese women [9]. In addition, a vast majority of those who had not sought treatment in the present study perceived that nocturia was not a significant medical issue to seek treatment. This appears consistent with finding by Low and colleagues who reported that majority of women in Northern Malaysia did not seek treatment for LUTS due to low level of disease awareness [11]. These findings could be attributed to poor knowledge pertaining to nocturia among Malaysians. As such, addressing the misconceptions about nocturia can help to increase the awareness, enhance treatment-seeking behaviour and also improve the overall quality of life among people with nocturia. Interestingly, this study revealed that most women did not seek treatment for nocturia as compared to men. This is in contrast with the finding from a study conducted in the primary care setting in Malaysia, which revealed the higher tendency for women to seek treatment when compared to men [44]. Further investigation is required to identify the sex difference in treatment-seeking behaviour among nocturia patients.

In the present study, convenience sampling was conducted instead of stratified sampling to define the population in Malaysia. Despite this limitation, the pool of subjects sampled were closely reflecting the real population in Malaysia. Although there was slightly difference between the sample and population in terms of age and sex, these differences were adjusted in the statistical analysis. Hence, the outcomes of this study are valuable to provide sights into prevalence of nocturia among Malaysians.

Conclusions

The prevalence of nocturia among Malaysian adults is high and strongly influenced by age, sex, race and comorbidities. There is a significant correlation between frequency of nocturnal voids with sleep disturbance and degree of bother. However, the awareness among Malaysians pertaining to nocturia being a health issue was generally poor. This affects treatment-seeking behaviour as many are not aware that it is a symptom that requires medical attention. Contrary to common belief that it is a natural physiological symptom associated with ageing, nocturia as a condition deserves public attention, given its profound impact on quality of life that may be associated with increased morbidity and mortality. The findings from this study may serve as impetus to better address this issue via educational intervention.

Abbreviations

ICS: International Continence Society; LUTS: Lower urinary tract symptoms; SD: Standard deviation; OR: Odd ratio; CI: Confidence interval.

Acknowledgements

The authors thank Prof. Dr. Charles Anthony Rhodes, School of Medicine, Taylor's University, Malaysia for his support in checking the English version of the questionnaire.

Authors' contributions

We declare that this work was done by the authors named in this article and all liabilities pertaining to claims relating to the content of this article will be borne by them. YHY, JTJL, MCW, OTA, ZMZ, TCC, NKS, GEH and ANF developed the idea to conduct this research. YHY, EWF, JTJL and MCW designed and planned the research and pilot study, as well as performed the literature search. YHY, JTJL, MCW and LSH conducted the data collection, YHY and MCW performed the data and statistical analyses. The manuscript was written and edited by YHY, and reviewed by all authors. All authors read and approved the final manuscript.

Competing interests

All authors declare that they have no competing interests. Ferring Pharmaceutical Malaysia provided financial support in respect of publication costs but had no influence on the content of the work.

Author details

[1]School of Pharmacy, Faculty of Health and Medical Sciences, Taylor's University (Lakeside Campus), Subang Jaya, Malaysia. [2]Ferring Pharmaceuticals Malaysia & Singapore, Kuala Lumpur, Malaysia. [3]School of Pharmacy, International Medical University, Kuala Lumpur, Malaysia. [4]Louis Bolk Institute, Bunnik, The Netherlands. [5]Urology Unit, Department of Surgery, Universiti Kebangsaan Malaysia, Kuala Lumpur, Malaysia. [6]Department of Urology, Hospital Selayang, Selangor, Malaysia. [7]Department of Surgery, Hospital Angkatan Tentera Tuanku Mizan, Kuala Lumpur, Malaysia. [8]Urology, Nephrology & Men's Health Clinic, Prince Court Medical Centre, Kuala Lumpur, Malaysia. [9]Department of Surgery, Faculty of Medicine, University of Malaya, 50603 Kuala Lumpur, Malaysia.

References

1. van Kerrebroeck P, Abrams P, Chaikin D, Donovan J, Fonda D, Jackson S, et al. The standardisation of terminology in nocturia: Report from the Standardisation Sub-committee of the International Continence Society. BJU Int. 2002;90:11–5.
2. International Continence Society. Terminology discussion: Nocturia. 2018. https://www.ics.org/committees/standardisation/terminologydiscussions/nocturia. Accessed 17 Mac 2020.
3. Bosch JL, Weiss JP. The prevalence and causes of nocturia. J Urol. 2010;184:440–6.
4. van Doorn B, Blanker MH, Kok ET, Westers P, Bosch JL. Once nocturia, always nocturia? Natural history of nocturia in older men based on frequency-volume charts: the Krimpen study. J Urol. 2011;186:1956–61.
5. Coyne KS, Zhou Z, Bhattacharyya SK, Thompson CL, Dhawan R, Versi E. The prevalence of nocturia and its effect on health-related quality of life and sleep in a community sample in the USA. BJU Int. 2003;92:948–54.
6. Asplund R, Marnetoft SU, Selander J, Akerström B. Nocturia in relation to somatic health, mental health and pain in adult men and women. BJU Int. 2005;95:816–9.
7. Weiss JP, Blaivas JG, Blanker MH, Bliwise DL, Dmochowski RR, Drake M, et al. The New England Research Institutes, Inc. (NERI) Nocturia Advisory Conference 2012: focus on outcomes of therapy. BJU Int. 2013;111:700–16.
8. Kupelian V, Fitzgerald MP, Kaplan SA, Norgaard JP, Chiu GR, Rosen RC. Association of nocturia and mortality: results from the Third National Health and Nutrition Examination Survey. J Urol. 2011;185:571–7.
9. Chen FY, Dai YT, Liu CK, Yu HJ, Liu CY, Chen TH. Perception of nocturia and medical consulting behavior among community-dwelling women. Int Urogynecol J Pelvic Floor Dysfunct. 2007;18:431–6.
10. Mariappan P, Turner KJ, Sothilingam S, Rajan P, Sundram M, Stewart LH. Nocturia, nocturia indices and variables from frequency-volume charts are significantly different in Asian and Caucasian men with lower urinary tract symptoms: a prospective comparison study. BJU Int. 2007;100:332–6.
11. Low BY, Liong ML, Yuen KH, Chong WL, Chee C, Leong WS, et al. Study of prevalence, treatment-seeking behavior, and risk factors of women with lower urinary tract symptoms in Northern Malaysia. Urology. 2006;68:751–8.
12. Wild D, Eremenco S, Mear I, Martin M, Houchin C, Gawlicki M, et al. Multinational trials—recommendations on the translations required, approaches to using the same language in different countries, and the approaches to support pooling the data: the ISPOR Patient Reported Outcomes Translation & Linguistic Validation Good Research Practices Task Force Report. Value Health. 2009;12:430–40.
13. Liew LC, Tiong HY, Wong ML, Png DC, Tan JK. A population study of nocturia in Singapore. BJU Int. 2006;97:109–12.
14. van Dijk L, Kooij DG, Schellevis FG. Nocturia in the Dutch adult population. BJU Int. 2002;90:644–8.
15. Zumrutbas AE, Bozkurt AI, Alkis O, Toktas C, Cetinel B, Aybek Z. The prevalence of nocturia and nocturnal polyuria: can new cutoff values be suggested according to age and sex? Int Neurourol J. 2016;20:304–10.
16. Choo MS, Ku JH, Park CH, Lee YS, Lee KS, Lee JG, et al. Prevalence of nocturia in a Korean population aged 40 to 89 years. Neurourol Urodyn. 2008;27:60–4.
17. Tikkinen KA, Tammela TL, Huhtala H, Auvinen A. Is nocturia equally common among men and women? A population based study in Finland. J Urol. 2006;175:596–600.
18. Kim SY, Bang W, Kim MS, Park B, Kim JH, Choi HG. Analysis of the prevalence and factors associated with nocturia in adult Korean men. Sci Rep. 2017;7:41714.
19. van Doorn B, Bosch JL. Nocturia in older men. Maturitas. 2012;71:8–12.
20. Mutalip MH, Kamarudin RB, Manickam M, Abd Hamid HA, Saari RB. Alcohol consumption and risky drinking patterns in Malaysia: findings from NHMS 2011. Alcohol Alcohol. 2014;49:593–9.
21. Fitzgerald MP, Litman HJ, Link CL, McKinlay JB. The association of nocturia with cardiac disease, diabetes, body mass index, age and diuretic use: results from the BACH survey. J Urol. 2007;177:1385–9.
22. Kupelian V, Link CL, Hall SA, McKinlay JB. Are racial/ethnic disparities in the prevalence of nocturia due to socioeconomic status? Results of the BACH survey. J Urol. 2009;181:1756–63.
23. Madhu C, Coyne K, Hashim H, Chapple C, Milsom I, Kopp Z. Nocturia: risk factors and associated comorbidities; findings from the EpiLUTS study. Int J Clin Pract. 2015;69:1508–16.
24. Yoshimura K, Terada N, Matsui Y, Terai A, Kinukawa N, Arai Y. Prevalence of and risk factors for nocturia: analysis of a health screening program. Int J Urol. 2004;11:282–7.
25. Feldstein CA. Nocturia in arterial hypertension: a prevalent, underreported, and sometimes underestimated association. J Am Soc Hypertens. 2013;7:75–84.
26. McKeigue PM, Reynard JM. Relation of nocturnal polyuria of the elderly to essential hypertension. Lancet. 2000;355:486–8.
27. Barua SK, Borah SJ, Rajeev TP. Current understanding of diabetes mellitus-induced lower urinary tract dysfunction. J Health Res Rev. 2019;6:50–6.
28. Hill SR, Fayyad AM, Jones GR. Diabetes mellitus and female lower urinary tract symptoms: a review. Neurourol Urodyn. 2008;27:362–7.
29. Fujimura T, Yamada Y, Sugihara T, Azuma T, Suzuki M, Nakagawa T, et al. Nocturia in men is a chaotic condition dominated by nocturnal polyuria. Int J Urol. 2015;22:496–501.
30. Wu MY, Wu YL, Hsu YH, Lin YF, Fan YC, Lin YC, et al. Risk of nocturia in patients with chronic kidney disease—do the metabolic syndrome and its components matter? J Urol. 2012;188:269–73.
31. Fukuda M, Motokawa M, Miyagi S, Sengo K, Muramatsu W, Kato N, et al. Polynocturia in chronic kidney disease is related to natriuresis rather than to water diuresis. Nephrol Dial Transplant. 2006;21:2172–7.
32. Espuña-Pons M, Blasco P, Pérez M, Rebollo P. Nocturia in patients with overactive bladder. Arch Esp Urol. 2010;63:363–72.

33. Tikkinen KA, Auvinen A, Johnson TM 2nd, Weiss JP, Keranen T, Tiitinen A, et al. A systematic evaluation of factors associated with nocturia—the population-based FINNO study. Am J Epidemiol. 2009;170:361–8.
34. Shiri R, Hakama M, Häkkinen J, Auvinen A, Huhtala H, Tammela TLJ, et al. The effects of lifestyle factors on the incidence of nocturia. J Urol. 2008;180:2059–62.
35. Yang DY, Lee WK. A current perspective on post-micturition dribble in males. Investig Clin Urol. 2019;60:142–7.
36. Boyle P, Robertson C, Mazzetta C, Keech M, Hobbs FDR, Fourcade R, et al. The prevalence of lower urinary tract symptoms in men and women in four centres. The UrEpik study. BJU Int. 2003;92:409–14.
37. Diokno AC, Brock BM, Brown MB, Herzog AR. Prevalence of urinary incontinence and other urological symptoms in the noninstitutionalized elderly. J Urol. 1986;136:1022–5.
38. Tikkinen KA, Johnson TM 2nd, Tammela TL, Sintonen H, Haukka J, Huhtala H, et al. Nocturia frequency, bother, and quality of life: how often is too often? A population-based study in Finland. Eur Urol. 2010;57:488–96.
39. Kim SC, Choi HS, Kim YJ, Kim HS, Hwang IS, Hwang EC, et al. Impact of nocturia on health-related quality of life and medical outcomes study sleep score in men. Int Neurourol J. 2011;15:82–6.
40. Ohayon MM. Nocturnal awakenings and comorbid disorders in the American general population. J Psychiatr Res. 2008;43:48–54.
41. Asplund R, Aberg H. Health of the elderly with regard to sleep and nocturnal micturition. Scan J Prim Health Care. 1992;10:98–104.
42. Welliver C, Sulaver R, Whittington A, Helfand BT, Çakır OO, Griffith JW, et al. Analyzing why men seek treatment for lower urinary tract symptoms and factors associated with nonimprovement. Urology. 2015;86:862–7.
43. Griffith JW, Messersmith EE, Gillespie BW, Wiseman JB, Flynn KE, Kirkali Z, et al. Reasons for seeking clinical care for lower urinary tract symptoms: a mixed methods study. J Urol. 2018;199:528–35.
44. Lim MT, Lim YMF, Tong SF, Sivasampu S. Age, sex and primary care setting differences in patients' perception of community healthcare seeking behaviour towards health services. PLoS ONE. 2019;14(10):e0224260.

14

Expression patterns of the immune checkpoint ligand CD276 in urothelial carcinoma

Wilhelm K. Aicher[1,3*], M. Korn[1], L. Reitnauer[1], F. B. Maurer[1], J. Hennenlotter[1], P. C. Black[2], T. Todenhofer[1], J. Bedke[1] and A. Stenzl[1]

Abstract

Background: CD276 is an immune checkpoint molecule. Elevated CD276 expression by urothelial carcinoma is associated with poor prognosis, but little is known about its expression across different tumor stages. We therefore investigated CD276 expression in bladder cancer (BC) cells and in tissue samples of BC stages from pT2 to pT4.

Methods: CD276 expression was explored in 4 urothelial cancer cell lines and 4 primary normal urothelial cell populations by quantitative RT-PCR, Western blot and flow cytometry. CD276 was investigated in bladder tumors from 98 patients by immunohistochemistry using a score (0–300) incorporating both, staining intensity and area of CD276 staining. Normal appearing urothelium in the bladder of the same patients served as controls.

Results: The urothelial carcinoma cell lines expressed significantly higher levels of CD276 on transcript ($p < 0.006$), total protein levels ($p < 0.005$), and on the cell surface ($p < 0.02$) when compared to normal urothelial cells. In pT2–T4 tumor tissue samples, CD276 was overexpressed (median score 185) when compared to corresponding healthy tissues from the same patients (median score 50; $p < 0.001$). No significant differences in CD276 expression were recorded in late, locally advanced ≥ pT3a tumors (median score 185) versus organ-confined < pT3a tumors (median score 190), but it was significantly lower in the normal urothelial tissue associated with ≥ pT3a tumors (median score 40) versus < pT3a tumors (median score 80; $p < 0.05$).

Conclusion: CD276 expression is significantly elevated in urothelial carcinoma cells in all stages but varies between individuals considerably. Reduced CD276 expression in normal urothelial cells may imply that these cells would be protected from CD276-mediated immuno therapies.

Keywords: Urothelial carcinoma, Immune check-point protein, CD276, B7-H3, Bladder tumor stages

Background

Bladder cancer ranks among the most common malignancies. Despite efforts in cancer research, the 5-year survival rates between 1996–2004 (80%) compared to 2008–2014 (77%) have not improved [1]. Therefore, additional tools for diagnosis and more effective therapies are urgently needed.

Recently active components to modulate immune responses have emerged as promising cancer therapies in bladder carcinoma [2]. These therapies mainly target the programmed death receptor 1 (PD-1) and its respective ligand PD-L1. PD1/PD-L1 immune checkpoint inhibitors have been approved in clinical settings for treatment of patients who are either cisplatin-refractory or cisplatin-ineligible based on the results of large phase II–III trials

*Correspondence: aicher@uni-tuebingen.de
[3] Department of Urology, Center for Medical Research, University of Tuebingen Hospital, Waldhoernlestrasse 22, 72072 Tübingen, Germany
Full list of author information is available at the end of the article

[3–5]. Other immune checkpoint receptors have been described and represent additional promising targets for therapy.

One such attractive therapeutic target is CD276 (alias B7-H3) which is over-expressed in many tumors [6–8] and often correlates with poor prognosis [9–11]. CD276 is a member of the B7/CD28 family of antigen independent co-stimulatory ligands. In mice, CD276 binds to the triggering receptor expressed on myeloid cells like transcript 2 (TLT-2) protein to modulate T-cell responses [12]. Elevated expression of CD276 enhances the TLT-2-mediated $CD8^+$ cytotoxic T-lymphocyte response to tumor in mice [13]. In another study, CD276 prevented activation of anti-tumor responses by blocking $CD4^+Th_1$-activation [14]. There is experimental evidence promising success of anti-CD276 tumor therapies [6, 14–16], and several clinical studies are underway or already completed (see https://clinicaltrials.gov).

Targeting CD276 directly on tumor cells is a promising strategy [6]. Such targeting would require knowledge about the amount of receptor on the cells and its distribution in the tissue. It has been estimated that 2000 CD276 ligands would be required per tumor cell for such a targeted therapy to be effective [6]. In this context, the objective of this study was to study the expression levels of CD276 on well-characterized human urothelial cancer cell lines and in tissue samples from bladder tumors as a function of the tumor staging.

Methods

Preparation and expansion of cells

Urothelial cancer cell lines (UCCLs) HT1197 (CRL-1473), TCCsup (HTB-5), RT4 (HTB-2), and 5637 (HTB-9) were purchased from ATCC (www.atcc.org). They were expanded in MEM medium enriched with bovine serum, non-essential amino acids, sodium pyruvate and antibiotics as recommended by the supplier. Normal urothelial cells (NUCs) were prepared from cancer-free ureteral tissue samples from 4 donors after informed and written consent, and expanded as previously described [17]. The integrity of each NUC culture was confirmed by immunohistochemistry with the pancytokeratin marker cytokeratin AE1/AE3 (not shown). Contamination of cultures by mycoplasma were excluded by PCR analysis following established protocols (Biontex). The study was approved by the Ethics Committee under file number 341/2002/BO.

Analysis of CD276 transcript and protein expression

Cells were expanded to reach confluence, washed with cold PBS, detached by mild proteolysis, lysed to isolate RNA (Qiagen RNeasy kit), and cDNA was synthesized by reverse transcription and oligo(dT) priming (Takara Bio). Quantitative RT-PCR was performed employing CD276 target gene primers. GAPDH and PPIAγ amplifications served as internal controls (Table 1) [18]. Proteins were detected in cell lysates after SDS-PAGE by immunoblotting (IB) [19] using monoclonal antibodies (mAb) or sera, followed by peroxidase-labelled secondary antibodies (Table 2), and quantified by a blot scanner (C-Digit, Licor). The CD276 signal intensities in each sample were normalized to β-actin signals of each sample.

Analysis of CD276 expression on cell surfaces

To quantify CD276 expression on UCCLs and NUCs, cells were grown to confluence, detached by mild proteolysis and washed twice by PBS. 5E05 cells were resuspended in PFEA buffer, incubated with anti-CD276 mAB and measured by flow cytometry (FC) as described (LSR II, Becton Dickinson) [20]. Staining of cells with a mAB to KLH served as isotype control (Table 2). Signal intensities were normalized to COMP-beads (Becton Dickinson) and the KLH isotype controls in each experiment.

Detection of CD276 in paraffin sections of tissue microarrays

Tissue microarrays (TMA) were assembled from 0.6 mm bladder tissue punches after radical cystectomy of 98 BC patients after informed and written consent as described [21]. 98 tissue punches were obtained from pathologically confirmed tumor areas. In addition, from the same bladders, 47 tissue punches were prepared from tumor adjacent but healthy appearing areas, which were pathologically confirmed as normal tissue. For immunohistochemistry (IHC), TMA sections were incubated with anti-CD276 mAb (1 h, 20 °C; Table 2), washed three times with 0.1% Tween 120 in PBS and counterstained by OptiView DAB IHC detection kit as described by the supplier (Ventana, Roche, Switzerland). To confirm histology, samples were stained after IHC by hematoxylin and eosin (HE). Antibody staining intensities (no = 0, weak = 1, middle = 2, strong = 3) and the percent area of staining per TMA (0–100%) were recorded by microscopy to generate scores ranging from "0" (no antibody

Table 1 Primers for quantitative RT-PCR

Gene	Primer	Sequence (5′ → 3′)
CD276	Forward	TTTCCTTTCCCCTCC
	Reverse	TGTGACCAGCACATG
GAPDH	Forward	GAGTCAACGGATTTGGTCGT
	Reverse	TTGATTTTGGAGGGATCTCG
PPIAγ	Forward	TTCATCTGCACTGCCAAGAC
	Reverse	TCGAGTTGTCCACAGTCAGC

Table 2 Antibodies to human antigens and detection reagents for immunoblotting (IB), flow cytometry (FC), and immunohistochemistry (IHC)

Target	Antibody/label	Species	Clone	Dilution	Source	Order #
IB						
CD276	IgG1 mAB	Mouse	6A1	1:600	abcam	ab105922
CD276	serum	Rabbit	⌀	1:500	abcam	ab226256
β actin	serum	Rabbit	⌀	1:1000	abcam	ab8227
Mouse IgG	serum/HRP	Rabbit	⌀	1:2000	Dako	P0260
Rabbit Ig	serum/HRP	Goat	⌀	1:2000	Dako	20034870
FC						
CD276	IgG1 mAB/PE	Mouse	MIH42	1:20	BioLegend	B7RP2
KLH	IgG1 mAB/PE	Mouse	X40	1:20	BD	345816
IHC						
CD276	IgG1 mAB	Mouse	6A1	1:300	abcam	ab105922

stain) to "300" (maximal staining intensity in the whole TMA) [21].

Statistics

Experimental results were processed by spreadsheet (Excel®, Microsoft) and statistics software (JMP®, SAS Institute Inc., Cary, USA). P values less than 0.05 were considered significant and marked in the figures accordingly.

Results

Expression of CD276 in urothelial carcinoma cell lines in vitro

Transcript amounts encoding CD276 were enumerated in UCCLs and NUCs by quantitative RT-PCR. CD276 mRNA was detected in both populations but the mean expression in the 4 UCCLs was significantly higher than in the 4 NUCs (threefold, $p < 0.006$, Fig. 1a). Similarly, immunoblotting revealed a significantly higher expression of CD276 protein in UCCLs compared to NUCs (fivefold, $p < 0.005$, Fig. 1b). The mean fluorescence intensity (MFI) of cell surface CD276 expression as determined by flow cytometry was increased 3.7-fold in UCCLs (MFI: 13,302 ± 2163) when compared to NUCs (MFI: 3591 ± 2080; $p < 0.012$; Fig. 2).

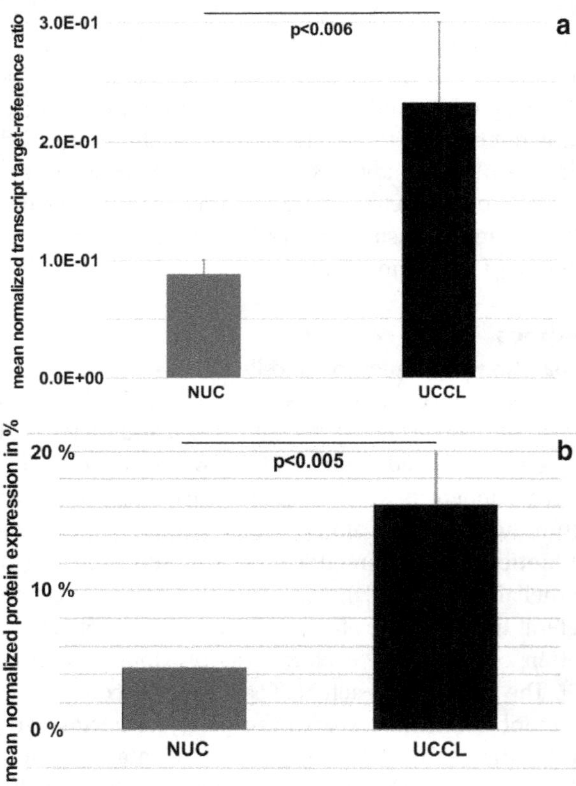

Fig. 1 CD276 transcript and protein expression. **a** Steady state mRNA amounts encoding CD276 were enumerated by qRT-PCR in four normal urothelial cells (NUCs) and four urothelial cancer cell lines (UCCLs). The graph shows the mean transcript levels ± standard deviations normalized to two housekeeping genes. **b** The total protein expression was investigated by immuno blotting of SDS-PAGEs. The mean expression of CD276 ± standard deviation of the four NUCs and four UCCLs is normalized to β-actin expression in each individual sample. UCCLs express significantly more CD276 transcripts ($p < 0.006$) and protein ($p < 0.005$) when compared to NUCs

Expression of CD276 in bladder tumor tissue samples

Tissue microarrays (TMA) were assembled from samples of 28 stage pT2, 46 stage pT3, 23 stage pT4 tumors and one additional BC tumor sample with unknown stage. The clinical and pathologic characteristics of the patient cohort are summarized in Table 3. Paraffin sections from tissue samples of these patients were stained with anti-CD276 antibody to determine the expression pattern of this immune checkpoint protein (Fig. 3). CD276 expression was found in urothelial cells but not in the

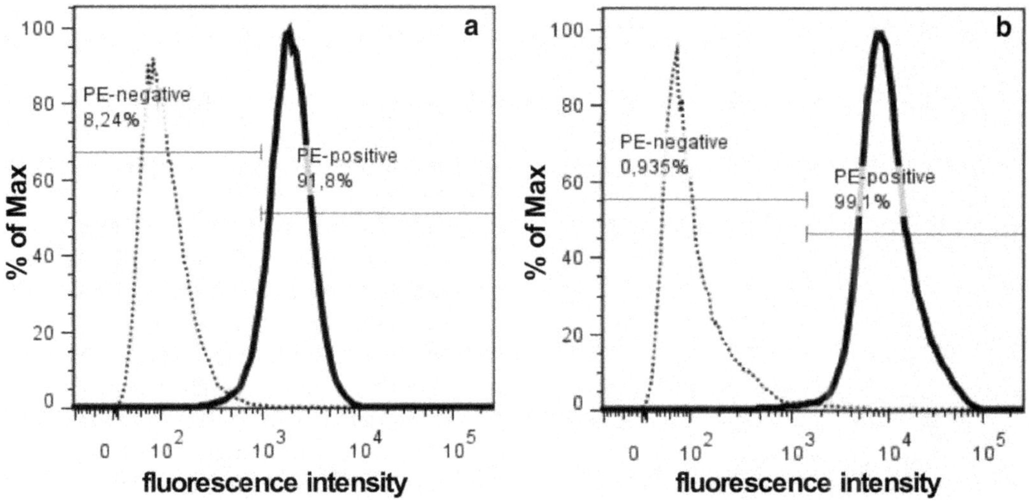

Fig. 2 Cell surface expression of CD276. The density of CD276 on cell surfaces was enumerated by flow cytometry on normal urothelial cells (NUCs) and urothelial cancer cell lines (UCCLs). **a** The representative NUC (HL19/17) shows a mean fluorescence intensity (MFI) of 2E03 and 91.8% of cells were gated positive for CD276 (solid histogram). **b** The representative tumor cell line HT1197 shows a MFI of 1.12E04 and 99.1% of cells were gated CD276 positive. Dotted histograms present isotype controls. The x-axis denotes the fluorescence intensity, the Y-axis the number of cells recorded as % of the maximum

connective tissue layers of histologically normal appearing bladder in bladder cancer patients (Fig. 3a). Low and dispersed CD276 expression was noted in some tumor samples (Fig. 3b), while its expression was high in other tumor samples (Fig. 3c). When comparing CD276 expression in healthy versus tumor tissue obtained from the 98 patient's bladders, its median expression was significantly lower in normal appearing tissue surrounding the tumors (score 50, n=47) when compared to the bladder tumors themselves (score 185, n=98; $p<0.0001$, Fig. 4). However, the CD276 expression scores were quite variable in both areas, in the tumors as well as the surrounding benigne tissue: the benign samples scored between 0 and 160, and tumor samples scored between 0 and 300.

However, the range of the CD276 score of benign samples surpassed the lowest quartile of the range of CD276 scores of the tumor samples (i.e., score 125) in only 3 of 47 cases (i.e., in 6.3%). In 12 of 47 benign samples (25%) CD276 expression was not observed at all (Fig. 4). Only 8 of 98 BC tumor samples (8.1%) scored within the range of the 3 lower quartiles of the benign samples (i.e., score < 90; Fig. 4).

When correlating the CD276 expression to the tumor stage, elevated expression was found in all bladder tumor stages from T2a to T4b (Fig. 5a) when compared to the median expression score of normal appearing urothelial samples from the same patients (Fig. 4). The peak median expression intensity of 210 was measured in samples obtained from pT2b tumors (Fig. 5a). No significant differences were observed in CD276 expression when comparing organ-confined (< pT3a, median score 190) with locally advanced tumors (≥ pT3a, median score 185; $\chi2=0.86$; Fig. 5B). However, a significant drop in the mean expression of CD276 was noted in the histologically normal tissue samples when stratified by the T stage of the tumor in the same specimen (< pT3a vs. ≥ pT3a, $p<0.042$; Fig. 6). The median score of CD276 expression dropped from 80 in benign urothelium from < pT3a patients to 40 in stage ≥ pT3a samples (Fig. 6).

Discussion

Elevated expression of CD276 in bladder cancer samples was reported previously [22] and success of experimental anti-CD276 antibody therapies raised hope for a new immune checkpoint therapy [6, 15, 16]. Our in vitro data using the well-established bladder cancer cell lines HT1197, TCCsup, RT4, and 5637 in comparison to four urothelial cell populations generated from explants from healthy ureters corroborated a significant overexpression of CD276 in BC cell lines. Significant overexpression of CD276 was also noted by immunohistochemistry in bladder tumors samples when compared to benign urothelium obtained from the same bladders. Slightly elevated CD276 scores in benigne samples from early-stage BC tumor patients could be caused by a moderate activation of CD276 expression in a few cells surrounding the tumor without showing the typical histology of a BC tumor by microscopy. CD276 transcript analyses of the corresponding malignant and benigne areas of BC samples could explore this hypothesis. Of note, healthy

Table 3 Patient characteristics

BC patients	98 total
Tumor samples—n (%)	98 (100.0)
Benigne samples—n (%)	47 (100.0)
Gender—n (%)	
Female	23 (23.5)
Male	75 (76.5)
Age, years	
Median (range)	69 (32–84)
pT-Stage—n (%)	
2a	15 (15.5)
2b	13 (13.6)
3a	22 (22.7)
3b	24 (24.7)
4a	17 (17.5)
4b	6 (6.2)
Unknown	1
Grading—n (%)	
1	0
2	23 (23.5)
3	75 (76.5)
Concomitant CIS—n (%)	
Yes	28 (30.1)
No	65 (69.9)
Unknown	5
cN-Stage—n (%)	
0	56 (59.5)
1	23 (24.5)
2	13 (13.7)
3	2 (2.3)
Unknown	4
cM-Stage—n (%)	
0	85 (90.4)
1	9 (9.6)
Unknown	4
R-Stage—n (%)	
0	80 (81.6)
1	15 (15.3)
2	3 (3.1)

bladder tissue from healthy volunteers was not available. Therefore, mechanisms of CD276 regulation in normal appearing tissue surrounding tumors versus healthy tissue are beyond the focus of the current study.

When analyzing the association between CD276 expression and tumor stage by immunohistochemistry in sample subsets, the highest median scores were observed in T2b and T3a tumors, followed by a minor, non-significant decline in higher stages (T3b and T4). In contrast, in benign urothelium from samples of patients with later stage tumors (≥ T3a) mean CD276 was significantly reduced when compared to benign sites in sample from patients with early-stage tumors (< T3a).

Expression of CD276 in bladder tissue samples from cancerous and adjacent healthy areas was determined by immunohistochemistry but not, for instance, by transcriptomics or other molecular analyses. Therefore, the mechanisms contributing to the significant changes in CD276 expression in situ in the normal tissue remained obscure. Total protein expression is often regulated on the transcript level and tumor grade-depended elevation of CD276 transcripts and CD276 total protein were found in BC [22]. However, other mechanisms may contribute to the changes in CD276 expression observed as well. For instance, protease-mediated release of soluble CD276 was described on activated leukocytes [23]. Blocking the protease activity caused an accumulation of CD276 on these leukocytes [23]. Based on this finding we hypothesize that elevated expression of proteases by the bladder tumor cells may play a role in degradation of even little CD276 from the surface of the benign cells surrounding the actual tumor. This mechanism may act on bladder tumors as well, and thereby contribute to the minor reduction of the mean CD276 score observed in the pT4 samples. This hypothesis is in line with the finding that elevated expression of CD276 correlated with elevated expression of matrix metalloproteinases -2 and-9 [22].

We noted considerable variations of CD276 expression in individual samples from all stages of bladder tumors. This may be in part associated with changes in cell surface versus cytoplasmic expression of CD276. Such a conversion of CD276 expression has been observed in clear cell renal cell carcinoma [24]. Tumors with pronounced cytoplasmic expression were associated with worse prognosis when compared to those with membrane expression. But degradation of CD276 by proteases as mechanism to generate the cytoplasmic CD276 phenotype was not investigated in that study [24]. In other studies, tumor therapy by a PD-1 inhibitor reduced the expression of CD276 on bladder cancer carcinoma cells significantly in about 67% of samples investigated [25]. These findings indicated that CD276 expression may change its levels and patterns during the course of disease and/or depending on the therapy. However, the patients included in our study were not treated by immune checkpoint inhibitors.

A technical challenge is of course the fact that histology yields in many cases the sum of protein expression in the cytoplasm and on the cell surface. For the interaction with T lymphocytes as well as the direct binding of anti-CD276 antibodies or alike, the presentation of CD276 on the cells surface is critical. Therefore, additional studies need to determine the correlation

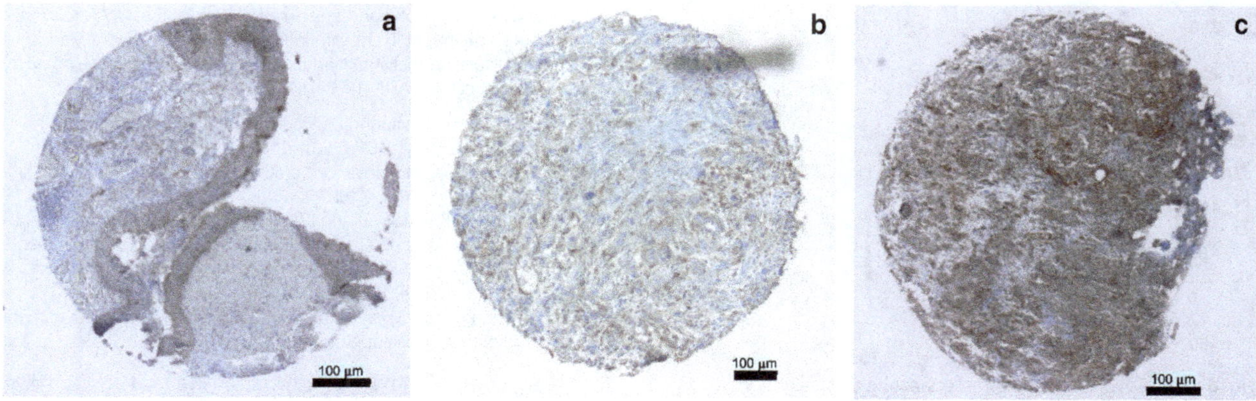

Fig. 3 Detection of CD276 in tissue samples by immunohistochemistry. Representative tissue samples of benign urothelium (**a**), low expressing tumor tissue (**b**) and high expressing tumor tissue (**c**) were assessed for expression of CD276 on a tissue microarray by immunohistochemistry. Sections were counterstained with hematoxylin and eosin to visualize tissue structure. Size bars = 100 µm

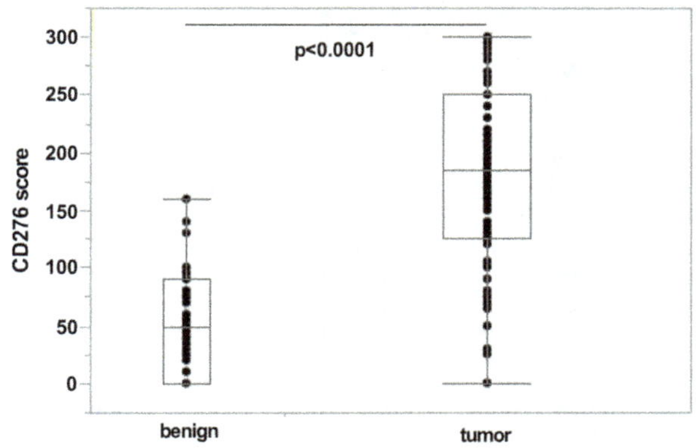

Fig. 4 Expression of CD276 in normal appearing versus malignant bladder tissue. Paraffin sections of tissue samples from bladder cancer patients of all stages were reacted with anti-CD276 antibody and then counterstained by hematoxylin. The median CD276 expression score was significantly lower in areas surrounding the tumor and appearing healthy (score 50) when compared to the areas confirmed by an expert pathologist as tumor tissue (score 185, $p < 0.0001$). A considerable scatter of individual CD276 scores was noted in both cohorts

between total protein expression in bladder tumor tissue in comparison to the CD276 density on tumor cell surfaces [22, 24, 25].

Conclusions

Median expression of CD276 is significantly elevated in bladder carcinoma tissue but presents with a high inter-individual variability among patient samples. Diagnosis or therapy utilizing CD276 as target molecule should therefore be considered and evaluated with care, especially in late-stage patients.

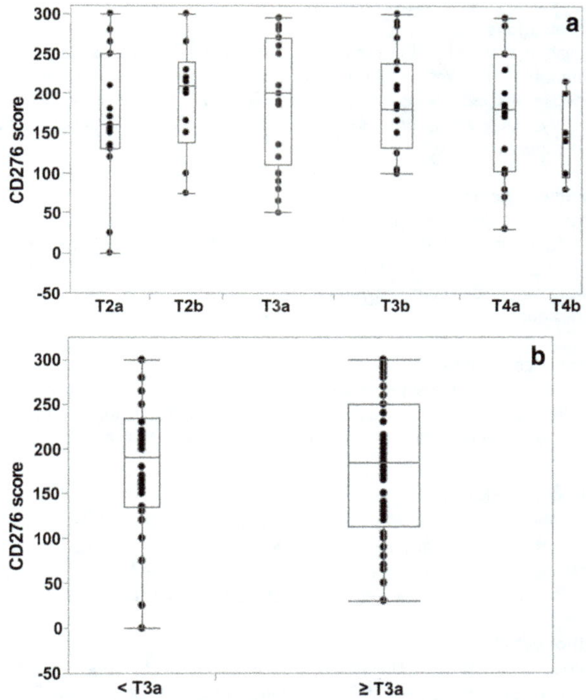

Fig. 5 Expression of CD276 in bladder tumors in different tumor stages. **a** Bladder tumor samples from patients at stages T2a to T4b were investigated for CD276 expression and are presented as function of the clinical tumor stage. The median CD276 expression peaked in stage T2b samples (score 210), slightly declined throughout later stages to drop in tumor tissue samples obtained from late-stage patients at T4b to a median score of 145. **b** Bladder tumor samples of patients in all stages were investigated for CD276 expression and correlated to the tumor stages < pT3a versus ≥ pT3a. Significant differences in expression of CD276 in < pT3a (median score 190) versus ≥ pT3a tumors (median score 185; $\chi2 = 0.86$) were not observed

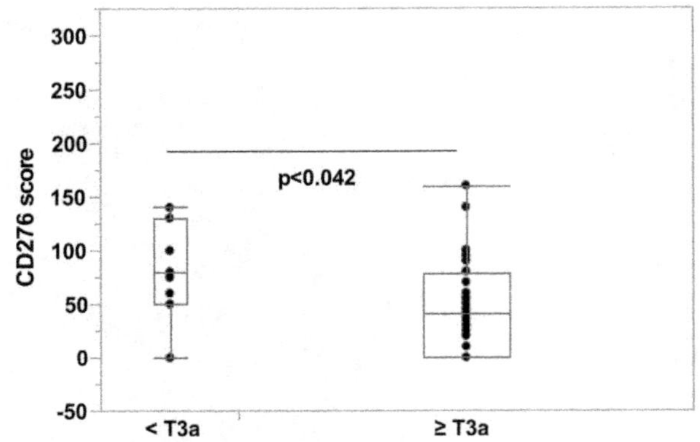

Fig. 6 CD276 expression in normal appearing urothelium from bladder tumor patients. Expression of CD276 was evaluated by immunohistochemistry in areas presenting with normal histology and samples obtained from patients at earlier (< pT3a) versus later T stages (≥ pT3a) were compared. In confirmed normal urothelium from patients of tumor stages < pT3a, CD276 expression scored with a median of 80. In confirmed normal urothelium from tumor patients at stages ≥ pT3a CD276 dropped significantly to a median of 40

Abbreviations

BC: Bladder cancer; FC: Flow cytometry; HRP: Horse reddish peroxidase; IB: Immunoblot, alias Western blot; IHC: Immunohistochemistry; KLH: Keyhole limped hemocyanin; mAB: Monoclonal antibody; MFI: Mean fluorescence intensity; NUCs: Normal urothelial cells; TMA: Tissue micro array; UCCL: Urothelial carcinoma cell line.

Acknowledgements

The authors express their gratitude to T. Neumann for expert help with statistics, Conny Bock and Tanja Abruzzese for excellent technical support and training of the students, A. Knoll for support of NUC analyses, Falko Fend for sharing expertise in pathology, and Chaim Goziga for support in preparation of the figures.

Authors' contributions

WKA, AS: study design, supervision, data evaluation, manuscr pt writing; MK, LR, FBM: lab experiments, data evaluation; JH, PCB, TT, JB: providing tumor sample or cell lines, data evaluation, manuscript writing; WKA, AS, TT: funding.

Competing interest

The authors declare that (1) they do not have any competing interests, and that (2) this study and all parts of it have not been published yet, nor are they considered for or submitted for publication anywhere else. All authors have seen the manuscript and agree with its publication in ***BMC Urology***.

Author details

[1] Department of Urology, University of Tuebingen Hospital, Hoppe-Seyler-Str. 3, 72076 Tübingen, Germany. [2] Vancouver Prostate Centre, University of British Columbia, Level 6, 2775 Laurel St, Vancouver, BC V5Z 1M9, Canada. [3] Department of Urology, Center for Medical Research, University of Tuebingen Hospital, Waldhoernlestrasse 22, 72072 Tübingen, Germany.

References

1. Siegel RL, Miller KD, Jemal A. Cancer statistics, 2019. CA Cancer J Clin. 2019;69(1):7–34.
2. Sharpe AH. Introduction to checkpoint inhibitors and cancer immunotherapy. Immunol Rev. 2017;276(1):5–8.
3. Sharma P, Retz M, Siefker-Radtke A, Baron A, Necchi A, Bedke J, Plimack ER, Vaena D, Grimm M-O, Bracarda S, et al. Nivolumab in metastatic urothelial carcinoma after platinum therapy (CheckMate 275): a multicentre, single-arm, phase 2 trial. Lancet Oncol. 2017;18(3):3 2–22.
4. Balar AV, Galsky MD, Rosenberg JE, Powles T, Petrylak DP, Bellmunt J, Loriot Y, Necchi A, Hoffman-Censits J, Perez-Gracia JL, et al. Atezolizumab as first-line treatment in cisplatin-ineligible patients with locally advanced and metastatic urothelial carcinoma: a single-arm, multicentre, phase 2 trial. The Lancet. 2017;389(10064):67–76.
5. Bellmunt J, de Wit R, Vaughn DJ, Fradet Y, Lee J-L, Fong L, Vogelzang NJ, Climent MA, Petrylak DP, Choueiri TK, et al. Pembrolizumab as second-line therapy for advanced urothelial carcinoma. N Engl J Med. 2017;376(11):1015–26.
6. Seaman S, Zhu Z, Saha S, Zhang XM, Yang MY, Hilton MB, Morris K, Szot C, Morris H, Swing DA, et al. Eradication of tumors through simultaneous ablation of CD276/B7-H3-positive tumor cells and tumor vasculature. Cancer Cell. 2017;31(4):501-515.e508.
7. Dong P, Xiong Y, Yue J, Hanley SJB, Watari H. B7H3 as a promoter of metastasis and promising therapeutic target. Front Oncol. 2018;8:264.
8. Li P, Yang Y, Jin Y, Zhao R, Dong C, Zheng W, Zhang T, Li J, Gu Z. B7-H3 participates in human salivary gland epithelial cells apoptosis through NF-κB pathway in primary Sjögren's syndrome. J Transl Med. 2019;17(1):268.
9. Xylinas E, Robinson BD, Kluth LA, Volkmer BG, Hautmann R, Kufer R, Zerbib M, Kwon E, Thompson RH, Boorjian SA, et al. Association of T-cell co-regulatory protein expression with clinical outcomes following radical cystectomy for urothelial carcinoma of the bladder. Eur J Surg Oncol. 2014;40(1):121–7.
10. Ye Z, Zheng Z, Li X, Zhu Y, Zhong Z, Peng L, Wu Y. B7-H3 overexpression predicts poor survival of cancer patients: a meta-analysis. Cell Physiol Biochem. 2016;39(4):1568–80.
11. Xu ZL, Zhang Y, Wang L, Li F, Man HW, Li PF, Shan BE. B7-H3 promotes malignant progression of muscle-invasive bladder cancer. Oncol Rep. 2018;40(5):2722–33.
12. Loos M, Hedderich DM, Friess H, Kleeff J. B7-H3 and its role in antitumor immunity. Clin Dev Immunol. 2010;2010:683875.
13. Kobori H, Hashiguchi M, Piao J, Kato M, Ritprajak P, Azuma M. Enhancement of effector CD8+ T-cell function by tumour-associated B7-H3 and modulation of its counter-receptor triggering receptor expressed on myeloid cell-like transcript 2 at tumour sites. Immunology. 2010;130(3):363–73.
14. Suh WK, Gajewska BU, Okada H, Gronski MA, Bertram EM, Dawicki W, Duncan GS, Bukczynski J, Plyte S, Elia A, et al. The B7 family member B7-H3 preferentially down-regulates T helper type 1-mediated immune responses. Nat Immunol. 2003;4(9):899–906.
15. Lee YH, Martin-Orozco N, Zheng P, Li J, Zhang P, Tan H, Park HJ, Jeong M, Chang SH, Kim BS, et al. Inhibition of the B7-H3 immune checkpoint limits tumor growth by enhancing cytotoxic lymphocyte function. Cell Res. 2017;27(8):1034–45.
16. Ma W, Ma J, Ma P, Lei T, Zhao M, Zhang M. Targeting immunotherapy for bladder cancer using anti-CD3x B7-H3 bispecific antibody. Cancer Med. 2018;7(10):5167–77.
17. Nagele U, Maurer S, Feil G, Bock C, Krug J, Sievert K-D, Stenzl A. In vitro investigations of tissue-engineered multilayered urothelium established from bladder washings. Eur Urol. 2008;54(6):1414–22.
18. Pfaffl MW. Quantification strategies in real-time PCR. In: Bustin SA, editor. A-Z of quantitative PCR. La Jolla, CA: International University Line; 2004. p. 87–112.
19. Ausubel FM, Brent R, Kingston RE, Moore DD, Seidman JG, Smith JA, Struhl K. Short protocols in molecular biology. New York: Wiley; 2002.
20. Pilz GA, Braun J, Ulrich C, Felka T, Warstat K, Ruh M, Schewe B, Abele H, Larbi A, Aicher WK. Human mesenchymal stromal cells express CD14 cross-reactive epitopes. Cytometry A. 2011;79(8):635–45.
21. Semilia M, Hennenlotter J, Pavone C, Bischoff T, Kuhs U, Gakis G, Bedke J, Stenzl A, Schwentner C, Todenhofer T. Expression patterns and prognostic role of transketolase-like 1 in muscle-invasive bladder cancer. World J Urol. 2015;33(10):1403–9.
22. Li Y, Guo G, Song J, Cai Z, Yang J, Chen Z, Wang Y, Huang Y, Gao Q. B7-H3 promotes the migration and invasion of human bladder cancer cells via the PI3K/Akt/STAT3 signaling pathway. J Cancer. 2017;8(5):816–24.
23. Zhang G, Hou J, Shi J, Yu G, Lu B, Zhang X. Soluble CD276 (B7-H3) is released from monocytes, dendritic cells and activated T cells and is detectable in normal human serum. Immunology. 2008;123(4):538–46.

24. Saeednejad Zanjani L, Madjd Z, Axcrona U, Abolhasani M, Rasti A, Asgari M, Fodstad Ã, Andersson Y. Cytoplasmic expression of B7-H3 and membranous EpCAM expression are associated with higher grade and survival outcomes in patients with clear cell renal cell carcinoma. Ann Diagn Pathol. 2020;46:151483.
25. Necchi A, Anichini A, Raggi D, Briganti A, Massa S, Luciano R, Colecchia M, Giannatempo P, Mortarini R, Bianchi M, et al. Pembrolizumab as neoadjuvant therapy before radical cystectomy in patients with muscle-invasive urothelial bladder carcinoma (PURE-01): an open-label, single-arm, phase II study. J Clin Oncol. 2018;36(34):3353.

15

Surgical findings in cryptorchidism in children with Zika-related microcephaly

Rômulo A. L. de Vasconcelos[3*], Ricardo A. A. Ximenes[3,4], Adriano A. Calado[3], Celina M. T. Martelli[1], Andreia V. Gonçalves[3,4], Elizabeth B. Brickley[2], Thalia V. B. de Araújo[4], Maria A. W. Rocha[3] and Demócrito de B. Miranda-Filho[3*]

Abstract

Background: Complications in the urinary tract related to congenital Zika syndrome have recently been reported. One complication, cryptorchidism, has been reported by the Microcephaly Epidemic Research Group/MERG, in Pernambuco/Brazil. The present article describes for the first time the surgical findings in a case series of boys with Zika-related microcephaly and cryptorchidism, who underwent surgical testicular exploration as a contribution to better understand the possible mechanisms involved in gonads formation and descent.

Methods: A total of 7 children (11 testicular units), aged 3 to 4 years, were submitted to inguinal or scrotal orchidopexy for the treatment of palpable cryptorchidism between August 2019 and January 2020. Characteristics of the gonads and its annexes related to appendixes, testis-epididymis dissociation, gubernacular insertion, and associated hydroceles and/or hernias were described. Measures in centimetres were taken for volume calculate.

Results: We found a low prevalence of testicular and epididymal appendix (66.7%), a high prevalence of testis-epididymis dissociation (55.6%), low mean testicular volume for their ages (lower for older boys) and ectopic gubernacular insertion in all cases. There was no evidence of associated hydroceles and/or hernias in any case. No surgical complication was registered or reported, and all explored gonads were properly placed in the scrotal sac.

Conclusions: We herein describe the surgical findings of these children's orchidopexies and discuss the possible mechanisms of viral action in embryogenesis and postnatal growth and development of the testes and annexes. These children need to be followed over time due to the higher risk of testicular atrophy and malignancy. Surgical timing seems to be relevant to avoid loss of testicular volume.

Keywords: Congenital Zika syndrome, Cryptorchidism, Microcephaly, Zika virus, Orchiopexy, Surgery, Case series

Background

Although neurodevelopmental impairments and structural brain defects are amongst the most common features in children with Zika-related microcephaly (ZRM), the condition has also been increasingly associated with abnormalities across a range of organ systems [1]. It is now recognized that a high frequency of children with ZRM may present with cryptorchidism [2]. Cryptorchidism is known to be associated with testicular cancer, infertility, and hypogonadism [3]. Here, we provide the first report on the findings of testicular surgical exploration in a case series of 7 male children, aged 3 to 4 years, with ZRM and cryptorchidism participating in the Microcephaly Epidemic Research Group (MERG) Paediatric Cohort, in Pernambuco, Brazil (Study Protocol:

*Correspondence: romulo.alv@hotmail.com; demofilho@gmail.com
[3] Universidade de Pernambuco, Rua Arnóbio Marques, 310 – Santo Amaro, Recife, PE 50100-130, Brazil
Full list of author information is available at the end of the article

http:/www.cpqam.fiocruz.br/merg/) [4]. As main objective to better understand the possible mechanisms involved in this syndrome and its influences over gonads formation and descent.

Methods

Between August/2019 and January/2020, a MERG paediatric urologist assessed 31 males with microcephaly (i.e., totalling 62 testicular units), using the criteria of the 2018 paediatric guidelines of the European Association of Urology, and the results have been previously described [5]. Twelve boys were diagnosed with true cryptorchidism (36.4%), while a further eleven had retractile testes (35.4%). Of the 12 boys identified as having cryptorchidism, eight underwent testicular surgical exploration. Five were operated on by a team of paediatric urologists from MERG, two by a paediatric surgeon from a private health service that was not part of the research group, and one by a paediatric surgeon at the same institution where follow-up of the MERG cohort is undertaken (NB: this child underwent surgery at age two and was subsequently recruited to the cohort, but was not included in this case series due to lack of information on surgical findings).

Laterality was defined during medical consultations by physical examination. The records regarding the aspect of the testes and annexes, gonadal volume, gubernacular insertion, and associated findings (hernias, hydroceles, and persistent peritoneal vaginal conduit) were obtained by in-surgery measurement and photographs taken by the research group during the surgical procedures. TED classification is confusing and not standardized, so it was classified in two groups: partial (head or tail attachment) or complete failure (even if attached to any structure distinct to the testis, like the gubernaculum) [6]. The location of the insertion of the gubernaculum was assessed by pulling at the gubernaculum and determining where the retraction occurred. Testicular volume was calculated using the formula: volume $(\text{cm}^3) = 0.523 \times \text{length} \times \text{height} \times \text{width}$ (cm), while the volume expected for age was obtained from the formula: volume $(\text{cm}^3) = 0.004 \times (\text{age in months}) + 0.438$ [7]. Data on the two children who underwent surgery in the private service were obtained through telephone contact with the responsible surgeon.

All parents/guardians signed an informed consent form. This study was approved by the Oswaldo Cruz Hospital Ethical Committee (CAAE: 94544518.2.0000.5192).

Results

Four children presented bilateral cryptorchidism with palpable gonads in the inguinal regions, two presented with palpable cryptorchidism in the left inguinal region only, and the last presented with palpable cryptorchidism in the right inguinal region only. In all cases, either inguinal or scrotal testicular exploration was performed. In one patient with bilateral cryptorchidism, exploration of the right side was not undertaken due to the occurrence of respiratory distress, which led us to curtail the surgery, following the recommendation of the anaesthesiologist. Following surgery, the child developed febrile illness, which was attributed to a respiratory viral infection, but went on to fully recover. In one of the patients with bilateral cryptorchidism submitted to surgery in the private service, exploration on the left side was not undertaken, as the attending physician decided that the surgery should be undertaken in two steps. In total, nine testes were submitted to orchidopexy. None of the children experienced complications related to surgical manipulation (Table 1).

Table 1 Characterization of a case series of cryptorchidism in children with ZRM submitted to surgical exploration

Patient	Age at surgery (years)	Laterality	Aspect on surgical exploration	Volume (cm^3)	Gubernacular insertion	Associated findings
1	3	Right	Ncrmal	Missing	Pubic	Absence
2	3	Left	TED	0.53	Pubic	TA
3	3	Bilateral	TED (both)	Right: 0.53 Left: 0.56	Pubic (both)	TA (both)
4	4	Bilateral	Right: not operated Left: TED	Right: not operated Left: 0.51	Right: not operated Left: pubic	Right: not operated Left: EA
5	3	Bilateral	Normal (both)	Right: 0.48 Left: 0.49	Pubic (both)	Right: EA Left: absence
6	4	Left	TED	0.43	Pubic	TA
7	4	Bilateral	Right: normal Left: not operated	Right: missing Left: not operated	Right: pubic Left: not operated	Right: absence Left: not operated

TED testis-epididymis dissociation, *TA* testicular appendix, *EA* epididymal appendix

Five testes (55.6%) presented with testis-epididymis dissociation (TED), which was partial in one case and complete in the other four (Fig. 1). Among the testes of the children operated on 3-years of age with available data (Patients 2, 3, and 5), the mean testicular volume observed was $0.52cm^3$ ($0.48–0.56cm^3$), lower than the expected mean volume of $0.60cm^3$ ($0.58–0.63cm^3$). For the testes of the 4-year-old group with available data (Patients 4 and 6), the mean testicular volume was $0.47cm^3$ ($0.43–0.51cm^3$), lower than the mean expected volume of $0.62cm^3$ ($0.63–0.67cm^3$). In two children (Patients 1 and 7), it was not possible to obtain data for calculating testicular volume. The testicular appendix was identified in four units operated on (44.5%) and in two epididymis (22.2%). In the cases that underwent surgery by the MERG surgeons and in the two patients included from the private health service, there was no identification or reports of persistent peritoneum-vaginal canal, hydrocele, or hernia. In all five cases operated on by the MERG surgeons and in the two from the private service, the gubernaculum presented an ectopic insertion in the pubic region (Table 2).

Discussion

The surgical findings we presented in this paper provide additional information to our previously reported case series and enlightens the possible mechanisms related to this condition [2]. The occurrence of TED was very high in this group of boys (5 occurrences—55.6%), and was complete in 4 cases. The expected frequency of this anomaly is only 0.9% in normal children and up to 8% in patients with cryptorchidism [8]. In our series, none of the boys presented with abnormalities of the peritoneum-vaginal canal. Our children are comparable to

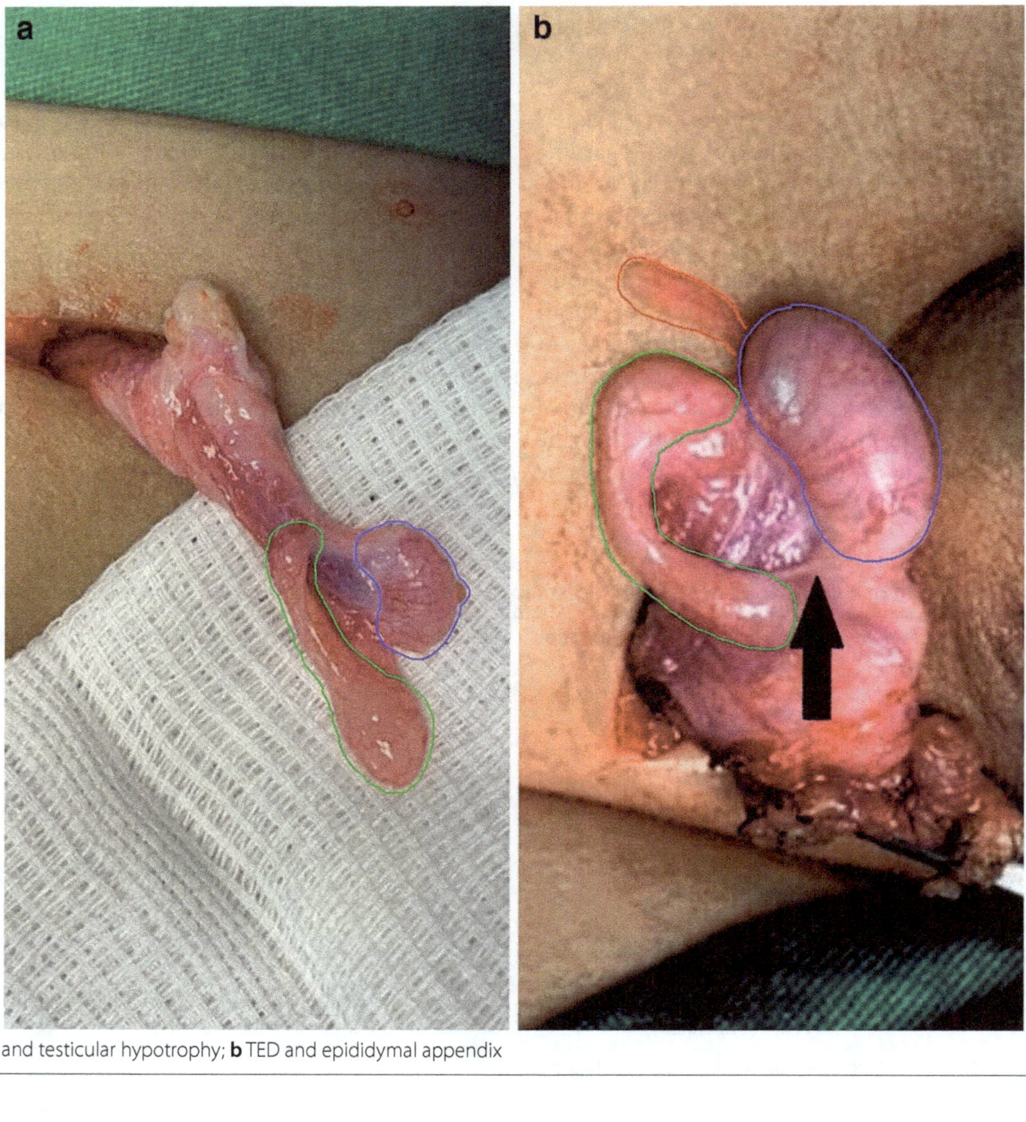

Fig. 1 **a** TED and testicular hypotrophy; **b** TED and epididymal appendix

Table 2 Findings of orchiopexies of a case series of cryptorchidism in children with ZRM

Mean testicular volume (n = 9 testicular units)		
3 years (5 testicular units)	0.52 cm^3	(0.48–0.56 cm^3)
4 years (2 testicular units)	0.47 cm^3	(0.43–0.51 cm^3)
Missing	2	
Testicular aspect (n = 9 testicular units)		
Normal	4	44.4%
TED	5	55.6%
Gubernacular insertion (n = 9 testicular units)		
Pubic	9	100%
Associated findings (n = 9 testicular units)		
Absence	3	33.3%
Appendix testis	4	44.5%
Appendix epididymis	2	22.2%

TED testis-epididymis dissociation

those of cerebral palsy in relation to brain damage and high frequency of undescended testicles (36.4% in our children and 24% in children with cerebral palsy), however differ in relation to the frequency of inguinal hernias (none in our case series versus 56% in cerebral palsy) [2, 9].

Our understanding of the pathogenesis of cryptorchidism in children with ZRM is developing, and this case series provides findings that can help to better understand this physiopathologic process. Although the mechanisms of testicular descent are multi-factorial, given the high prevalence of TED and absence of anomalies of the peritoneum-vaginal conduit, it is plausible to suggest that congenital ZIKV infections should be considered as a possible explanation for the interferences on the formation mechanisms of the testis and epididymis during embryogenesis. Transmission of the Zika virus through the seminal fluid has been identified [10], which leads us to assume that there is a possible tropism of the virus to the gonadal and adnexal tissue. This possibility needs to be explored further in cadaver parts or testes submitted to orchiectomy. The frequency of gonadal appendix in our series (44.5% in the testes and 22.2% in the epididymes) was lower than the reported by Zdizvic [11], who described a frequency of 78.7% in gonads located close to the external inguinal ring in 89 normal boys. All operated testes of our series were palpable close to the external inguinal ring. Testicular appendixes are remnants of the paramesonephric ducts, but their role in testicular descent has not been well established. The function of the gubernaculum, on the other hand, is to guide the descent of the testicles in the second phase (inguinoscrotal), through the action of testosterone and the genitofemoral nerve associated with abdominal pressure, and has been well documented [12]. The finding of 100% ectopic gubernacular insertion in the pubic position could point this as being a possible mechanism responsible for the complete non-descent of these gonads and could also explain a lower, extra-abdominal location. The prevalence of ectopic gubernacular insertion in congenital cryptorchidism reported in the literature is low. Favorito [13] found no gubernacular ectopic insertion in 101 patients with cryptorchidism with a mean age of 6.4 years. Meijde Vries [14], describing surgical findings in congenital cryptorchidism in 76 testes, found 17% of gubernacular insertion in the bottom of the scrotum and 57% in the upper scrotum, totalling 74% scrotal gubernacular insertion. Due to their location, the non-descending gonads in the children with ZRM would be subjected to thermal stress, which could contribute to a progressive loss of testicular mass and volume. In this series, children operated at three years presented with abnormally low testicular volume, and the reduction in volume was even greater in children operated at four years. Delayed surgery (i.e., beyond the recommended maximum of 18 months of age) [5] may explain the lower testicular volume in the children with ZRM.

Conclusions

Our finding of a significant loss of testicular volume, attributed to late surgical correction, reinforces the importance of providing early attention to this anomaly. There is no apparent association with abnormalities of the peritoneum-vaginal canal, frequently seen in other children with cryptorchidism, even with cerebral palsy. The gubernaculum has an uncommon pubic insertion. A high frequency of TED calls attention to possible interference within gonadal formation, but further studies with a larger number of cases, histological examination and exploration of neuronal and hormonal abnormalities should be performed to better analyse these findings.

Abbreviations

ZRM: Zika-related microcephaly; MERG: Microcephaly Epidemic Research Group; TED: Testis-epididymis dissociation.

Acknowledgements

We extend our thanks to the Unipeclin/UPE and to the Zika virus research field team for helping with data collection and for providing support for the children and caregivers during their clinical consultations.

Author contributions

RALV: made substantial contributions to the conception, design of the work, acquisition, analysis, interpretation of data and has drafted the work. RAAX: made substantial contributions to the interpretation of data and has substantially revised it. AAC: made substantial contributions to the conception, design of the work and acquisition of data. CMTM: made substantial contributions to the interpretation of data and has substantially revised it. AVG: made substantial contributions to the interpretation of data and has substantially revised it. EBB: made substantial contributions to the interpretation of data and has substantially revised it. TVBA: made substantial contributions to the interpretation of data and has substantially revised it. MAWR: made substantial contributions to the interpretation of data and has substantially revised it. DBMF: made substantial contributions to the conception, design of the work, analysis, interpretation of data and has drafted the work. All authors read and approved the final manuscript.

Competing interests
None of the authors have competing interest that could be perceived to bias this work.

Author details
[1] Instituto de Pesquisa Aggeu Magalhães – Fiocruz, Recife, Pernambuco, Brazil. [2] London School of Hygiene and Tropical Medicine, London, UK. [3] Universidade de Pernambuco, Rua Arnóbio Marques, 310 – Santo Amaro, Recife, PE 50100-130, Brazil. [4] Universidade Federal de Pernambuco, Recife, Brazil.

References
1. Melo A, Aguiar R, Amorim M, et al. Congenital Zika virus infection. JAMA Neurol. 2016. https://doi.org/10.1001/jamaneurol.2016.3720.
2. de Vasconcelos R, Ximenes R, Calado A, et al. Cryptorchidism in children with Zika-related microcephaly. Am J Trop Med Hyg. 2020. https://doi.org/10.4269/ajtmh.19-0753.
3. Gurney J, McGlynn K, Stanley J, et al. Risk factors for cryptorchidism. Nat Rev Urol. 2017. https://doi.org/10.1038/nrurol.2017.90.
4. França G, Schuler-Faccini L, Oliveira W, et al. Congenital Zika virus syndrome in Brazil: a case series of the first 1501 livebirths with complete investigation. The Lancet. 2016. https://doi.org/10.1016/s0140-6736(16)30902-3.
5. Radmayr C, et al. EAU guidelines on paediatric urology. 2018. https://uroweb.org/guideline/paediatric-urology/. Accessed 1 Feb 2020.
6. Qin K, Morley C, Nataraja R, Pacilli M. The spectrum of testicular-epididymal fusion anomalies in children with cryptorchidism: personal experience, systematic review and meta-analysis. J Pediatr Urol. 2020. https://doi.org/10.1016/j.jpurol.2019.12.016.
7. Shin H, Yoon H, Lee Y, et al. Normal changes and ranges of pediatric testicular volume and shear wave elasticity. Ultrasound Med Biol. 2019. https://doi.org/10.1016/j.ultrasmedbio.2019.02.026.
8. Sharma S, Sen A. Complete testicular epididymal dissociation in the abdominal cryptorchid testis. J Pediatr Urol. 2013. https://doi.org/10.1016/j.jpurol.2013.02.017.
9. Barthold J, Wintner A, Hagerty J, Rogers K, Hossain M. Cryptorchidism in boys with cerebral palsy is associated with the severity of disease and with co-occurrence of other congenital anomalies. Front Endocrinol (Lausanne). 2018. https://doi.org/10.3389/fendo.2018.00151.
10. Mansuy J, Dutertre M, Mengelle C, et al. Zika virus: high infectious viral load in semen, a new sexually transmitted pathogen? Lancet Infect Dis. 2016. https://doi.org/10.1016/s1473-3099(16)00138-9.
11. Zvizdic Z, Zivkovic D, Sabanovic J, Milisic E. The role of the appendix testis in normal testicular descent: is there a connection? Biomed Res Int. 2018. https://doi.org/10.1155/2018/3078031.
12. Niedzielski J, Oszukowska E, Słowikowska-Hilczer J. Undescended testis—current trends and guidelines: a review of the literature. Arch Med Sci. 2016. https://doi.org/10.5114/aoms.2016.59940.
13. Favorito L, Klojda C, Costa W, Sampaio F. Is there a relationship with anomalous insertions of the distal gubernaculum testis and testicular ectopia? Analysis in human fetuses and patients with cryptorchidism. J Urol. 2003. https://doi.org/10.1097/01.ju.0000070436.98851.46.
14. Meij-de Vries A, Hack W, Heij H, Meijer R. Perioperative surgical findings in congenital and acquired undescended testis. J Pediatr Surg. 2010. https://doi.org/10.1016/j.jpedsurg.2010.02.121.

16

Clinical efficacy of retrograde urethrography-assisted urethral catheterization after failed conventional urethral catheterization

Si Hyun Kim, Hee Jo Yang, Doo Sang Kim, Chang Ho Lee, Youn Soo Jeon and Ki Hong Kim*

Abstract

Background: Several approaches for urethral catheterization after the failure of initial urethral catheterization have been introduced. However, standard procedures regarding what should be done after failed conventional urethral catheterization have been not established. Therefore, we investigated the clinical efficacy of retrograde urethrography (RGU)-assisted urethral catheterization after failed conventional urethral catheterization.

Methods: Between July 2015 and July 2018, 136 patients who underwent RGU-assisted urethral catheterization after failed conventional urethral catheterization were included in this retrospective study. Patients' clinical data, such as age, catheterization site, and previous history of urologic operations, were collected and assessed via chart review. Univariate and multivariate logistic regression analyses were performed to identify predictive factors for the failure of this procedure.

Results: Of the 136 patients, 94 (69.1%) experienced successful RGU-assisted urethral catheterization. Having a previous history of urologic operations, such as urethrotomy and transurethral prostatectomy, was identified as an independent predictive factor for the failure of RGU-assisted urethral catheterization (odds ratio = 9.453, 95% confidence interval = 2.703–33.063, $p < 0.001$).

Conclusions: RGU-assisted urethral catheterization can be one of the modalities for providing successful catheterization after failed conventional urethral catheterization. We believe that RGU-assisted urethral catheterization can be an effective procedure if patients have no previous history of urologic operations, such as urethrotomy and transurethral prostatectomy.

Keywords: Retrograde urethrography, Urethral catheterization, Urethral injury

Background

Urethral catheterization is one of the most common urologic procedures. For various reasons, this procedure is performed on about a quarter of inpatients [1]. However, clinicians are sometimes faced with unexpected difficulties during urethral catheterization (DDUCs). Although DDUCs are not common, if this is not properly handled, they could cause critical problems, such as urethral injury [2]. Complications associated with urethral injury are significant hazards of urinary catheterization. This causes patients to unnecessarily increase hospitalization and pay extra-medical expenses [3]. A recent study has reported that urethral catheter-related injuries occur in 1.4% of urethral catheterization patients [4], and the cost of managing these injuries was about $371,790 [5].

Further, there are many factors that can cause failed catheterization [6]. Common causes of DDUCs for normal urethras include tight external sphincters caused by anxiety in patients and poor catheterization technique.

*Correspondence: urokim@schmc.ac.kr
Department of Urology, Soonchunhyang University Cheonan Hospital, Soonchunhyang University College of Medicine, 31 Suncheonhyang 6-gil, Dongnam-gu, Cheonan 31151, Korea

Additionally, pathologic causes include urethral stricture, phimosis, edema, bladder neck contracture, prostate cancer, false passages, and benign prostatic hypertrophy, among others [7]. Among them, most urethral injuries, particularly false passages, occur during initial catheterization. This is because external sphincter contraction occurs when the catheter enters the bulbous membranous urethra. Injuries are sometimes caused by the balloon when the catheter is not fully inserted or the catheter tip itself causes incorrect passage [4]. In these cases, the retrial of catheterization with conventional blind technique could further damage the urethra [8].

Several approaches for urethral catheterization after the failure of initial urethral catheterization have been introduced [7]. However, standard procedures regarding what should be done after failed conventional urethral catheterization have been not established. Therefore, we investigated the clinical efficacy of urethral catheterization under retrograde urethrography (RGU) guidance after failed conventional urethral catheterization and attempted to identify factors for the success of this procedure.

Methods

Study design

A total of 136 consecutive male patients who underwent urethral catheterization under RGU guidance between July 2015 and July 2018 were included in this retrospective study. All patients underwent RGU-assisted urethral catheterization after failed conventional urethral catheterization. After institutional review board approval (No. 2018-08-021) was granted for this study, we conducted a retrospective chart review of the included patients. All patients received written informed consent and agreed prior to the procedure. All procedures in this study were performed in accordance with the ethical standards of the institutional and national research committee and with the 1964 Helsinki declaration.

RGU-assisted urethral catheterization procedure

RGU using a fluoroscope was performed during urethral catheterization. Urethral catheterization was performed using a 18 French sized three-way Foley catheter with a hole that was used for continuous irrigation. Prior to the procedure, the operator wore protective equipment against radiation exposure. To start the procedure, a fluoroscope was placed in front of patients. Then, a hydrophilic guide wire (Terumo Radiofocus® Guide wire Angled, 0.35″, 150 cm) was inserted into bladder through the hole of the catheter under fluoroscopic guidance. Next, a 60-mL enema syringe was filled with 1:2 mixture of contrast solution and normal. Under RGU guidance, the syringe was then connected at the drainage hole of the Foley catheter and pressure was applied to the urethra. Finally, catheterization was completed through this guide wire (Fig. 1).

Patients' clinical data and statistical analysis

The following clinical data were assessed: age, past history, previous history of urologic operations, medication for lower urinary tract symptoms, site of catheterization, reason for catheterization, history of trauma, and RGU finding. Baseline characteristics were compared via ANOVA for continuous variables and via chi-square test for categorical variables. Univariate and multivariate logistic regression analyses were performed to identify predictive factors for the failure of RGU-assisted urethral catheterization. The two-sided p-values of <0.2 and <0.005 were considered statistically significant for the univariate and multivariate analyses, respectively. All statistical analyses were performed using SPSS Statistics version 20.0.0 (IBM Corp., Armonk, NY, USA).

Results

In total, 136 patients underwent RGU-assisted urethral catheterization. Of these 136, 94 (69.1%) experienced successful RGU-assisted urethral catheterization and 42 (30.9%) experienced failed RGU-assisted urethral catheterization. Moreover, 18 (13.2%) patients required suprapubic percutaneous catheterization or cystoscopy-assisted urethral catheterization after failed RGU-assisted urethral catheterization, and 15 (11.0%) were treated via urethral sound dilatation after successful RGU-assisted urethral catheterization.

Patients' baseline clinical characteristics are presented in Table 1. In our study, 18 (13.2%) patients had a previous history of urologic operations, including transurethral prostatectomy, radical prostatectomy, and endoscopic urethrotomy. Most events happened in the emergency room, and most of urethral catheterizations were performed for checking urine output, absolute bed rest or operation. Definite urethral injury under RGU was identified in 33 (24.3%) patients.

The complete results of our univariate and multivariate analyses are presented in Table 2. These analyses identified a previous history of urologic operations as an independent predictor of failed RGU-assisted urethral catheterization (odds ratio = 9.453, 95% confidence interval = 2.703–33.063, $p < 0.001$).

Discussion

Since the Seldinger technique, which involves using a guide wire to obtain safe access to blood vessels, was introduced [9], it has been applied as a second-line method after failed initial urethral catheterization [2, 10–17]. The Seldinger technique safely to indwell urethral

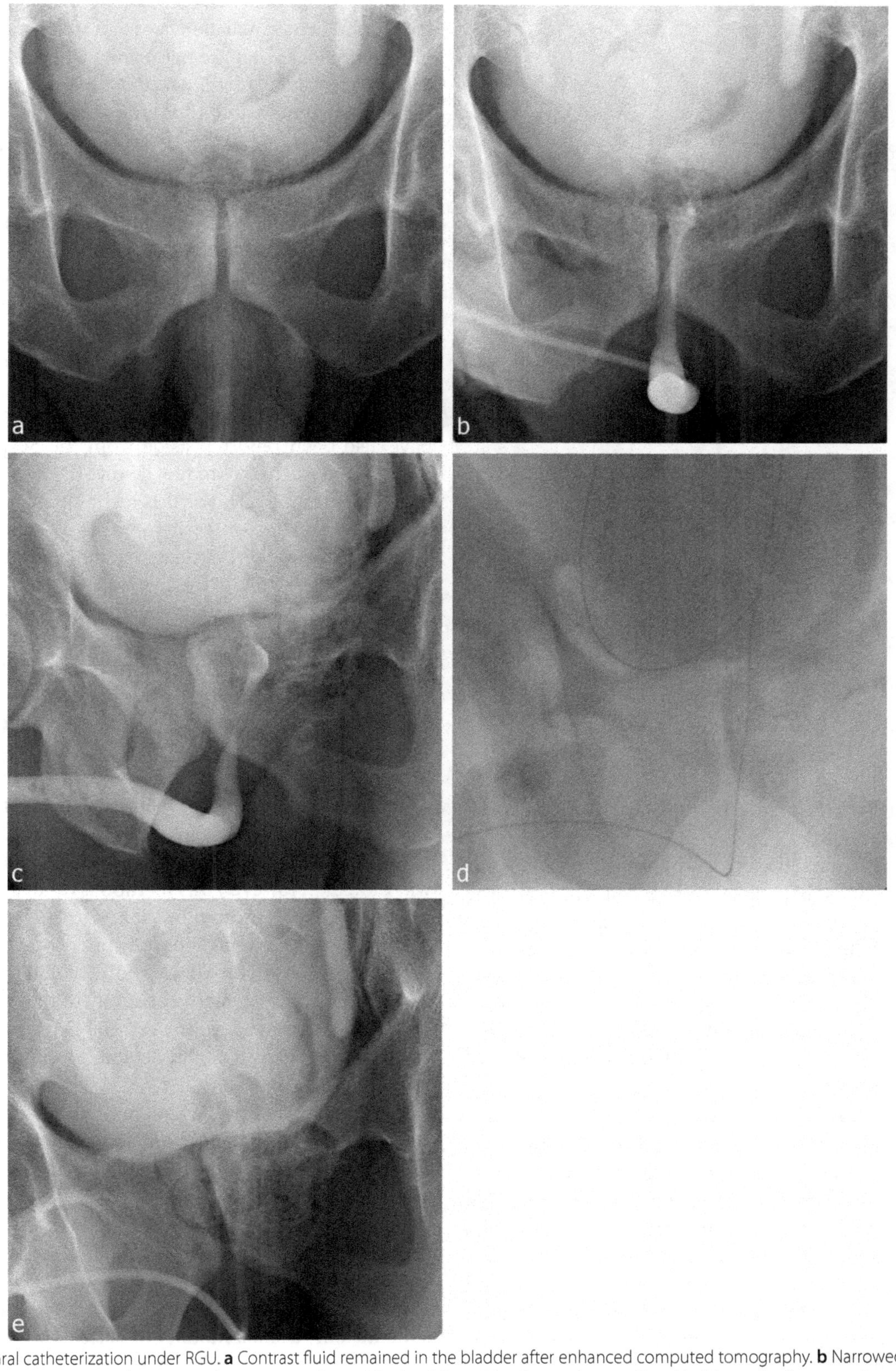

Fig. 1 Urethral catheterization under RGU. **a** Contrast fluid remained in the bladder after enhanced computed tomography. **b** Narrowed prostatic urethra. **c** An oblique image of a narrowed prostatic urethra. **c** A hydrophilic guide wire was inserted into bladder under fluoroscopic guidance. **d** Foley catheter was inserted into the bladder using a hydrophilic guide wire

Table 1 Patients characteristics

Age	**76.0 (65.0–81.0)**
Past history	
Cerebral vascular disease	29
Heart disease	28
Pulmonary disease	47
Diabetes	20
Hypertension	50
Chronic renal failure	10
Previous urologic procedure	18
Medication for LUTS	56
Site	
ER	89
Ward	47
Reason for catheterization	
AUR	23
Routine catheterization	113
Trauma	
Perineal	122
None	11
Others	3
RGU finding	
Except urethral rupture	103
Urethral rupture	33

catheter can be classified according to whether cystoscopy is used or not.

Urethral catheterization using only hydrophilic guide wires for DDUCs has been introduced [11–17]. The insertion of a hydrophilic guide wire, which helps to lead the urethral catheter to the correct location, can be performed without causing trauma to the urethra and with minimal pain to the patient [13]. Unfortunately, this technique is often unsuccessful making a false passage or tissue damage, because the location of guide wire could not be affirmed [11].

Recently, a novel Foley catheter that integrates a hydrophilic guide wire has also been introduced [2]. Physicians have advocated for the use of this device by reporting that it is relatively simple to use and its use results in high success rates with a 0% incidence rate of adverse events for nurse-led male urethral catheterization. However, it is difficult to guarantee a 100% success rate for the general population because this novel catheter has not been used in cases where slight resistance during urethral catheterization was present.

There have also been several reports about performing urethral catheterization via the Seldinger technique with a flexible cystoscope [10, 18]. The authors of such a report stated that the success rate of this method was 96% [10]. Further, Villanueva et al. reported on the common approaches that are performed when initial urethral catheterization fails [19]. Based on an online survey, urologic residents most commonly resorted to flexible cystoscopy as opposed to the blind placement of guide wires or filiforms/followers after trying one or more urethral catheters. However, Villanueva et al. mentioned that urethral catheterization with flexible cystoscopy assistance is limited in terms of economics and time saving. Further, it is important to consider the learning curve for performing flexible cystoscopy. MacKenzie et al. reported that acceptable flexible cystoscopy was achieved by the 122nd procedure [20]. In other words, this procedure can only be performed with a certain level of expertise.

Other second-line urethral catheterization techniques have also been reported aside from the Seldinger technique. One such technique involves using pressure to open the urethra [21]. For this technique, a syringe filled with normal saline or sterile water is attached to behind of a typical catheter, drainage channel. By pressing the plunger of the syringe, the hydrostatic effect of the fluid helps to separate the prostatic lobes, thereby providing the tip of the catheter easier passage into the bladder [21].

Moreover, Kameda et al. attempted using trans-abdominal ultrasonography as a second-line urethral catheterization method [22]. They evaluated whether trans-abdominal ultrasonography could show the tip of a urethral catheter and whether trans-abdominal ultrasound-guided catheterization with transrectal pressure could result in successful catheterization for male patients in whom performing standard catheterization was difficult. However, this method is difficult to perform without an experienced physician.

Minagawa et al. reported that trans-rectal ultrasonography can be useful for DDUCs [6]. It could provide more clear findings regarding the anatomy of the male urethra. However, this procedure can only be performed by experienced physicians who understand trans-rectal ultrasound findings.

In a study including 10 patients, Athanasopoulos et al. suggested that using a ureteral access sheath for urethral dilation was helpful for the catheterization of difficult urethral strictures [23]. They mentioned that the use of both a hydrophilic guide wire and ureteral sheath proved their technique's efficacy and resulted in the atraumatic characteristics observed within the ureteral lumen. However, while successful catheterization was achieved in all patients, only a small number of patients were enrolled.

RGU-assisted urethral catheterization is a method that combined the following techniques: the Seldinger technique, fluoroscopy, and the application of hydrostatic pressure to the urethra. Therefore, the greatest advantage

Table 2 Predictive factors for the failure of urethral catheterization under RGU

Univariate analysis		
Variables	**OR**	***p* value**
Age		
Continuous	0.985 (0.957–1.014)	0.311
Categorized	1.198 (0.578–2.481)	0.627
Past history		
Cerebral vascular disease	1.175 (0.488–2.830)	0.718
Heart disease	1.024 (0.416–2.518)	0.959
Pulmonary disease	0.603 (0.271–1.340)	0.214
Diabetes	0.657 (0.221–1.953)	0.450
Hypertension	1.187 (0.554–2.545)	0.659
Chronic renal failure	0.219 (0.027–1.794)	**0.157**
Previous urologic procedure	8.200 (2.671–25.177)	**< 0.001**
Medication for LUTS	0.746 (0.349–1.597)	0.451
Site (ER vs GW)	0.674 (0.306–1.485)	0.328
Reason for catheterization (AUR vs routine)	0.514 (0.205–1.289)	**0.156**
Perineal trauma (vs none)	0.472 (0.098–2.287)	0.351
RGU finding (others vs rupture)	0.640 (0.261–1.568)	0.329
Multivariate analysis		
Variables	**OR**	***p* value**
Chronic renal failure	0.211 (0.022–2.021)	0.177
Previous urologic procedure	9.453 (2.703–33.063)	**< 0.001**
Reason for catheterization (AUR vs routine)	0.805 (0.279–3.320)	0.688

of this method is that it allows clinicians to clearly identify the anatomy of the urethra and evaluate the position of the guide wire. Moreover, the catheter tip could be easily inserted into the bladder because the application of hydrostatic pressure of the mixture of contrast solution and normal saline during RGU, to the urethra helped to separate the prostatic lobes. In summary, RGU-assisted urethral catheterization is a method that provides a combination of the advantages of previously reported methods. This procedure is relatively simple to implement, whereas urethral catheterization through flexible cystoscopy requires an experienced urologist.

Previous urological procedures were identified as an independent predictor for the failure of this method in multivariate analysis. Prostate transurethral resection, visual internal urethral resection, prostate holmium laser resection, and simple or radical prostatectomy are common surgeries in this category. The authors contend that these procedures resulted in an anatomical change in the urethra that the Foley catheter or guide wire could not pass through. If the patient has no history mentioned above, this method is worth considering clinically.

Our study is limited because it is retrospective in nature, it assessed only single-center data, and it did not include a large number of patients. Therefore, the results of our study must be confirmed and validated with a prospective large-scale multi-center study. Further, radiation exposure was not evaluated in our study, and a successful catheterization rate of 69.1% may not be satisfactory. However, high success rates can be expected after appropriate patient selection, as a history of previous urologic operations was identified as an independent predictor of failed RGU-assisted urethral catheterization.

Conclusions

RGU-assisted urethral catheterization can be considered one of the methods for providing successful catheterization after failed conventional urethral catheterization. In particular, if there is no previous history of urologic operations, such as urethrotomy and transurethral prostatectomy, RGU-assisted urethral catheterization can be an effective procedure for DDUCs.

Abbreviations

RGU: Retrograde urethrography; DDUC: Difficult during urethral catheterization; BPH: Benign prostatic hypertrophy; LUTS: Lower urinary tract symptoms; ER: Emergency room; AUR: Acute urinary retention.

Acknowledgements

This manuscript was prepared with the assistance of EDITAGE, an English-language scientific editing company.

Authors' contributions

Si Hyun Kim: Conceptualization, Data curation, Methodology, Validation, Investigation, Writing-original draft. Hee Jo Yang, Doo Sang Kim, Chang Ho Lee, Youn Soo Jeon: Data curation, Validation, Investigation. Ki Hong Kim: Conceptualization, Data curation, Methodology, Validation, Investigation, Writing-original review & editing. All authors read and approved the final manuscript.

Competing interests

The authors declare that they have no competing interests.

References

1. Jain P, Parada JP, David A, Smith LG. Overuse of the indwelling urinary tract catheter in hospitalized medical patients. Arch Intern Med. 1995;155(13):1425–9.
2. Bugeja S, Mistry K, Yim IHW, Tamimi A, Roberts N, Mundy AR. A new urethral catheterisation device (UCD) to manage difficult urethral catheterisation. World J Urol. 2019;37(4):595–600.
3. Kashefi C, Messer K, Barden R, Sexton C, Parsons JK. Incidence and prevention of iatrogenic urethral injuries. J Urol. 2008;179(6):2254–7.
4. Wagner KR, Bird ET, Coffield KS. Urinary catheterization: a paradigm shift in difficult urinary catheterization. Curr Urol Rep. 2016;17(11):82.
5. Davis NF, Quinlan MR, Bhatt NR, Browne C, MacCraith E, Manecksha R, Walsh MT, Thornhill JA, Mulvin D. Incidence, cost, complications and clinical outcomes of iatrogenic urethral catheterization injuries: a prospective multi-institutional study. J Urol. 2016;196(5):1473–7.
6. Minagawa T, Suzuki T, Domen T, Yokoyama H, Ishikawa M, Hirakata S, Nagai T, Nakazawa M, Ogawa T, Ishizuka O. Modified sonourethrography assists urethral catheterization. J Med Ultrasonics (2001). 2016;43(3):443–8.
7. Villanueva C, Hemstreet GP 3rd. Difficult male urethral catheterization: a review of different approaches. IntBraz J Urol. 2008;34(4):401–11.
8. Manalo M Jr, Lapitan MC, Buckley BS. Medical interns' knowledge and training regarding urethral catheter insertion and insertion-related urethral injury in male patients. BMC Med Educ. 2011;11:73.
9. Seldinger SI. Catheter replacement of the needle in percutaneous arteriography; a new technique. Acta Radiologica (Stockholm, Sweden: 1987). 1953;39(5):368–76.
10. Beaghler M, Grasso M 3rd, Loisides P. Inability to pass a urethral catheter: the bedside role of the flexible cystoscope. Urology. 1994;44(2):268–70.
11. Blitz BF. A simple method using hydrophilic guide wires for the difficult urethral catheterization. Urology. 1995;46(1):99–100.
12. Pachler J, Frimodt-Moller C. A comparison of prelubricated hydrophilic and non-hydrophilic polyvinyl chloride catheters for urethral catheterization. BJU Int. 1999;83(7):767–9.
13. Zammit PA, German K. The difficult urethral catheterization: use of a hydrophilic guidewire. BJU Int. 2004;93(6):883–4.
14. Levy B, Charkin A. A revised guide-wire technique for urethral catheter insertion. Ann R Coll Surg Engl. 2006;88(2):228–9.
15. Tang VC, Bott SR. A better way to insert urethral catheter with guide-wire. Ann R College Surg Engl. 2006;88(7):693.
16. Kaynar M, Akand M, Goktas S. A novel cannulation technique for difficult urethral catheterization. Associazione Ricerche Urol. 2016;88(1):60–1.
17. Yuminaga Y, Kam J, Louie-Johnsun M. Multi-centre, prospective evaluation of the Seldinger technique for difficult male urethral catheter insertions by non-urology trained doctors. BJU Int. 2017;120(Suppl 3):21–7.
18. Krikler SJ. Flexible urethroscopy: use in difficult male catheterisation. Ann R Coll Surg Engl. 1989;71(1):3.
19. Villanueva C, Hemstreet GP 3rd. The approach to the difficult urethral catheterization among urology residents in the United States. Int Braz J Urol. 2010;36(6):710–5.
20. MacKenzie KR, Aning J. Defining competency in flexible cystoscopy: a novel approach using cumulative Sum analysis. BMC Urol. 2016;16(1):31.
21. Harkin DW, Hawe M, Pyper P. A novel technique for difficult male urethral catheterization. Br J Urol. 1998;82(5):752–3.
22. Kameda T, Murata Y, Fujita M, Isaka A. Transabdominal ultrasound-guided urethral catheterization with transrectal pressure. J Emerg Med. 2014;46(2):215–9.
23. Athanasopoulos A, Liatsikos EN. The use of a ureteral access sheath for the urethral dilatation and catheterization of difficult urethral strictures. Urol Int. 2009;83(3):359–61.

Optimal treatment for penile verrucous carcinoma

Dong In Jo[1], Song Hyun Han[1], Soon Heum Kim[1], Hye Young Kim[2], Hong Chung[3] and Hong Sup Kim[3*]

Abstract

Background: Verrucous carcinoma, a rare low-grade well-differentiated squamous cell carcinoma, is known for its favorable biological behavior and lack of metastatic potential. However, aggressive resection is problematic in terms of compromised function and aesthetics. Hence, more conservative treatments are needed. Methods: To identify the up-to-date general biological behavior, diagnosis, and treatment trends, we searched PubMed using the keyword "penile verrucous carcinoma" without restrictions on publication date. Results: Current treatments for penile verrucous carcinoma include wide surgical excision, seldom preventive lymphadenectomy, and conservative chemotherapy without surgery or local excision with safe margins. Despite the advent of partial penectomy to minimally impact function and aesthetics, affected patients experience psychosexual problems. Local excision can be used to save the penile shaft and glans penis without preventive lymphadenectomy or adjuvant therapy and can achieve good clinical prognosis with rare recurrence. Conclusions: To preserve the functional and cosmetic aspects, we recommend local excision, especially for tumors measuring < 3 cm and classified as stage T1 according to the 2016 tumor node metastasis clinical and pathological classification for penile cancer.

Keywords: Local excision, Penile verrucous carcinoma, Squamous cell carcinoma

Background

Verrucous carcinoma, a rare low-grade well-differentiated squamous cell carcinoma (SCC), is known for its slowly compressive expanding warty growth and rare metastasis [1–3]. Aggressive treatment, such as penectomy, has been suggested based on the concept that penile verruca carcinoma (PVC) is malignant. In contrast, less aggressive treatment, such as local excision without preventive lymphadenectomy, has been suggested based on the concept that the biological behavior of PVC resembles that of a benign tumor. In patients who had undergone aggressive wide surgical excision of the glans penis and penile shaft, many functional, cosmetic, and psychosexual problems have been reported. To date, surgical treatment trends have been unclear regarding the use of preservation surgery. Here we reviewed the literature to determine the most effective treatment for PVC and suggest best practices for treatment guidelines.

Methods

To summarize the prevalence, causative factors, diagnostic methods, treatment methods, clinical behaviors, diagnostic imaging techniques, and prognosis of PVC, we searched PubMed for relevant studies using the keyword "penile verrucous carcinoma" without restrictions on publication year and retrieved abstracts published in English that mentioned PVC diagnosis and treatment. The abstracts were screened according to inclusion and exclusion criteria. The inclusion criteria were presented cases and the corresponding treatment methods, microscopic diagnosis of PVC, availability of full text articles, and publication in English. The exclusion criteria were lack of tumor staging information and tumor staging beyond T2 (Stage T2 penile cancers are different from penile verrucous carcinoma and defined as invasive

*Correspondence: hskim@kku.ac.kr
[3] Department of Urology, Konkuk University School of Medicine, Gukwon-daero 82, 27376 Chungju, Chungbuk, Republic of Korea
Full list of author information is available at the end of the article

cancers such as squamous cell carcinoma and others). To check the association between treatment method and conditions of cases, the treatments were categorized into 2 groups—the less aggressive treatment group included shaving, local excision, and no surgery and the aggressive treatment group included glansectomy, partial penectomy, and total penectomy. Individual factors included age, case history, tumor size, tumor shape, tumor location, tumor stage, adjuvant treatment, lymph node metastasis, disease-free status, recurrence, human papilloma virus (HPV) infection status, and treatment trends over time.

The statistical analysis was performed using SPSS for Windows version 25 (SPSS Inc., Chicago, IL, USA). We hypothesized that aggressive treatment is more effective and investigated the difference in efficacy between the 2 treatments. We performed a t-test, a chi-squared test, and Fisher's exact test to ensure data accuracy and a regression analysis to examine whether the individual factors were correlated in the 2 groups.

Results

A total of 276 articles were retrieved from PubMed. Among them, 68 abstracts that mentioned PVC diagnosis and/or treatment and were published in English were selected. The studies were published between 1969 and February 2019. Most of the studies were published in English; other publication languages included Spanish (14), Chinese (3), French (3), Japanese (2), Bulgarian (1), Israeli (1), and Italian (1). Several studies mentioned regarding PVC treatment and were simple case reports [4–47]. Its rarity is supported by the fact that 1 case in a 10-year period and 13 cases in a 30-year period were reported [10, 48–51]. Among the 68 studies retrieved, 28 met the inclusion criteria. Of those, 9 were excluded according to the exclusion criteria. Thus, a total of 19 studies were subjected to full-text review (Fig. 1) [4–7, 10, 11, 20, 23, 31, 32, 35, 37–40, 43, 45–47].

The studies comprised a total of 58 cases of PVC (Table 1). The patients were 28–86 years of age. The case histories were 1–204 months long. The tumor sizes were 0.8–10 cm. Fifty-4 of the cases included a description of tumor shape: papillary cauliflower in 30, keratotic horn-like in 3, and warty verrucous in 21. The tumors involved the glans in 33 cases, coronoid sulcus in 4, shaft in 4, prepuce in 7, prepuce and glans in 4, glans and coronoid sulcus and shaft in 1, prepuce and coronoid sulcus in 2, glans and coronoid sulcus in 2, and coronoid sulcus and shaft in 1. A total of 10 cases involved the coronoid sulcus, an area in which penile carcinoma would more rapidly infiltrate the penile fascia. Regarding staging, 52 cases were classified as stage Ta, 4 were classified as T1, and 2 were classified as T1a. Regarding treatment, no surgery was performed in 4 cases, local excision was performed in 10, shaving in 3, Mohs surgery was performed in 2, circumcision was performed in 1, glansectomy was performed in 3, partial penectomy was performed in 29, and total penectomy was performed in 6. Thus, 20 cases involved less aggressive treatment and 38 cases involved aggressive treatment. Fifteen cases of adjuvant treatment were reported, including 1 of radiotherapy, 6 of chemotherapy, 2 of chemoradiotherapy, and 6 of local therapy (CO_2 laser, cryotherapy, intralesional interferon, and topical fluorouracil). There was only 1 case of lymph node metastasis. The reported lymphadenopathies were revealed as inflammation without metastasis [4–6]. One case of bilateral lymph node metastasis, which was suspected as a mixed tumor condition with moderately differentiated SCC, was reported [35]. The follow-up period was 6–228 months (19 years). There were 7 cases of tumor recurrence: 5 in the less aggressive treatment group and 2 in the aggressive treatment group. All cases except 2 achieved tumor-free status. The other 2 patients died due to other malignant conditions [35, 47]. Six cases were associated with the following diseases: anaplastic spindle cell carcinoma suggestive of malignant transformation after radiotherapy, hybrid verrucous SCC, moderately differentiated SCC, lichen sclerosis, pseudoepitheliomatous keratotic and micaceous balanitis, and human immunodeficiency virus infection. HPV infection status was described as negative in 8 cases; the others were not specified. The reported cases following the year of issue categorized in 10-year increments: 1 in the 1970s, 14 in the 1980s, 2 in the 1990s, 15 in the 2000s, and 26 in the 2010s. The main diagnostic method was biopsy. Chest x-ray, HPV polymerase chain reaction (PCR), ultrasonography, and computed tomography were optional. The best diagnostic method was biopsy and HPV PCR. Ultrasonography, computed tomography, and magnetic resonance imaging (MRI) offered more precise information about tumor anatomy and regional lymphadenopathy. Two reports mentioned surgical treatment guidelines according to tumor size [8] and depth [17]. Concerning surgical excision, the main treatment was radical surgery, including at least partial penectomy [4–47], even with the relatively small tumor size (<3 cm) [8]. The surgical margins were 2 cm in cases of partial penectomy and 0.3–1 cm in cases of local excision (Table 2) [5, 6]. In contrast, some studies have emphasized the good clinical results of local excision because of the favorable clinical behavior of PVC [5, 6, 11, 15, 17, 31, 32, 37, 39, 40, 43, 45–47].

The results of the t-test using categories of age, case history, and tumor size and the result of the cross-sectional analysis of the categories of tumor shape, disease-free status, and HPV status were excluded since some

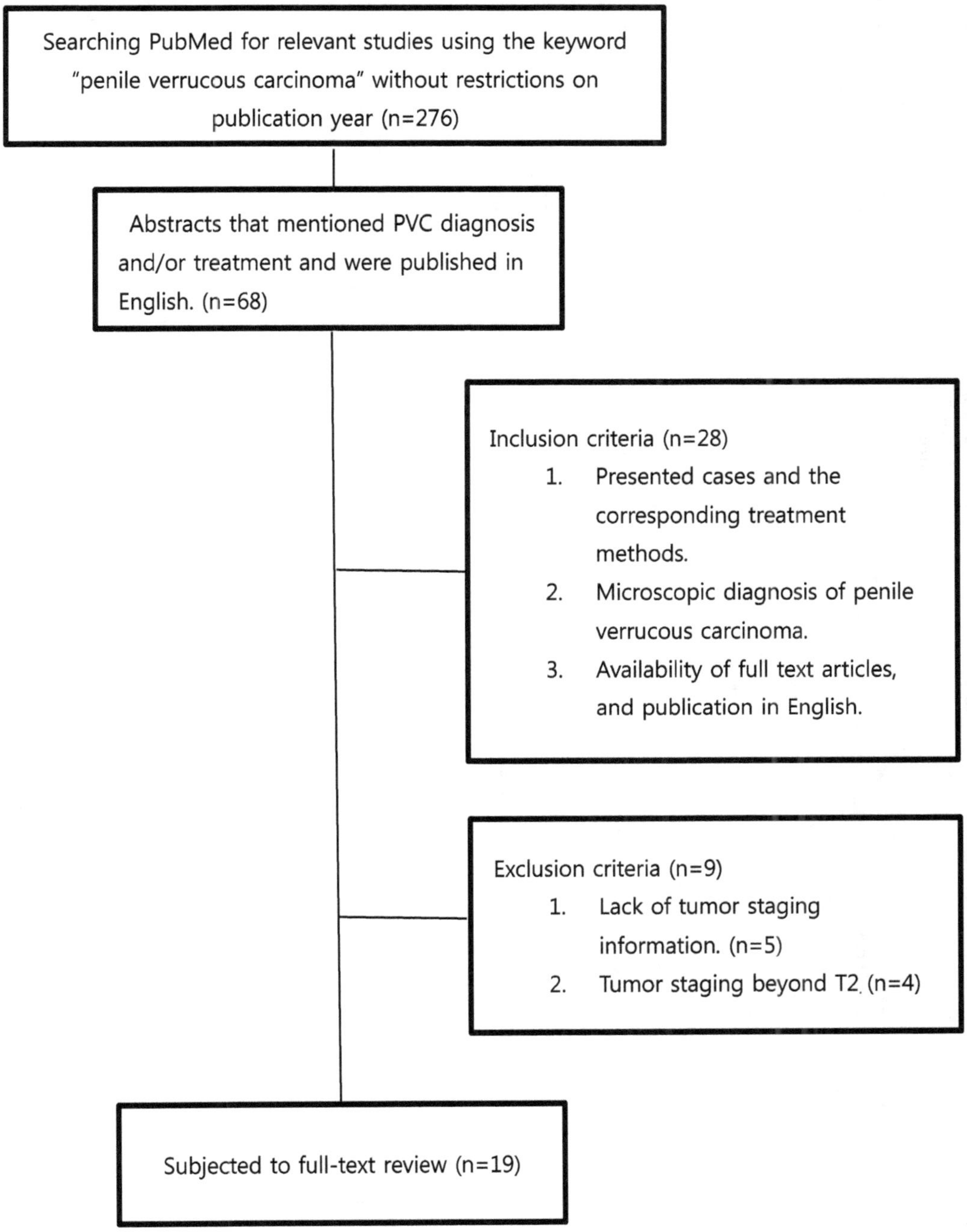

Fig. 1 The study flow chart

individual data for each case were missing (data not shown). In the cross-sectional analysis, tumor location, tumor stage, and recurrence were not significantly associated with either treatment. Regarding the clinical results, all but 2 patients (who died of other malignant conditions) achieved disease-free status. Regarding treatment efficacy, the recurrence rates did not differ significantly between the less aggressive and aggressive treatments. Patients who received adjuvant therapy tended to ultimately receive less aggressive treatment. Regarding the test statistics, the X^2 was 21.926 and the probability was 0.000. Thus, the results were statistically significant. Regarding differences in treatment trends over time, the X^2 was 12.549 and the probability was 0.005. Thus, the result was statistically significant (Table 3).

Table 1 Clinical manifestations of penile verrucous carcinoma

Case (Ref.)	Age (years)	Case history (months)	Tumor size (Cm)	Tumor shape	Tumor location	Stage (TNM)	Operation	Adjuvant threatment	Lymphnode metasatsis	Follow up (months) /disease free	Recurrence (months after)	Associated disease	HPV	Year of issue
1(47)	49	12	5 × 4.5 x 2	Papillary cauliflower	Glans, coronoid sulcus,	Ta	local excision	Systemic bleomycine, methotrexate,	none	48/no	24	Anaplastic spindle cell carcinoma	Negative	1994
					shaft			Radiotherapy				Malignant transformation after Radiotherapy		
2(46)	62	3	3	Cauliflower-like	Prepuce, coronal sulcus	Ta	Local excision	None	None	54/yes	26	Hybrid verrucous-squamous cell carcinoma	Negative	2000
3(45)	42	4	7	Cauliflower-like	Prepuce, glans	Ta	Local excision	CO_2 laser	None	36/yes	None	None	?	2008
4(43)	51	24	?	Verrucous	Glans, coronary sulcus	Ta	Recurred mass	Liquid nitrogne, topical 5% fluorouracil	None	42/yes	None	None	?	1978
							after local excision							
							and skin graft							
							after local excision							
5(40)	60	?	?	?	Glans	Ta	Shaving	Intralesional interferone	None	30/yes	None	None	Negative	2000
6(39)	69	24	1	Keratotic	Glans	Ta	Shaving	Cryosurgery with liquid nitrogen	None	36/yes	None	None	?	2002
7(39)	69	24	1.5	Keratotic	Glans	Ta	Shaving	Cryosurgery with liquid nitrogen	None	36/yes	None	None	?	

Table 1 (continued)

Case (Ref.)	Age (years)	Case history (months)	Tumor size (Cm)	Tumor shape	Tumor location	Stage (TNM)	Operation	Adjuvant threatment	Lymphnode metasatsis	Follow up (months) /disease free	Recurrence (months after)	Associated disease	HPV	Year of issue
8(38)	27	12	5 × 5	Verrucous	gLans	Ta	None	Intra-aortic infusion with metho-trexate	None	214/yes	None	None	?	2003
9(38)	65	3	4 × 3	Warty	Glans	Ta	None	Intra-aortic infusion with metho-trexate	None	165/yes	None	None	?	
10(38)	31	48	5 × 5	?	Shaft	Ta	Total penec-tomy	Intra-aortic infusion with metho-trexate	None	149/yes	36/partial	None	?	
							due to partial response and unbara-ble pain				Response			
11(38)	75	120	2 × 2	?	Glans	Ta	None	Intra-aortic infusion with metho-trexate	none	104/yes	None	None	?	
12(37)	70	?	?	Verrucous	Shaft, base of penis	T1	Mohs sur-gery and FTSG	Cisplatin and fluo-rouracil with radio-therapy	none	36/yes	16	None	negative	2009
							after recur-rence (local excision)							
13(35)	47	3	4 × 3	?	Prepuce, glans	Ta	Total penec-tomy	Intra-aortic infusion with metho-trexate	Bilateral	37/no	18/partial	Moderately differ-entiated squamous cell	?	2010

Table 1 (continued)

Case (Ref.)	Age (years)	Case history (months)	Tumor size (Cm)	Tumor shape	Tumor location	Stage (TNM)	Operation	Adjuvant threatment	Lymphnode metasatsis	Follow up (months) /disease free	Recurrence (months after)	Associated disease	HPV	Year of issue
							due to partial response				Response	Carcinoma, malignant transfor-mation?		
14(35)	28	72	5 × 4.5x2	Verrucous	Prepuce, glans	Ta	None	Intra-aortic infusion with metho-trexate	None	45/yes	None	None	?	
15(32)	42	?	1	Warty	Glans	Ta	Mohs sur-gery	None (healed by secondary intention)	None	12/yes	None	Lichen sclerosus	?	1987
16(31)	74	12	2 × 1.5	Warty	Glans	Ta	Local exci-sion	Failed cryo-therapy with liquid nitrogen	None	48/yes	None	Pseudoepi-thelioma-tous	negative	2000
				Nodule			(surgical margin 2 cm)					Keratotic and micaceous balanitis		
17(23)	60	7	3 × 3	Verrucous, ulcerative	Prepuce, glans	Ta	Partial penec-tomy	None	None	24/yes	None	Human immuno-deficiency virus infec-tion	negative	2015
18(20)	71	6	2.8 × 1.6	Keratotic hornlike	Glans	T1a	Partial penec-tomy	None	None	10/yes	None	None	Negative	1990
							total penec-tomy	(due to residual tumor on the resection margins)						
19(11)	61	?	7 × 4	Cauliflower-like	Shaft	T1a	Local exc-sion, skin graft	None	None	36/yes	None	None	?	2019

Table 1 (continued)

Case (Ref.)	Age (years)	Case history (months)	Tumor size (Cm)	Tumor shape	Tumor location	Stage (TNM)	Operation	Adjuvant threatment	Lymphnode metasatsis	Follow up (months) /disease free	Recurrence (months after)	Associated disease	HPV	Year of issue
20(10)	30 to 86	at least 12	1 to 8	Warty or fungating	11 glans	10 Ta	9 partial penectomy	All none but	All	72 to 228	All	All none	All	1985
	mean 47	in 10 cases	mean 3.6	(multiple nodules	2 prepuce	3 T1	3 total penectomy	1 radiotherapy	none	/yes	none		?	
		(in 5 cases		in 7 cases)			1 circumcision	(before total penaectomy)						
	13 cases	2,2,4,8,17 years)												
		in 3 cases												
32(10)		(1,2,4 months)												
33(7)	40 to 63	8 to 25	2.5 to 6.2	Cauliflower-like	Glans	Ta	Glansectomy	None	None	18 to 65	None	None	?	2001
	mean 54 ± 7						with frozen section			mean 38 ± 14				
34(7)				Cauliflower-like	Glans	Ta	Glansectomy	None	None	/Yes	None	None	?	
35(7)				Cauliflower-like	Glans	Ta	Partial penectomy after	None	None		3	None	?	
							glansectomy							
36(7)				Cauliflower-like	Glans	Ta	Glansectomy	None	None		None	None	?	
37(6)	73	12	3	Verrucous	coronary sulcus, shaft	Ta	Local excision	None	None	24/yes	None	None	Negative	2017
38(5)	52	96	6	All	coronoid sulcus	all	Partial penectomy	All none	All	6 to 60	All	Squamous atypical hyperplasia	All	2011
39(5)	85	48	3	Exophytic papillary	Glans	Ta	Local excision		None	mean 36	None	None	?	
40(5)	55	24	5	Cauliflower-like	Coronoid sulcus		Partial penectomy			/yes		None		

Table 1 (continued)

Case (Ref.)	Age (years)	Case history (months)	Tumor size (Cm)	Tumor shape	Tumor location	Stage (TNM)	Operation	Adjuvant threatment	Lymphnode metasatsis	Follow up (months) /disease free	Recurrence (months after)	Associated disease	HPV	Year of issue
41(5)	64	3	2		Glans		Partial penec-tomy					None		
42(5)	74	3	3		Glans		Local exci-sion					Squamous papilloma		
43(5)	56	12	2		Glans		Local exc-sion					Squamous atypical hyperpla-sia		
44(5)	52	3	2.5		Coronoid sulcus		Partial penec-tomy					None		
45(5)	55	24	10		Shaft		Partial penec-tomy					Squamous atypical hyperpla-sia		
46(5)	68	60	2		Coronoid sulcus		Circumci-sion,	Surgical margin 2 cm for partial penec-tomy				None		
							Partial penec-tomy	0.5–1 cm for local excision						
47(5)	70	6	4.5		Glans		Partial penec-tomy	Acknowl-edging excessive resection in 3 cases				None		
48(5)	49	3	3		Glans		Partial penec-tomy	For the small-sized mass limited to glans				None		
49(4)	35 to 72	All ?	0.8 to 4	All	5 prepuce	All	All	All none	All	8 to 108	All	All	All	2015

Table 1 (continued)

Case (Ref.)	Age (years)	Case history (months)	Tumor size (Cm)	Tumor shape	Tumor location	Stage (TNM)	Operation	Adjuvant threatment	Lymphnode metasatsis	Follow up (months) /disease free	Recurrence (months after)	Associated disease	HPV	Year of issue
50(4)	mean 51.5			Cauliflower-like	1 prepuce, coronoid sulcus	Ta	Partial penec-tomy		None	/Yes	but 1 case	but 1 squamous metapla-sia with	?	
51(4)					1 glans, coronoid sulcus						36, 60, 84	partial hyperkera-tosis		
52(4)					3 glans									
53(4)														
54(4)	10 cases													
55(4)														
56(4)														
57(4)								8 Biopsy before surgical treatment						
58(4)								2 circum-cision before surgical treatment						

?; missing individual data, Ref.; reference number

Table 2 Cumulative data of clinical presentations and treatments

Total cases	58
Age (years)	28–86
Case History (months)	1–204
Size (Cm)	0.8–10
Tumor shape	
Papillary cauliflower	30
Keratotic hornlike	3
Warty verrucous	21
Unknown	4
Location (cases)	
Glans	33
Coronoid sulcus	4
Shaft	4
Prepuce	7
Prepuce and glans	4
Glans and coronoid sulcus and shaft	1
Prepuce and coronoid sulcus	2
Glans and coronoid sulcus	2
Coronoid sulcus and shaft	1
Coronoid sulcus involvement	10
Stage (cases)	
Ta	52
T1	6
Treatment (cases)	
No surgery	4
Local excision	10
Shaving	3
Mohs surgery	2
Circumcision	1
Glansectomy	3
Partial penectomy	29
Total penectomy	6
Adjuvant treatment (cases)	
Radiotherapy	1
Chemotherapy	6
Chemoradiotherapy	2
Local therapy (CO_2 laser, cryotherapy, intralesional interferon, and topical fluorouracil)	6
Lymphnode metastasis (cases)	1
Follow up period (months)	6–228
Recurrence (cases)	7
Disease free (cases)	56
Surgical margin (Cm)	0.3–2
Cases following the year of issue (cases)	
1970s	1
1980s	14
1990s	2
2000s	15
2010s	26

According to the regression analysis of age, case history, tumor size, tumor shape, tumor location, tumor stage, adjuvant treatment, tumor recurrence, and treatment trends over time did not appear to have a significant negative or positive effect (data not shown).

In summary, the associations between tumor location and treatment method and tumor depth and treatment method were not statistically significant. Adjuvant therapy tended to be performed alone or with local excision preventing a penectomy or glansectomy. Partial penectomy cases (aggressive treatment group) were predominantly reported in the 2010s. No intergroup differences were seen in clinical results. Therefore, our hypothesis that aggressive treatment is more effective was rejected.

Discussion

Some studies have reported that PVC is observed in approximately 2.4–24% of all penile cancers and 20% of verruciform lesions of the penis; PVC is also observed in patients with Buschke–Löwenstein, warty carcinoma, and papillary SCC [1–3]. Several cases have been reported during the past 2–3 decades among many countries due to its rarity [10, 48–51]. PVC primarily occurs in the glans penis, and phimosis and redundant prepuce are 2 of its important causes [2, 52]. Lichen sclerosus and pseudoepitheliomatous, keratotic, and micaceous balanitis are other possible causes [31–33, 53]. Local squamous epithelial hyperplasia and hyperkeratosis may be important in the development of PVC [54, 55]. Clinically, they do not cause significant pain, but they grow slowly and uninhibited, sometimes invading the shaft over the glans. In most cases, the patients present with a slow-growing mass with multiple papillary lesions [4–6].

Biopsy and HPV PCR tests are basic diagnostic tools for differentiating PVC from HPV-related tumors. Increased immunohistochemical expression of markers such as Mdm2 and Ki67 and low expression of Bcl-2 may be useful for the detection of PVC [56–58]. Microscopically, the hematoxylin- and eosin-stained sections shows extension of the epithelium downward into the underlying tissues in a bulbous or drumstick process, while the tumor exhibits clear boundaries and rich lymphocytic infiltration into the surrounding mesenchyme [4–6].

To avoid misdiagnosis, repeated deeper biopsies are recommended that include the basement membrane of the papillomatous tumor, especially in cases in which PVC is highly suspected. However, because the gross morphology of PVC is very similar to that of condyloma acuminatum, it can be difficult to identify. HPV is known to be closely associated with penile cancer and condyloma acuminatum in most cases [8]. In contrast, in all PVC cases, the pathogenesis is not associated with HPV infection [3, 59–61]. Thus, an HPV-negative status may be the key in the differential diagnosis of PVC. In our study, the differential diagnosis from condyloma acuminatum was confirmed in only 8 cases. We assume that diagnostic biopsy played a decisive role since HPV infection status was unknown.

Table 3 Cross analysis (chi-square) with Fisher's exact test

			Operation		Total	χ^2 (p)
			Less aggressive treatment	Aggressive treatment		
Tumor location	Glans	Case	11	22	33	2.532 (.686)
		%	55.0%	57.9%	56.9%	
	Coronoid sulcus involvement	Case	4	6	10	
		%	20.0%	15.8%	17.2%	
Stage	Ta	Case	17	35	52	.713 (.405)
		%	85.0%	92.1%	89.7%	
	T1	Case	3	3	6	
		%	15.0%	7.9%	10.3%	
Adjuvant treatment	none	Case	8	35	43	21.926** (.000)
		%	40.0%	92.1%	74.1%	
	Radiotherapy	Case	0	1	1	
		%	0.0%	2.6%	1.7%	
	Chemotherapy	Case	4	2	6	
		%	20.0%	5.3%	10.3%	
	Chemoradiotherapy	Case	2	0	2	
		%	10.0%	0.0%	3.4%	
	Local therapy	Case	6	0	6	
		%	30.0%	0.0%	10.3%	
Recurrence	No	Case	17	34	51	.247 (.619)
		%	85.0%	89.5%	87.9%	
	Yes	Case	3	4	7	
		%	15.0%	10.5%	12.1%	
Treatment trends over time following the year of issue	1970s	Case	1	0	1	12.549** (.005)
		%	5.0%	0.0%	1.7%	
	1980s	Case	2	12	14	
		%	10.0%	31.6%	24.1%	
	1990s	Case	1	1	2	
		%	5.0%	2.6%	3.4%	
	2000s	Case	10	5	15	
		%	50.0%	13.2%	25.9%	
	2010s	Case	6	20	26	
		%	30.0%	52.6%	44.8%	

*$p < 0.05$, **$p < 0.01$

Surgical treatments reported in other studies focused on aggressive treatments, including glansectomy and partial or total penectomy with a 4–20-mm surgical margin [4, 5, 7, 8]. Partial penectomy with a 2-cm margin has traditionally been the suggested treatment for tumors involving the glans penis, with total penectomy being indicated when the tumor involves a larger portion of the penile shaft [49].

However, since PVC has a relatively rare incidence and is termed carcinoma despite its favorable behavior, surgeons often lack of experience treating such cases and decide to unnecessarily remove part or all of the penis. Moreover, wide excision was commonly performed for relatively small masses (≤3 cm) [5]. However, since the 1980s, local excision has been advised to preserve the penis [4–6],15,17. Mohs surgery was adopted in cases of PVC showing favorable behavior [15, 62]. The authors agree that local excision should be the first choice of treatment because of the favorable biological behavior of PVC. Treatments have been suggested according to 2 general concepts: penectomy is mandatory because PVC is malignant; and less aggressive treatment as local excision is sufficient because the biological behavior of PVC resembles that of a benign tumor.

This review revealed that the glans was the area most often involved in cases of PVC. We expected that distal and local lesions would be treated less aggressively. However, as a result, tumor location did not affect treatment aggressiveness. Interestingly, the coronoid sulcus involvement suggests that, in the absence of a dartos layer, penile carcinoma would more rapidly infiltrate the penile fascia, a known low-resistance pathway for local spread; thus, clinicians would expect a higher risk of tumor recurrence and inguinal involvement as well as a worse outcome. Thus, we expected that coronoid sulcus involvement would require more aggressive treatment. However, our results demonstrated 11 cases in the less aggressive treatment group versus 22 cases in the aggressive treatment group, respectively. Although there were more cases in the latter than the former group, the intergroup difference was insignificant.

Regarding tumor depth, PVC is defined as a superficial stage Ta lesion by the 2016 Tumor Node Metastasis (TNM) classification, a so-called non-invasive verrucous carcinoma. Although no statistically significant intergroup difference was noted, aggressive treatments were more often applied than less aggressive treatments for superficial lesions. However, 20 cases of the less aggressive treatment group showed good clinical results. Stage T1 tumors were seen, even in cases of deeper lesions. This means that less aggressive treatments with careful follow-up of stage T1 tumors can also result in good post-treatment results.

Even if a case of PVC is malignant, it may present as a benign tumor. Thus, to preserve functional and cosmetic results, we recommend that local excision with minimal surgical margins followed by careful observation be the first-line choice of treatment, especially for tumors measuring < 3 cm and classified as stage T1. In other conditions, the tumor should be considered not PVC and the excision should be widened. In our study, we excluded tumor staging beyond T2. Stage T2 penile cancers are different from PVC and defined as invasive cancers such as squamous cell carcinoma and others with bad prognosis. In these cases, aggressive treatment is recommended.

Regarding adjuvant therapy, preventive inguinal lymphadenectomy was hardly used because of rarity of evident lesions [4, 5, 9, 34, 35, 63, 64]. Conservative systemic chemotherapy without surgery was reported [35, 38]. Other adjuvant therapies for the verrucous lesion have been introduced, such as topical aminolevulinic acid–photodynamic therapy; topical, systemic, or intralesional interferon; cryotherapy; laser therapy; and radiation [35–45, 65, 66]. Our results demonstrated that adjuvant treatments were more predominantly applied when less aggressive treatment was administered. This finding supports that conservative surgery could be the first choice of treatment. However, the 4 cases treated with intralesional interferon and 1 case of cryotherapy with good clinical results could not be evaluated due to the absence of information on tumor stage [25, 41, 42].

This literature review revealed that inguinal lymphadenectomy was performed in certain patients; however, no evident lesions were found in such cases [4, 5, 9, 34, 35, 63, 64]. The 1 case of lymph node metastasis reported was suspected to be a combined lesion with moderately differentiated SCC [35]. Thus, we agree that inguinal lymphadenectomy is not an appropriate prophylactic treatment. For lymphadenopathy, treatment with anti-inflammatory drugs may be the treatment of choice, followed by a lymph node biopsy as needed. Thus, if a case of PVC is confirmed by biopsy and no signs of inguinal lymphadenopathy are seen on physical examination, further workups such as computed tomography or ultrasonography could be postponed initially, and high-end MRI saved for later and then used if needed to investigate tumor depth [67].

As for tumor behavior, complicated microlesions of invasive SCC, a certain number of which eventually progressed to other invasive types, have been observed in < 30% of the reported cases of PVC [46, 68]. There was one case of recurrent SCC after anaplastic transformation following radiation therapy [47]. Therefore, close follow-up for the early detection of any sign of recurrence requiring additional resection is essential after a less aggressive treatment, such as local excision. In our study, all but 2 cases achieved tumor-free status during long follow-up periods despite 7 cases of recurrence. Regarding those 2 cases, 1 was suspected as malignant transformation after radiotherapy to anaplastic spindle cell carcinoma [47] and the other was the previously mentioned lymph node metastasis case that eventually failed treatment and required total penectomy due to partial response after chemotherapy [35].

Despite the favorable clinical behavior of PVC and the many studies emphasizing less aggressive treatments, the use of aggressive treatment was predominantly reported in the 2010s. However, we do not think that this reflects the recent treatment trends because the timing of the reported treatment does not represent the actual clinical practice at the time.

However, information is still lacking about the association between treatment and tumor condition, evidence of which could lead us to define an appropriate guideline. Due to the limitations of a literature review, controllable factors were often undetermined. Thus, we recommend that future studies always include a unified scale for multiple factors including tumor condition and functional outcome. This mission will require long discussions and consensus of many experts. Despite this limitation, we believe that our findings are meaningful since this is the first review of diagnostic and treatment trends of PVC, a rare condition.

Conclusion

The review performed here revealed that PVC tends not to recur or metastasize after resection but that surgical treatment tends to remove too much tissue. However, in most cases of local excision, the wound heals well and local recurrence rarely occurs. Therefore, considering the ability of local excision with minimal surgical margins to spare the functional and cosmetic aspects of the penile shaft and glans penis, we recommend it as the first-line choice of treatment with observation, especially for tumors measuring < 3 cm and classified as stage T1 according to the 2016 tumor node metastasis clinical and pathological classification for penile cancer.

Abbreviations

HPV: Human papilloma virus; MRI: Magnetic resonance imaging; PCR: Polymerase chain reaction; PVC: Penile verruca carcinoma; SCC: Squamous cell carcinoma; TNM: Tumor node metastasis.

Acknowledgements

We would like to thank Editage (www.editage.co.kr) for English language editing.

Authors' contributions

HK have made substantial contributions to the conception of the work; SH, SK, HYK and HC have made substantial contributions to the acquisition and analysis of data; DJ have made substantial contributions to the design of the work and the interpretation of data and have drafted the work and substantively revised it. All authors have read and approved the final manuscript.

Competing interests

The authors declare no conflicts of interest.

Author details

[1] Department of Plastic and Reconstructive Surgery, Konkuk University School of Medicine, Chungju, Republic of Korea. [2] Department of Anesthesiology and Pain Medicine, Konkuk University School of Medicine, Chungju, Republic of Korea. [3] Department of Urology, Konkuk University School of Medicine, Gukwon-daero 82, 27376 Chungju, Chungbuk, Republic of Korea.

References

1. Chaux A, Velazquez EF, Algaba F, et al. Developments in the pathology of penile squamous cell carcinoma. Urology. 2010;76(2 Suppl 1):S7-14.
2. Schwartz RA. Verrucous carcinoma of the skin and mucosa. J Am Acad Dermatol. 1995;32(1):1–21.
3. Stankiewicz E, Kudahetti SC, Prowse DM, et al. HPV infection and immunochemical detection of cell-cycle markers in verrucous carcinoma of the penis. Mod Pathol. 2009;22(9):1160–8.
4. Li F, Xu Y, Wang H, et al. Diagnosis and treatment of penile verrucous carcinoma. Oncol Lett. 2015;9(4):1687–90.
5. Chuanyu S, Ke X, Jie Z, et al. Surgical treatment for 11 cases of penile verrucous carcinoma. Ann Dermatol. 2011;23(Suppl 3):S346-349.
6. Dong In Jo, Hong Sup Kim, et al. Local excision for the treatment of penile verrucous carcinoma. Urology Case Reports 2017;13:16–18.
7. Hatzichristou DG, Apostolidis A, Tzortzis V, et al. Glansectomy: an alternative surgical treatment for Buschke-Löwenstein tumors of the penis. Urology. 2001;57:966–9.
8. Chen GX, Li ZH, Zhang XS, Ding DG, Zhu XB, Chen X. Clinicopathological features and management of penile verrucous carcinoma. Zhonghua Nan Ke Xue. 2018;24(1):62–6.
9. Bañón Pérez V, Nicolás Torralba JA, Valdelvira Nadal P, Martínez Barba E, Server Pastor G, López Cubillana P, Prieto González A, Pérez AM. Penile verrucous carcinoma. Arch Esp Urol. 1999;52(9):937–40.
10. Johnson DE, Lo RK, Srigley J, Ayala AG. Verrucous carcinoma of the penis. J Urol. 1985;133(2):216–8.
11. Philippou P, Kitsios C, Miliatou M, Poullou C, Konstantinou P. Organ-sparing surgery for a giant verrucous carcinoma of the penile shaft: a case report and review of the literature. Case Rep Urol. 2019;2019:1537379. https://doi.org/10.1155/2019/1537379.
12. Wang ZL, Ou MR, Sun XL, Wang XF, Zhang JF, Sun LJ, Zhao P, Ji XR. Diagnosis and treatment of penile verrucous carcinoma: a report of 4 cases. Zhonghua Nan Ke Xue. 2007;13(6):527–30.
13. Venkov G. Verrucous carcinoma of the penis. Khirurgiia (Sofiia). 2003;59(6):22–4.
14. Sánchez Zalabardo D, Toledo Santana G, Arocena García-Tapia J, Sanz Pérez G, Diez-Caballero Alonso F, Martín-Marquina Aspiunza A, Rosell CD. Verrucous carcinoma of the penis: report of 2 cases. Arch Esp Urol. 2001;54(1):76–9.
15. Muro Vidaurre I, Hernáez Manrique I, Sanz Jaka JP, Rekarte Barriola JA, Lluch CA. Verrucous carcinoma of the penis: local excision with the Mohs micrographic technique. Arch Esp Urol. 1996;49(9):959–64.
16. Llarena Ibarguren R, Pérez García A, Zabala Egurrola JA, Arruza EA. Verrucous carcinoma of the penis: apropos of 2 cases. Arch Esp Urol. 1989;42(1):30–2.
17. Graziotti P, Maio G, Aragona F, Dal Bianco M, Cisternino A, Dante S. Verrucous carcinoma of the penis. 2 cases and review of the literature. J Chir (Paris). 1988;125(5):364–366.
18. Yaman I, Bozdag AD, Derici H, Tansug T, Reyhan E. Verrucous carcinoma arising in a giant condyloma acuminata (Buschkelowenstein Tumour): ten-year follow-up. Ann Acad Med Singapore. 2011;40(2):104–5.
19. Zhu JW, Luo D, Li CR, Lu Y, Ji X, Zhu J, Ming YL, Shen CH. A case of penile verrucous carcinoma associated with cutaneous horn. Clin Exp Dermatol. 2007;32(2):213–4.
20. Yeager JK, Findlay RF, McAleer IM. Penile verrucous carcinoma. Arch Dermatol. 1990;126(9):1208–10.
21. Castillo Jimeno JM, Queron Nasarre I, Cea Rey SA, Paredero Paredero S, Jaso López AC, Córdoba A. Verrucous carcinoma of the penis: report of two cases. Arch Esp Urol. 1996;49(7):757–60.
22. Beddouche A, Kallat A. Penile verrucous carcinoma. Pan Afr Med J. 2016;24:188.
23. Noronha TM, Girisha BS, Bhat SP, Christy CM, Handattu S, Fernandes MS. A rare case of verrucous carcinoma of penis in an human immunodeficiency virus- infected patient. Indian J Sex Transm Dis AIDS. 2015;36(2):192–4.
24. Fujimoto N, Nakanishi G, Ushida H, Okada Y, Tanaka R, Fujimoto W, Jo Y, Hara R, Tanaka T. Penile verrucous carcinoma arising in HPV-negative condylomatous papules. Eur J Dermatol. 2011;21(3):436–8.
25. Kanik AB, Lee J, Wax F, Bhawan J. Penile verrucous carcinoma in a 37-year-old circumcised man. J Am Acad Dermatol. 1997;37(2 Pt 2):329–31.
26. Vesga Molina F, Llarena Ibarguren R, Acha Pérez M, Albisú Tristán A, Blasco de Villalonga M, Arruza Echevarría A, Pertusa Peña C. Verrucous carcinoma of the penis: our caseload. Arch Esp Urol. 1993;46(1):23–25.
27. Rossi M, Giustina A, Tonetti F, Gorini P, Mina A, Dutto C, Nobili U. Verrucous carcinoma of the penis. A case report and review of the literature. Minerva Chir. 1991;46(18):999–1002.
28. Castiñeiras Fernández J, López Múñoz A, Cabello Torres P, Vilches TJ. Verrucous carcinoma of the penis. Actas Urol Esp. 1991;15(2):169–72.
29. Shah PJ, Abrams PH, Gaches CG, Ashken MH, McCann BG. Verrucous carcinoma of the penis or Buschke-Löwenstein tumour. Eur Urol. 1981;7(2):78–80.
30. Smith RB, Young HH 2nd, Chaffey BT. Verrucous carcinoma of the penis: report of a case and review. Br J Urol. 1969;41(3):327–31.
31. Child FJ, Kim BK, Ganesan R, Southern SA, Herrington CS, Calonje E. Verrucous carcinoma arising in pseudoepitheliomatous keratotic and micaceous balanitis, without evidence of human papillomavirus. Br J Dermatol. 2000;143(1):183–7.
32. Weber P, Rabinovitz H, Garland L. Verrucous carcinoma in penile lichen sclerosus et atrophicus. J Dermatol Surg Oncol. 1987;13(5):529–32.

33. Barbagli G, Palminteri E, Mirri F, Guazzoni G, Turini D, Lazzeri M. Penile carcinoma in patients with genital lichen sclerosus: a multicenter survey. J Urol. 2006;175(4):1359–63.
34. Seixas AL, Ornellas AA, Marota A, et al. Verrucous carcinoma of the penis: retrospective analysis of 32 cases. J Urol. 1994;152:1476–9.
35. Sheen MC, Sheu HM, Jang MY, et al. Advanced penile verrucous carcinoma treated with intra-aoritc infusion chemotherapy. J Urol. 2010;183(5):1830–5.
36. He X, Zhang J, Tan L, Wang W, Song Y, Wang H, Zhang X, Kou H1, Lu Y. Treatment of verrucous carcinoma in penis with topical aminolevulinic acid photodynamic therapy: An effective and safe treatment method. Photodiagnosis Photodyn Ther. 2018;24:232–236.
37. Eliason M, Bowen G, Bowen A, Hazard L, Samlowski W. Primary treatment of verrucous carcinoma of the penis with fluorouracil, cis-diamino-dichloro-platinum and radiation therapy. Arch Dermatol. 2009;145(8):950–2.
38. Sheen MC, Sheu HM, Huang CH, Wang YW, Chai CY, Wu CF. Penile verrucous carcinoma successfully treated by intra-aortic infusion with methotrexate. Urology. 2003;61(6):1216–20.
39. Michelman FA, Filho AC, Moraes AM. Verrucous carcinoma of the penis treated with cryosurgery. J Urol. 2002;168(3):1096–7.
40. Gómez De La Fuente E, Castaño Suarez E, Vanaclocha Sebastian F, Rodriguez-Peralto JL, Iglesias Díez L. Verrucous carcinoma of the penis completely cured with shaving and intralesional interferon. Dermatology. 2000;200(2):152.
41. Maiche AG, Pyrhonen S. Verrucous carcinoma of the penis: three cases treated with interferon-alpha. Br J Urol. 1997;79(3):481–3.
42. Pyrhönen S, Maiche AG, Mäntyjärvi R. Verrucous carcinoma of the penis successfully treated with interferon. Br J Urol. 1991;68(1):102–4.
43. Carson TE. Verrucous carcinoma of the penis. Successful treatment with cryosurgery and topical fluorouracil therapy. Arch Dermatol. 1978;114(10):1546–1547.
44. Ilkay AK, Chodak GW, Vogelzang NJ, Gerber GS. Buschke-Lowenstein tumor: therapeutic options including systemic chemotherapy. Urology. 1993;42(5):599–602.
45. Martin JM, Molina I, Monteagudo C, Marti N, Lopez V, Jorda E. Buschke-Lowenstein tumor. J Dermatol Case Rep. 2008;2(4):60–2.
46. Kato N, Onozuka T, Yasukawa K, Kimura K, Sasaki K. Penile hybrid verrucous-squamous carcinoma associated with a superficial inguinal lymph node metastasis. Am J Dermatopathol. 2000;22(4):339–43.
47. Fukunaga M, Yokoi K, Miyazawa Y, Harada T, Ushigome S. Penile verrucous carcinoma with anaplastic transformation following radiotherapy. A case report with human papillomavirus typing and flow cytometric DNA studies. Am J Surg Pathol. 1994;18(5):501–505.
48. Korczak D, Siegel Y, Lindner A. Verrucous carcinoma of the penis. Harefuah. 1989;117(12):436–7.
49. Zheng FF, Liang YY, Guo YS, Dai YP, Zheng KL. Diagnosis and therapy for penile cancer: a report of 46 cases with literature review. Ai Zheng. 2008;27(9):962–5.
50. Heyns CF, van Vollenhoven P, Steenkamp JW, Allen FJ. Cancer of the penis–a review of 50 patients. S Afr J Surg. 1997;35(3):120–4.
51. Bañón Pérez VJ, Nicolás Torralba JA, Valdelvira Nadal P, Server Pastor G, Martínez Barba E, Gómez Gómez G, Prieto González A, López Cubillana P, Pérez AM. Malignant neoplasms of the penis. Actas Urol Esp. 2000;24(8):652–8.
52. Chen MF, Chen WC, Wu CT, et al. Contemporary management of penile cancer including surgery and adjuvant radiotherapy: an experience in Taiwan. World J Urol. 2004;22:60–6.
53. Alvarez Alvarez C, Meijide Rico F, Rodríguez González L, Antón Badiola I, Zungri Telo E, Antonio Ortiz-Rey J. Verrucous carcinoma of the penis arising from a lichen planus. A true preneoplastic lesion? Actas Urol Esp. 2006;30(1):90–92.
54. Chaux A, Cubilla AL. The role of human papillomavirus infection in the pathogenesis of penile squamous cell carcinomas. Semin Diagn Pathol. 2012;29:67–71.
55. Velazquez EF, Chaux A, Cubilla AL. Histologic classification of penile intraepithelial neoplasia. Semin Diagn Pathol. 2012;29:96–102.
56. Ouban A1, Dellis J, Salup R, Morgan M.: Immunohistochemical expression of Mdm2 and p53 in penile verrucous carcinoma. Ann Clin Lab Sci. 2003 Winter;33(1):101–106.
57. Medina Pérez M, Valero Puerta J, Martínez Igarzabal MJ. Verrucous carcinoma of the penis with intense basal expression of Ki 67. Arch Esp Urol. 1999;52(9):983–5.
58. Saeed S, Keehn CA, Khalil FK, Morgan MB. Immunohistochemical expression of Bax and Bcl-2 in penile carcinoma. Ann Clin Lab Sci. 2005 Winter;35(1):91–96.
59. Masih AS, Stoler MH, Farrow GM, Wooldridge TN, Johansson SL. Penile verrucous carcinoma: a clinicopathologic, human papillomavirus typing and flow cytometric analysis. Mod Pathol. 1992;5(1):48–55.
60. Chan KW, Lam KY, Chan AC, Lau P, Srivastava G. Prevalence of human papillomavirus types 16 and 18 in penile carcinoma: a study of 41 cases using PCR. J Clin Pathol. 1994;47(9):823–6.
61. KIMBERLY L. BRADY, MD, MARY GAIL MERCURIO, MD, AND MARC D. BROWN, MD. Malignant Tumors of the Penis. Dermatol Surg. 2013;39:527–547.
62. Shindel AW, Mann MW, Lev RY, Senge lmann R, Petersen J, Hruza GJ, Brandes SB. Mohs micrographic surgery for penile cancer: management and long-term follow up. J Urol. 2007;178(5):1980–1985.
63. López Alcina E, Rodrigo Aliaga M, Martínez Sarmiento M, Monserrat Monfort JJ, Rivas Rodero S, Jiménez CF. Verrucous carcinoma of the penis. Actas Urol Esp. 1996;20(6):560–3.
64. Ricós Torrent JV, Casanova Ramón-Borja J, Iborra Juan I, Monros Lliso JL, Dumont Martínez R, Solsona Nárbon E. Verrucous carcinoma of the penis. Report of 8 cases. Actas Urol Esp. 1990;14(6):410–412.
65. Clemente Ramos LM, Maganto Pavón E, García González R, Burgos Revilla FJ, Fernández Cañadas S, Crespo Martínez L, Castañeda Casanova A, Escudero Barrilero A. Verrucous carcinoma of the penis. A report of 6 new cases and a review of the diagnostic and therapeutic aspects. Actas Urol Esp. 1997;21(4):372–376.
66. Hughes PS. Cryosurgery of verrucous carcinoma of the penis (Buschke-Lowenstein tumor). Cutis. 1979;24(1):43–5.
67. Nishikawa Y, Maruoka M, Miyauchi T, Nagayama T, Komatsu T, Matsuzaki O. Verrucous carcinoma of the penis: a case report and MRI findings. Hinyokika Kiyo. 1993;39(6):573–5.
68. Shimizu A, Tamura A, Ishikawa O. Invasive squamous cell carcinoma arising from verrucous carcinoma. Recognition of verrucous carcinoma of skin as an in situ carcinoma. Eur J Dermatol 2006;16(4):439–442.

18

Health-related quality of life in the randomized phase 3 study of ramucirumab plus docetaxel versus placebo plus docetaxel in platinum-refractory advanced urothelial carcinoma (RANGE)

Andrea Necchi[1*], Hiroyuki Nishiyama[2], Nobuaki Matsubara[3], Jae-Lyun Lee[4], Daniel P. Petrylak[5], Ronald de Wit[6], Alexandra Drakaki[7], Astra M. Liepa[8], Huzhang Mao[8], Katherine Bell-McGuinn[8] and Thomas Powles[9]

Abstract

Background: To evaluate patient-reported outcomes with ramucirumab plus docetaxel, a regimen which improved progression-free survival in platinum-refractory advanced urothelial carcinoma (aUC).

Methods: RANGE—a randomized, double-blinded, phase 3 trial in patients with platinum-refractory aUC. Ramucirumab (10 mg/kg) plus docetaxel (75 mg/m^2) or placebo plus docetaxel were administered every 21 days until disease progression or unacceptable toxicity. Patients received maximum 10 cycles of docetaxel. European Organization for Research and Treatment of Cancer Quality of Life Questionnaire C30 (EORTC QLQ-C30) and EuroQoL five-dimensions (EQ-5D-5L) were administered at baseline, start of each cycle, and 30-day follow-up visit. A ≥ 10-point change in QLQ-C30 scores was considered meaningful. Rates of improved/stable scores were compared between treatment arms using Fisher's exact test. Time to deterioration (TtD) was estimated and compared using Kaplan–Meier estimation and log-rank test.

Results: Of the 530 patients, ~ 97% patients in each arm provided baseline QLQ-C30 data. On-treatment compliance was ≥ 88% for first 8 cycles. Mean baseline QLQ-C30 scores were similar between arms, with global quality of life (QoL), fatigue, pain, and insomnia having greatest impairment. Postbaseline rates of improved/stable QLQ-C30 scores were similar between treatment arms except for greater improvement in pain score with ramucirumab. TtD of QLQ-C30 scales favored ramucirumab arm. Baseline EQ-5D-5L index and visual analogue scale scores were similar between arms, followed by relatively stable on-treatment scores. EQ-5D-5L scores worsened at post-discontinuation follow-up visit.

Conclusions: Ramucirumab plus docetaxel did not negatively impact QoL compared with docetaxel alone in platinum-refractory aUC. Improved TtD and tumor associated rates of pain favored ramucirumab treatment.

*Correspondence: andrea.necchi@istitutotumori.mi.it

[1] Department of Medical Oncology, Fondazione IRCCS Istituto Nazionale Dei Tumori, 20133 Milan, Italy

Full list of author information is available at the end of the article

Keyword: Antiangiogenesis, Bladder cancer, Neoplasm metastatsis, Patient-reported outcomes, Quality of life, Ramucirumab, Urinary bladder neoplasm, Urothelial carcinoma

Background

Advanced/metastatic urothelial carcinoma (UC), including carcinomas arising in the bladder, urethra, ureter, and/or renal pelvis, has a poor prognosis. Median survival is approximately 12–14 months with standard first-line platinum-based chemotherapy for advanced/metastatic disease [1]. Despite approvals of various targeted therapies for platinum-refractory advanced UC, most patients have limited treatment options as they experience disease progression. Ramucirumab plus docetaxel has shown higher response rate and improved progression-free survival (PFS) compared to placebo plus docetaxel in the platinum-refractory population [2, 3]. In the refractory setting, quality of life (QoL) is an important factor in the treatment decision-making process for patients with cancer where symptom palliation is the primary goal of therapy [4, 5]. Monitoring of QoL via patient-reported symptoms is also associated with better outcomes than observed with usual care [6].

UCs overexpress the vascular endothelial growth factor (VEGF) ligand and its receptor, vascular endothelial growth factor receptor (VEGFR)-2 [7, 8]. Ramucirumab (a human IgG1 monoclonal antibody and a VEGFR-2 antagonist) [9, 10] plus docetaxel improved PFS (hazard ratio [HR] = 0.757; 95% confidence interval [CI] [0.607, 0.943]) compared with placebo plus docetaxel in the randomized phase 3 trial for platinum-refractory advanced UC (RANGE; NCT02426125) [2]. Whereas other antiangiogenic drugs have failed thus far in refractory UC [1, 11, 12]. Patients treated in the ramucirumab arm also had a numerically higher objective response rate (24.50%, 95% CI [18.80, 30.30] vs 14.0%, 95% CI [9.40, 18.60]) [2]. Although not statistically significant, overall survival (OS) at the final analysis favored the ramucirumab arm (HR = 0.887; 95% CI [0.724, 1.086]; $p = 0.25$) [3]. The most frequent adverse events (AEs) of any grade reported for both the ramucirumab and placebo arms were fatigue (39.1% vs 36.2%), alopecia (23.6% vs 30.6%), diarrhea (23.6% vs 16.6%), decreased appetite (22.1% vs 17.0%), nausea (22.1% vs 14.0%), and stomatitis (23.2% vs 9.0%). Of these AEs, only fatigue had an incidence of $\geq$ 5% for grade 3/4 (7.0% vs 6.0%). On-study, treatment-related deaths were relatively rare (8 [3.0%] and 5 [2.0%], respectively) [3]. Overall, the proportion of patients with AEs receiving ramucirumab plus docetaxel was similar to the proportion of patients with AEs in the placebo plus docetaxel arm. No new safety signals were detected for ramucirumab plus docetaxel, and the safety profile was considered manageable [2].

The impact of treatment on QoL is not widely reported in refractory advanced UC (aUC), particularly for chemotherapy and anti-VEGFR-2 drug combination therapies. Therefore, we assessed the patient-reported outcomes (PROs) as secondary endpoints in the RANGE trial to evaluate the benefit-risk profile of the addition of ramucirumab to docetaxel from the patient perspective [3]. We hypothesized that patients would experience more symptomatic improvement without experiencing detriment in QoL.

Methods

Study design

The RANGE trial design and the outcome of its primary endpoint were previously published [2]. The trial was conducted during July 2015 and April 2017 and approved by appropriate review boards/ethics committees and followed the principles outlined in the Declaration of Helsinki. All patients provided written informed consent. This study adhered to the CONSORT guidelines.

Patient eligibility criteria

Eligibility criteria included patients with Eastern Cooperative Oncology Group (ECOG) performance status of zero or one and whose advanced disease progressed during or $\leq$ 14 months after first-line platinum-based chemotherapy. Patients may have also received one checkpoint inhibitor therapy prior to enrollment onto RANGE, in which case prior platinum-containing chemotherapy in $\leq$ 24 months was allowed. Patients were excluded if they had received a taxane previously [2].

Eligible patients were randomized to receive docetaxel (75 mg/m^2, intravenously [IV]) plus ramucirumab (10 mg/kg, IV) or docetaxel plus placebo, administered on day 1 of each 21-day cycle. Randomization was stratified by geographic region (North America, East Asia, or Europe/other), ECOG performance status at baseline (0 or 1), and visceral metastasis (present or absent). Ramucirumab treatment continued until there was documented disease progression, toxicity or intolerance requiring discontinuation, withdrawal of consent, or noncompliance. Docetaxel could continue, if no prespecified discontinuation criteria were met, for up to six cycles with an additional four cycles allowed if an adequate treatment response was observed. Tumor responses were assessed using Response Evaluation Criteria in Solid Tumors (RECIST) v1.1 [13].

Outcomes and assessments

Assessment of PROs, a secondary endpoint of the RANGE trial, was conducted through use of the European Organization for Research and Treatment of Cancer Quality of Life Questionnaire C30 (EORTC QLQ-C30), version 3 and the EuroQoL five-dimensions, 5 level (EQ-5D-5L) questionnaire, which measure QoL (functional domains and symptoms) and health status, respectively [14, 15]. Patients completed the questionnaires only if there were cross-culturally validated translations in which they were fluent. Prior to any extensive contact with clinical personnel, patients were asked to complete the questionnaires at baseline, prior to the start of each cycle, and within 30 days after treatment discontinuation (follow-up). QLQ-C30 data were scored according to the EORTC guidelines, using a 0–100 scale with higher scores for global QoL and functional scales representing better QoL and lower scores for symptom scales representing less burden. A ≥ 10-point change was considered clinically meaningful [16]. EQ-5D-5L index values were based on the value set for England with a range of -0.281 to 1, with zero representing death and one representing perfect health [17]. Additionally, patients indicated their current health status by marking on a visual analogue scale (VAS) ranging from 0 (worst-imaginable health state) to 100 (best-imaginable health state) [15].

Statistical analysis

Analyses were conducted in the intention-to-treat (ITT) population except for descriptive statistics that were limited to the number of patients who provided data at a given assessment. Compliance rates were calculated based on the number of patients expected to provide data at a given assessment (i.e., those patients still receiving study therapy). Descriptive statistics were used to summarize data, including change from baseline as well as for the EQ-5D-5L scores. QLQ-C30 scores were classified as improved or worsened if change from baseline was ≥ 10 points; change < 10 points was classified as stable. For each scale at each postbaseline assessment, the proportion of patients with improved or stable scores was compared using the Fisher's exact test. Time to sustained deterioration (TtD) was defined as time from randomization date to first worsening of ≥ 10 points with no subsequent non-worsened assessment relative to baseline. If there were no subsequent assessments, the patient was classified as deteriorated. The follow-up assessment after treatment discontinuation could not be considered as a subsequent non-worsened assessment. Patients without deterioration were censored at the last non-deteriorated assessment. Kaplan–Meier method was used to estimate the probability of TtD, and unstratified log-rank test was used to investigate significance between treatment groups. Univariable Cox regression analysis was performed to test the association of treatment with TtD. No adjustments were made for multiplicity, but *p*-values < 0.05 were used to identify potential trends. These analyses discussed here were performed on the ITT population at the time of the OS database lock [3]. All the analyses were conducted using SAS software (SAS, Version 9.1.2 or higher).

Results

RANGE patients and questionnaire compliance

In the randomly assigned patients (N = 530, ITT population) from the 727 screened for eligibility (Fig. 1), baseline characteristics were similar between treatment arms (Table 1). At baseline, 254 (96.6%) of patients in the ramucirumab arm and 260 (97.4%) in the placebo arm provided QLQ-C30 and EQ-5D-5L data (Table 2). For the first 8 cycles, compliance was ≥ 88% for both the QLQ-C30 and EQ-5D-5L, (Table 2). The most common reasons for noncompliance were failure by the site to administer and patient refusal to complete the questionnaires (Fig. 1). At the post-discontinuation follow-up visit, compliance was lower overall, with 52–54% of patients providing data. When grouped by those who provided data at follow-up and those who did not, the groups were similar in baseline patient characteristics, time on therapy, BOR, and reasons for discontinuation.

Descriptive summaries

Mean baseline scores for both questionnaires were similar between treatment arms (Table 3). With high scores being favorable for global QoL and functional domains of the QLQ-C30, the lowest mean scores were reported for global QoL, indicating the domain with greatest impairment at baseline. With low scores being favorable for symptoms, the highest mean scores were reported for fatigue, pain, and insomnia, indicating the symptoms of greatest burden at baseline.

When considering high-level assessment of QoL and health status, no clear differences were observed between the treatment arms for changes in mean scores from baseline of the QLQ-C30 global QoL scale, EQ-5D-5L index, and EQ-5D-5L VAS (Fig. 2a–c). Although scores within arms worsened over time, the mean changes for on-treatment assessments were small. Similar patterns of no differences between arms in changes from baseline were observed for the other QoL scales, with the exception of pain (Additional file 1: Figure S1). For the functional scales, worsened scores over time were observed for physical and role functioning. For symptom scales,

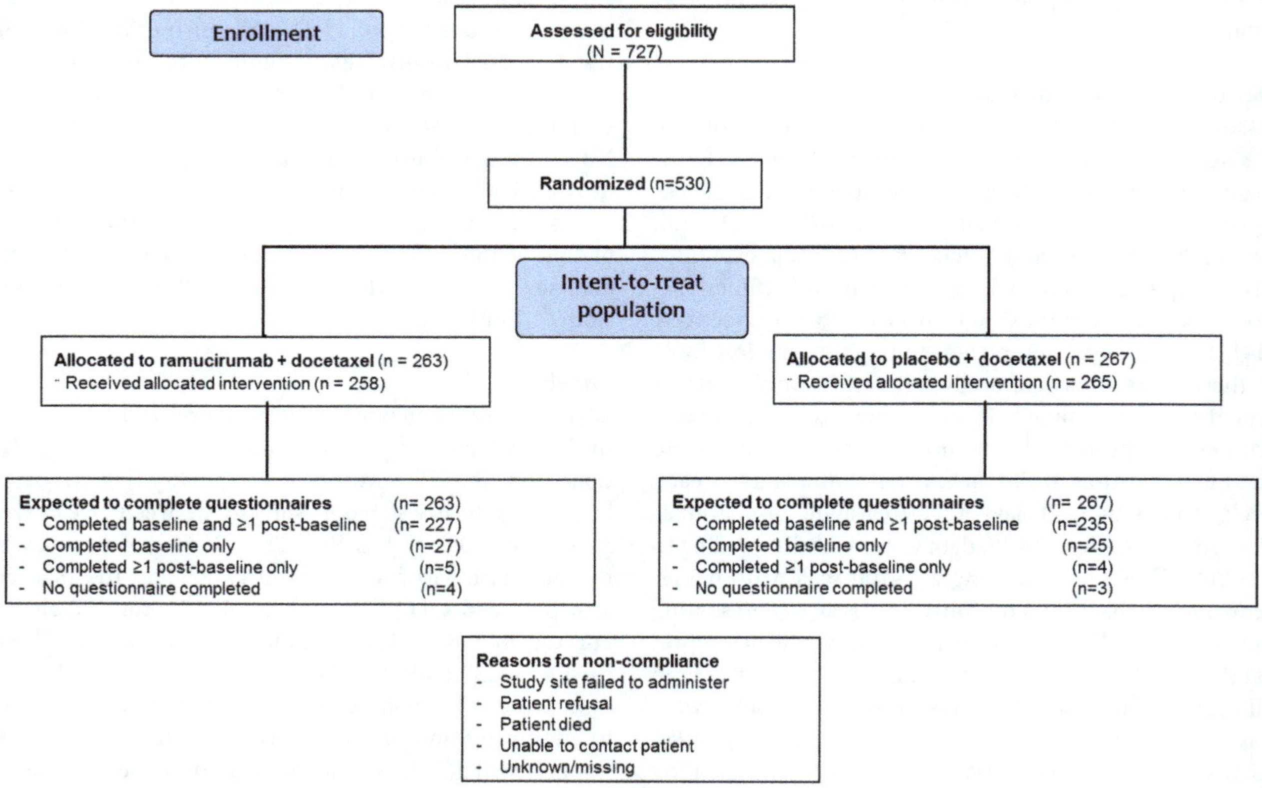

Fig. 1 Patient disposition. *n* = number of patients

fatigue, dyspnea, and diarrhea had the greatest worsening over time. In the case of pain, improved scores were observed in the ramucirumab arm over the first five cycles, while scores worsened in the placebo arm. Additional file 1: Figure S2 summarizes the distribution of EQ-5D-5L responses over time. At baseline, the highest levels of impairment (i.e., moderate or more severe) were reported for pain/discomfort. In general, the distributions of responses for all dimensions were similar over time for on-treatment assessments (Additional file 1: Figure S2A-E). For all scales, change from baseline was worst at the post-discontinuation follow-up assessment. Thus, in general, findings of the QLQ-C30 and the EQ-5D-5L were consistent.

Time to sustained deterioration

Results for TtD of QLQ-C30 scales are summarized in Fig. 3. The HR was < 1 for all scales (range 0.76–0.96), indicating a trend towards longer TtD in the ramucirumab arm. Kaplan–Meier figures are presented for those scales with ˂65% censoring of events (Additional file 1: Figure S3A-I). Median TtD for global QoL was 6.9 months (95% CI 4.2 months—8.9 months) vs. 4.6 months (95% CI 3.5 months—5.5 months) (HR 0.88, 95% CI 0.7–1.2).

Rates of improved or stable scores

The proportion of patients whose QoL scores improved, remained stable, or deteriorated from baseline at each postbaseline assessment are shown in Fig. 4, for the scales with the greatest impairment at baseline; Additional file 1: Figure S4 depicts these results for all other scales. For each scale, rates of improved/stable were similar between treatment arms in early cycles. Of note, a higher proportion of patients in the ramucirumab arm had either improved or stable pain scores at cycles 4, 5, and 7 compared to the placebo arm (Fig. 4d). Indeed, across all cycles, the pain scale, relative to the other scales (Fig. 3a and Additional file 1: S4), exhibited consistency with respect to having the greatest proportion of patients with improvement in pain within the ramucirumab arm.

Exploratory analyses

Considering all prespecified analyses, the consistency of the pain results prompted an exploratory analysis evaluating the association with best overall response to treatment (Fig. 5). Because the global QoL scale provides the most holistic assessment, it was similarly evaluated. During the first four cycles, the range of patients achieving complete response (CR)/partial response (PR) with

Table 1 Baseline demographics and disease characteristics

	RAM + DOC (n = 263)	PL + DOC (n = 267)
Median age, years (range)	65 (34–86)	66 (32–83)
Male	213 (81)	215 (81)
Race		
White	203 (77)	204 (76)
Asian	54 (20)	61 (23)
ECOG performance status		
0	121 (46)	125 (47)
1	139 (53)	142 (53)
Geography		
North America	24 (9)	24 (9)
East Asia	53 (20)	57 (21)
Europe/Other	186 (71)	186 (70)
Primary tumor site		
Bladder	180 (68)	177 (66)
Urethra	7 (3)	6 (2)
Renal pelvis	39 (15)	42 (16)
Ureter	33 (13)	37 (14)
Other	1 (< 1)	5 (2)
Sites of metastases		
Lymph node only	41 (16)	42 (16)
Visceral	182 (69)	188 (70)
Liver	78 (30)	69 (26)
Lung	98 (37)	121(45)
Bone	56 (21)	53 (20)
Hemoglobin < 10 g/dL	34 (13)	36 (13)
Patients with time since previous chemotherapy < 3mo	115 (44)	126 (47)
Bellmunt risk factors		
0	88 (33)	93 (35)
1	105 (40)	109 (41)
2	64 (24)	57 (21)
3	6 (2)	8 (3)
Prior neoadjuvant or adjuvant therapy	87 (33)	107 (40)
Prior platinum-based therapy:		
Cisplatin	161 (61)	189 (71)
Carboplatin	97 (37)	77 (29)
Prior immune checkpoint inhibitor	17 (7)	28 (10)

DOC docetaxel, *ECOG* Eastern Cooperative Oncology Group, *mo* months, *n* number of patients, *PL* placebo, *RAM* ramucirumab

Data are n (%), unless otherwise indicated

For a full list of patient demographics and disease characteristics at baseline in the intention-to-treat population [2]

improved global QoL was 17.6–25.0% for ramucirumab and 10.8–21.6% for placebo; the range for patients with stable disease (SD) was 9.6–17.3% for ramucirumab and 10.0–21.8% for placebo (Fig. 5a). During the first four cycles, the range of patients achieving CR/PR with

Table 2 EORTC QLQ-C30 and EQ-5D-5L compliance rates from baseline through cycle 8 and 30-day follow-up (ITT population)

Assessment time point	QLQ-C30		EQ-5D-5L	
	RAM + DOC (n = 263)	PL + DOC (n = 267)	RAM + DOC (n = 263)	PL + DOC (n = 267)
Baseline	254/263 (97)	260/267 (97)	254/263 (97)	260/267 (97)
Cycle 1	214/229 (93)	226/237 (95)	212/229 (93)	225/237 (95)
Cycle 2	159/165 (96)	159/165 (96)	158/165 (96)	159/165 (96)
Cycle 3	139/147 (95)	133/138 (96)	136/147 (93)	133/138 (96)
Cycle 4	114/126 (90)	100/105 (95)	114/126 (90)	100/105 (95)
Cycle 5	108/114 (95)	88/94 (94)	107/114 (94)	88/94 (94)
Cycle 6	79/87 (91)	64/71 (90)	83/87 (95)	63/71 (89)
Cycle 7	64/68 (94)	52/59 (88)	66/68 (97)	52/59 (88)
Cycle 8	52/56 (93)	36/41 (88)	51/56 (91)	36/41 (88)
Follow-up	116/215 (54)	119/231 (52)	113/215 (53)	121/231 (52)

DOC docetaxel, *EORTC QLQ-C30* European Organization for Research and Treatment of Cancer Quality of Life Questionnaire C30, *EQ-5D-5L* EuroQoL five-dimensions, *ITT* intention-to-treat, *PL* placebo, *RAM* ramucirumab

Data are presented as number/total number (%)

For compliance, the total number is the number expected to complete at the assessment time point

On-treatment compliance reporting is truncated at cycle 8, but similar rates were reported for later cycles

The median number of cycles administered in both treatment arms was 4

Table 3 Baseline Scores (Mean [standard deviation])

	RAM + DOC (n = 263)	PL + DOC (n = 267)
EORTC QLQ-C30 Scales[a]		
Global QoL	62.0 (22.9)	60.8 (21.4)
Physical functioning	75.9 (22.4)	74.2 (21.7)
Role functioning	73.3 (29.5)	72.1 (29.9)
Emotional functioning	76.0 (22.4)	75.0 (21.2)
Cognitive functioning	85.9 (18.3)	84.6 (20.3)
Social functioning	74.6 (28.8)	71.2 (30.2)
Fatigue	33.1 (25.9)	36.0 (24.8)
Nausea/vomiting	8.0 (16.1)	9.0 (17.5)
Pain	32.0 (31.1)	33.8 (30.7)
Dyspnea	17.4 (24.6)	17.9 (25.4)
Insomnia	27.7 (30.9)	28.8 (29.9)
Appetite loss	22.4 (29.2)	23.3 (31.9)
Constipation	21.0 (28.3)	24.6 (30.0)
Diarrhea	8.1 (16.6)	6.3 (16.0)
EQ-5D-5L Index Score[b]	0.77 (0.23)	0.78 (0.19)
EQ-5D-5L VAS	67.2 (21.7)	67.3 (18.7)

DOC docetaxel, *EORTC QLQ-C30* European Organization for Research and Treatment of Cancer Quality of Life Questionnaire C30, *EQ-5D-5L* EuroQoL five-dimensions, *n* number of patients, *PL* placebo, *QoL* quality of life, *RAM* ramucirumab, *SD* standard deviation, *VAS* visual analogue score

[a] For the EORTC QLQ-C30, high scores are favorable for functional domains and global QoL; low scores are favorable for symptoms

[b] For the EQ-5D-5L, high scores are favorable. The range for Index Score is -0.281 to 1 and the range for VAS is 0 to 100 (higher scores are favorable)

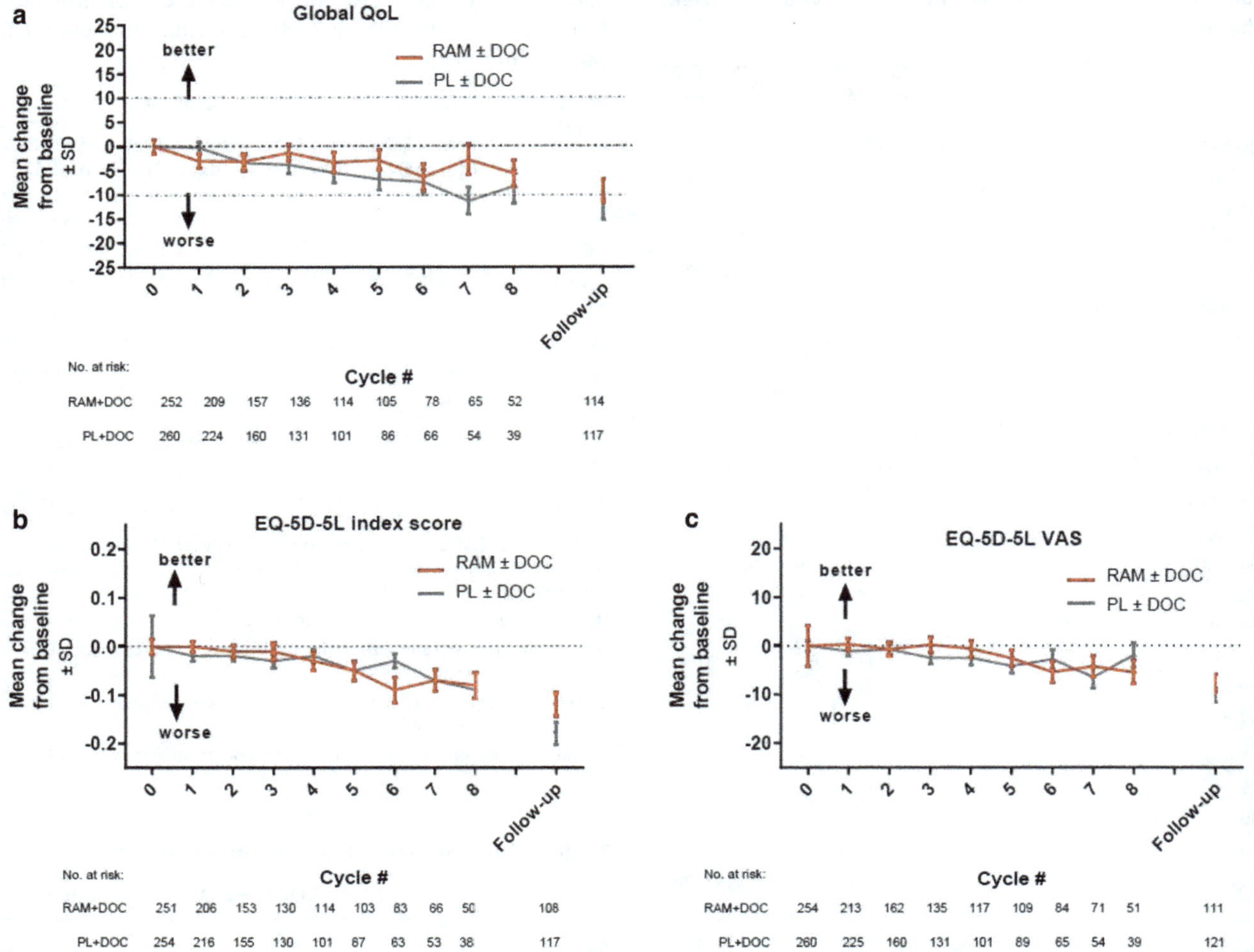

Fig. 2 Mean change from baseline in the mean scores of the EORTC QLQ-C30 global QoL scale (**a**), EQ-5D-5L index (**b**) and visual analogue scale scores (**c**). *DOC* docetaxel, *EORTC QLQ-C30* European Organization for Research and Treatment of Cancer Quality of Life Questionnaire C30, *EQ-5D-5L* EuroQoL five-dimensions, *RAM* ramucirumab, *SD* standard deviation, *VAS* visual analogue scale

improved pain was 29.4–30.9% for ramucirumab and 13.5–27.0% for placebo; the range for patients with SD was 17.3–28.8% for ramucirumab and 16.4–29.1% for placebo (Fig. 5b).

In general, a higher proportion of patients who achieved CR/PR had improved pain scores in the ramucirumab arm versus the placebo arm. No apparent difference in pain palliation was seen between arms for patients who achieved SD. Similar results were observed for improved global QoL between ramucirumab versus placebo arms in patients who achieved CR/PR and SD (Fig. 5).

Discussion

QoL is of utmost importance when considering therapeutic options for patients in the palliative setting [4, 18]. There can be concerns when a second agent is added to chemotherapy if gains in efficacy are also accompanied by increased toxicity [19], such as in the RANGE study where there were numerically higher rates of any-grade diarrhea, decreased appetite, nausea, and stomatitis in the ramucirumab plus docetaxel arm compared with the placebo plus docetaxel arm [3]. Thus, evaluating the effects on QoL through PROs when ramucirumab plus docetaxel was compared to placebo plus docetaxel was a key secondary endpoint in the RANGE trial. While on therapy, patients in the placebo plus docetaxel arm generally maintained global QoL and health status. Results were similar for the ramucirumab plus docetaxel arm, suggesting no detrimental impact. Worsening at the 30-day follow-up visit in both treatment arms was potentially associated with the negative impact of disease progression, which was the most common reason for treatment discontinuation. The longer PFS was consistent with trend for longer TtD in global QoL in the ramucirumab plus docetaxel arm. These findings may be

EORTC QLQ-C30 Scale	RAM+DOC (N = 263) # Events	PL+DOC (N = 267) # Events	Hazard Ratio (95% CI)
Global Health Status	101	104	0.882 (0.670−1.624)
Physical Functioning	121	133	0.806 (0.629−1.032)
Role Functioning	151	144	0.943 (0.750−1.187)
Emotional Functioning	71	80	0.776 (0.563−1.071)
Cognitive Functioning	105	104	0.852 (0.649−1.119)
Social Functioning	98	101	0.898 (0.679−1.186)
Fatigue	156	155	0.932 (0.744−1.166)
Nausea and Vomiting	76	78	0.809 (0.588−1.112)
Pain	112	119	0.793 (0.612−1.029)
Dypsnea	97	111	0.762 (0.579−1.001)
Insomnia	88	85	0.874 (0.647−1.181)
Appetite Loss	103	94	0.958 (0.723−1.270)
Constipation	67	73	0.757 (0.541−1.058)
Diarrhea	69	73	0.822 (0.590−1.146)

Hazard Ratio

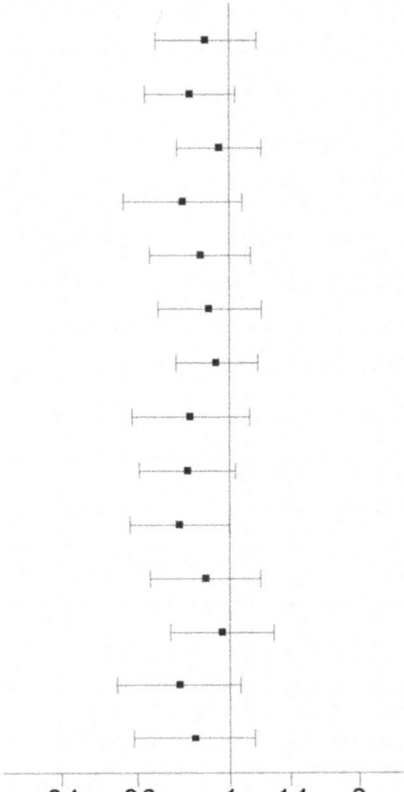

Fig. 3 Time to sustained deterioration of QLQ-C30 scales. *CI* confidence interval; *DOC* docetaxel, *EORTC QLQ-C30* European Organization for Research and Treatment of Cancer Quality of Life Questionnaire C30, *N* number of patients, *HR* hazard ratio, *PL* placebo, *QoL* quality of life; *RAM* ramucirumab. Forest plot of time to sustained deterioration, HRs (unstratified) for each functional and symptom scale are depicted. HRs were estimated using a Cox regression model. 2-sided p-values were based on normal approximation

helpful when considering the value of delaying disease progression and the balance of benefit and risk of combination therapy from the patient perspective.

In our study, all of the more specific aspects of QoL were at least maintained in the ramucirumab plus docetaxel arm relative to the placebo plus docetaxel arm. The strongest trend of delay in deterioration among the functional scales favoring ramucirumab plus docetaxel was for physical functioning which addresses mobility and self-care. Fatigue and insomnia were two of the most prominent symptoms reported by patients at baseline. Changes in fatigue were similar between arms, with patients more likely to report worsening. Insomnia scores generally remained similar both between and within arms.

Of all of the dimensions assessed by the QLQ-C30 and the EQ-5D-5L, pain may be the one most closely associated with disease symptoms and treatment efficacy, with less confounding by toxicity of treatment [20–22]. At baseline, the mean score for pain from the QLQ-C30 indicated high levels of pain and < 30% of patients reported no pain or discomfort on the EQ-5D-5L. All analyses of pain from the QLQ-C30 suggested a differential effect between arms. In the descriptive summaries, mean scores generally improved for the ramucirumab plus docetaxel arm, but worsened for the placebo plus docetaxel arm. At later cycles, more patients in the ramucirumab plus docetaxel arm reported improved or stable pain scores. The HR for TtD was 0.79 (95% CI 0.61, 1.0). In the exploratory analysis conducted, patients treated with ramucirumab plus docetaxel, who achieved a complete or partial response, often reported improvement in pain. The observed relative benefit in pain palliation may be associated with the greater extent of tumor shrinkage among responders and longer duration of response seen in the ramucirumab plus docetaxel arm. The association of symptom palliation with tumor response in other populations has been previously reported [23, 24].

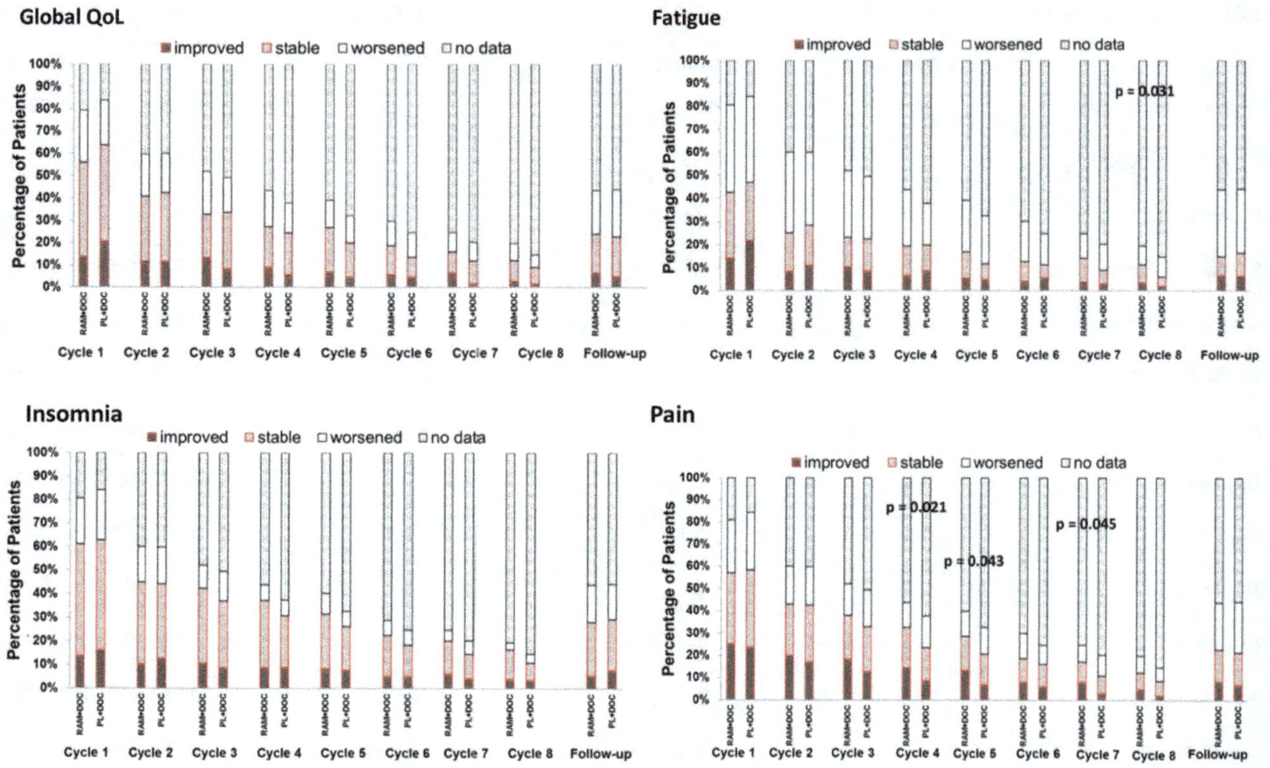

Fig. 4 Proportion of patients in ITT population with improved, stable or worsened QoL of the scales with greatest impairment at baseline. *QoL* quality of life, *ITT* intention-to-treat. For each scale at each postbaseline assessment, proportion of patients with improved or stable scores was compared using the Fisher's exact test

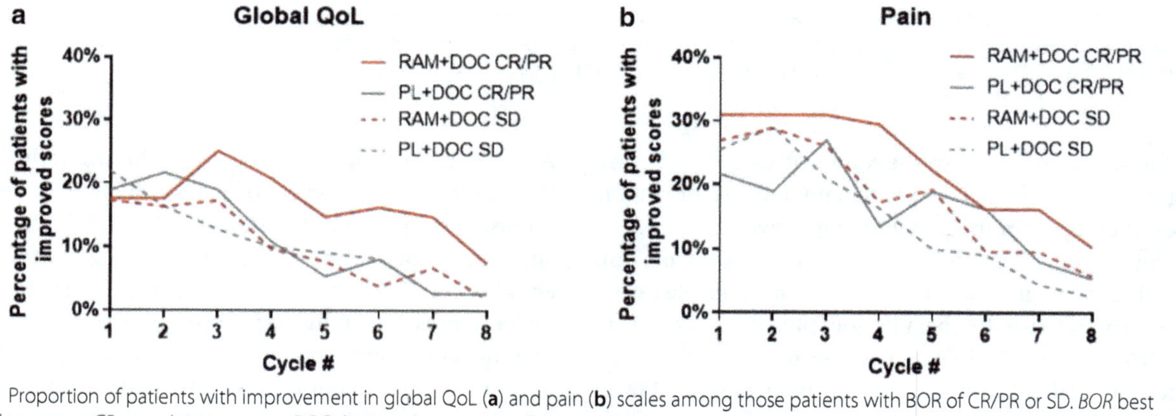

Fig. 5 Proportion of patients with improvement in global QoL (**a**) and pain (**b**) scales among those patients with BOR of CR/PR or SD. *BOR* best overall response, *CR* complete response, *DOC* docetaxel, *n* number of patients, *PL* placebo, *PR* partial response, *QoL* quality of life; *RAM* ramucirumab, *SD* stable disease. For each scale at each postbaseline assessment, proportion of patients with improved or stable scores between treatment and placebo arms was compared using the Fisher's exact test. PR/CR as BOR: RAM + DOC (n = 68) and PL + DOC (n = 37). SD as BOR: RAM + DOC (n = 104) and PL + DOC (n = 110)

Recent phase 3 studies of immune checkpoint inhibitors in similar study populations also assessed QoL [25, 26]. Although trial designs differed, the control arms were single-agent chemotherapy, and QoL was assessed with the QLQ-C30. However, different analysis approaches limit comparisons across the studies. In general, chemotherapy-based regimens were associated with within-arm worsening in global QoL over time and checkpoint inhibitors were associated with no within-arm improvement or worsening. In KEYNOTE-045, the HR for time to first deterioration in global QoL was0.72, indicating a longer time to first deterioration for pembrolizumab compared to chemotherapy [25]. In IMvigor211, the HR for time to sustained deterioration in global QoL was not reported, but median values were the same for atezoluzimab and chemotherapy [26].The HR for time to sustained deterioration in global QoL in RANGE was 0.887, trending for a longer time to deterioration for ramucirumab plus docetaxel compared to chemotherapy (docetaxel). In RANGE, the addition of ramucirumab to chemotherapy did not further worsen QoL but demonstrated within-arm improvements in pain scores. Both RANGE and KEYNOTE-045 [25] observed a worsening of QoL associated with disease progression. This supports our findings that disease-related symptoms may have a more prominent effect on QoL in this setting.

This study used robust analytical methods. The analysis was prespecified and completion rate of questionnaires was high during the study. The ramucirumab and placebo groups were similar at baseline in PROs and patient and disease characteristics. This study showed no deterioration of QoL with addition of ramucirumab, with consistency observed across QLQ-C30 global QoL scale, EQ-5D-5L index, and VAS scores. The completion rate at the post-discontinuation follow-up visit in our study was comparable to other studies in advanced cancer [27, 28]. In our study slightly more than half of patients provided post-discontinuation data, limiting the characterization of QoL and health status for that time period.

Limitations in the study include PRO instruments, patient characteristics, and incomplete follow-up data. Although cancer-specific and the most widely used in aUC trials, the QLQ-C30 is not specific to UC. No validated tumor-specific module to supplement the QLQ-C30 is available for use to assess additional concerns of aUC patients [29, 30]. With the baseline eligibility criterion of ECOG performance status of zero or one, there is less opportunity for patients to report improvements in PROs. As is common in advanced cancer trials, early discontinuation of patients results in non-random missing data; therefore, we attempted to minimize the impact by conducting cycle-by-cycle analysis to explore data trend instead of focusing on only certain cycle as a snapshot. We also made the general assumption that patients who discontinued therapy likely have worsened QoL, as might be expected with disease progression which was most common reason for study discontinuation. While PRO completion rates were lower at follow-up, characteristics and outcomes of patients who provided follow-up data were similar to those who did not. However, despite these limitations, trends in differences between arms were observed that were consistent with other clinical outcomes.

As the term itself suggests, PROs are reported by patients themselves without any interpretation from a physician or anyone else. PROs can be used to support evaluation of response to treatment and to increase clinician-patient engagement [31]. Integration of PROs to the care demonstrated a survival benefit in patients with cancer compared with patients undergoing usual care (median 31.2 months vs. median 26.0 months, $p=0.03$) [6]. In addition, PROs provide patients with a mechanism to self-report symptoms, minimize a decline in QoL, reduce hospitalization and emergency room admissions, and prolonged time on chemotherapy [32]. As newer agents become available for aUC, PRO/QoL data should be provided to help clinicians make informed treatment decisions [33–35].

Conclusions

In summary, QoL outcomes of the phase 3 RANGE trial presented here provided additional insights regarding no negative impact of ramucirumab plus docetaxel on QoL compared with placebo plus docetaxel. The association of pain palliation with tumor response and disease control observed in this study may be used when considering therapeutic choices for advanced UC.

Abbreviations

aUC: Advanced urothelial carcinoma; CI: Confidence interval; ECOG: Eastern Cooperative Oncology Group; EORTC QLQ-C30: European Organization for Research and Treatment of Cancer Quality of Life Questionnaire C30; EQ-5D-5L: EuroQoL five-dimensions, 5 level; HR: Hazard ratio; IV: Intravenously; OS: Overall survival; PRO: Patient-reported outcome; QoL: Quality of life; VEGF: Vascular endothelial growth factor; VEGFR: Vascular endothelial growth factor receptor.

Acknowledgements

We thank the patients and their caregivers for participating in this trial. We also thank the investigators and their support staff who generously participated in this work. Karan Sharma from Eli Lilly Services India Pvt. Ltd. provided medical writing and editing support.

Authors' contributions

Study Concept and Design: RdW, AML, DPP. Acquisition of Data: AN, HN, NM, JLL, RdW. Analysis and interpretation of data: AN, HN, NM, JLL, DPP, RdW, AD, AML, HM, KBM. Drafting of the manuscript: AN, HN, JLL, DPP, RdW, AML, KBM, TP. Critical revision of the manuscript for important intellectual content: All authors. Statistical analysis: HM. Administrative, technical, or material support: KBM. Supervision: KBM. All authors have read and approved the manuscript.

Competing interests

Andrea Necchi is consultant for: Merck, Roche, BMS, Bayer, GSK, Astellas, Janssen. Nobuaki Matsubara received research funding from Eli Lilly, AstraZeneca, Astellas, Bayer, Janssen, MSD and Sanofi. Daniel Petrylak received consulting fee from Ada Cap (Advanced Accelerator Applications), Amgen, Astellas, AstraZeneca, Bayer, Boehringer Ingelheim, Bristol Myer Squibb, Clovis, Eli Lilly, Exelixis, Incyte, Janssen, Pfizer, Pharmacyclics, Roche Laboratories, Seattle Genetics, Urogen. Grant support from Ada Cap (Advanced Accelerator Applications), Astellas, AstraZeneca, Bayer, Bristol Myer Squibb, Clovis, Eli Lilly, Endocyte, Genentech, Innocrin, MedImmune, Merck, Novartis, Pfizer, Progenics, Roche Laboratories, Sanofi Aventis, Seattle Genetics. Ronald de Wit received consultancy or speaker fees from Sanofi, Merck, Janssen, Roche, Clovis, and Bayer. Institutional grants from Sanofi, and Bayer. Alexandra Drakaki received grants from Eli Lilly, BMS, AstraZeneca, Seattle Genetics/Astellas. Astra M Liepa,

Huzhang Mao and Katherine-Bell McGuinn are employees and Shareholders in Eli Lilly and Company. Tom Powles received consultancy fee from AstraZeneca, BMS, Exelixis, Incyte, Ipsen, Merck/MSD, Novartis, Pfizer, Seattle Genetics. Received grant/funding from AstraZeneca and Roche. Strategic Advisory for Pfizer, AstraZeneca, Roche, and BMS.

Author details

[1] Department of Medical Oncology, Fondazione IRCCS Istituto Nazionale Dei Tumori, 20133 Milan, Italy. [2] University of Tsukuba, Tsukuba, Japan. [3] National Cancer Center Hospital East, Chiba, Japan. [4] Asan Medical Center, University of Ulsan College of Medicine, Seoul, Republic of Korea. [5] Yale University, New Haven, CT, USA. [6] Erasmus MC Cancer Institute, Rotterdam, Netherlands. [7] University of California Los Angeles, Los Angeles, CA, USA. [8] Eli Lilly and Company, Indianapolis, IN, USA. [9] Barts Cancer Institute, London, UK.

References

1. Cumberbatch K, He T, Thorogood Z, Gartrell BA. Emerging drugs for urothelial (bladder) cancer. Expert Opin Emerg Drugs. 2017;22(2):149–64.
2. Petrylak DP, de Wit R, Chi KN, Drakaki A, Sternberg CN, Nishiyama H, Castellano D, Hussain S, Flechon A, Bamias A, et al. Ramucirumab plus docetaxel versus placebo plus docetaxel in patients with locally advanced or metastatic urothelial carcinoma after platinum-based therapy (RANGE): a randomised, double-blind, phase 3 trial. Lancet. 2017;390(10109):2266–77.
3. Petrylak DP, de Wit R, Chi KN, Drakaki A, Sternberg CN, Nishiyama H, Castellano D, Hussain SA, Flechon A, Bamias A, et al. Ramucirumab plus docetaxel versus placebo plus docetaxel in patients with locally advanced or metastatic urothelial carcinoma after platinum-based therapy (RANGE): overall survival and updated results of a randomised, double-blind, phase 3 trial. Lancet Oncol. 2020;21:105–20.
4. Howie L, Peppercorn J. Early palliative care in cancer treatment: rationale, evidence and clinical implications. Ther Adv Med Oncol. 2013;5(6):318–23.
5. Orom H, Biddle C, Underwood W 3rd, Nelson CJ, Homish DL. What is a "good" treatment decision? decisional control, knowledge, treatment decision making, and quality of life in men with clinically localized prostate cancer. Med Decis Making. 2016;36(6):714–25.
6. Basch E, Deal AM, Dueck AC, Scher HI, Kris MG, Hudis C, Schrag D. Overall survival results of a trial assessing patient-reported outcomes for symptom monitoring during routine cancer treatment. JAMA. 2017;318(2):197–8.
7. Sato K, Sasaki R, Ogura Y, Shimoda N, Togashi H, Terada K, Sugiyama T, Kakinuma H, Ogawa O, Kato T. Expression of vascular endothelial growth factor gene and its receptor (flt-1) gene in urinary bladder cancer. Tohoku J Exp Med. 1998;185(3):173–84.
8. Xia G, Kumar SR, Hawes D, Cai J, Hassanieh L, Groshen S, Zhu S, Masood R, Quinn DI, Broek D, et al. Expression and significance of vascular endothelial growth factor receptor 2 in bladder cancer. J Urol. 2006;175(4):1245–52.
9. Lu D, Shen J, Vil MD, Zhang H, Jimenez X, Bohlen P, Witte L, Zhu Z. Tailoring in vitro selection for a picomolar affinity human antibody directed against vascular endothelial growth factor receptor 2 for enhanced neutralizing activity. J Biol Chem. 2003;278(44):43496–507.
10. Poole RM, Vaidya A. Ramucirumab: first global approval. Drugs. 2014;74(9):1047–58.
11. Aragon-Ching JB, Trump DL. Targeted therapies in the treatment of urothelial cancers. Urol Oncol. 2017;35(7):465–72.
12. Mazzola CR, Chin J. Targeting the VEGF pathway in metastatic bladder cancer. Expert Opin Investig Drugs. 2015;24(7):913–27.
13. Eisenhauer EA, Therasse P, Bogaerts J, Schwartz LH, Sargent D, Ford R, Dancey J, Arbuck S, Gwyther S, Mooney M, et al. New response evaluation criteria in solid tumours: revised RECIST guideline (version 1.1). Eur J Cancer. 2009;45(2):228–47.
14. Aaronson NK, Ahmedzai S, Bergman B, Bullinger M, Cull A, Duez NJ, Filiberti A, Flechtner H, Fleishman SB, de Haes JC, et al. The European Organization for Research and Treatment of Cancer QLQ-C30: a quality-of-life instrument for use in international clinical trials in oncology. J Natl Cancer Inst. 1993;85(5):365–76.
15. Herdman M, Gudex C, Lloyd A, Janssen M, Kind P, Parkin D, Bonsel G, Badia X. Development and preliminary testing of the new five-level version of EQ-5D (EQ-5D-5L). Qual Life Res. 2011;20(10):1727–36.
16. Osoba D, Rodrigues G, Myles J, Zee B, Pater J. Interpreting the significance of changes in health-related quality-of-life scores. J Clin Oncol. 1998;16(1):139–44.
17. Devlin NJ, Shah KK, Feng Y, Mulhern B, van Hout B. Valuing health-related quality of life: An EQ-5D-5L value set for England. Health Econ. 2018;27(1):7–22.
18. Kaasa S, Loge JH, Aapro M, Albreht T, Anderson R, Bruera E, Brunelli C, Caraceni A, Cervantes A, Currow DC, et al. Integration of oncology and palliative care: a Lancet Oncology Commission. Lancet Oncol. 2018;19(11):e588–653.
19. Yafi FA, North S, Kassouf W. First- and second-line therapy for metastatic urothelial carcinoma of the bladder. Curr Oncol. 2011;18(1):e25-34.
20. Taarnhoj GA, Johansen C, Pappot H. Quality of life in bladder cancer patients receiving medical oncological treatment; a systematic review of the literature. Health Qual Life Outcomes. 2019;17(1):20.
21. Serpentini S, Del Bianco P, Chirico A, Merluzzi TV, Martino R, Lucidi F, De Salvo GL, Trentin L, Capovilla E. Self-efficacy for coping: utility of the Cancer behavior inventory (Italian) for use in palliative care. BMC Palliat Care. 2019;18(1):34.
22. Huang W, Yang J, Liu Y, Liu C, Zhang X, Fu W, Shi L, Liu G. Assessing health-related quality of life of patients with colorectal cancer using EQ-5D-5L: a cross-sectional study in Heilongjiang of China. BMJ Open. 2018;8(12):e022711.
23. Geels P, Eisenhauer E, Bezjak A, Zee B, Day A. Palliative effect of chemotherapy: objective tumor response is associated with symptom improvement in patients with metastatic breast cancer. J Clin Oncol. 2000;18(12):2395–405.
24. Chau I, Fuchs CS, Ohtsu A, Barzi A, Liepa AM, Cui ZL, Hsu Y, Al-Batran SE. Association of quality of life with disease characteristics and treatment outcomes in patients with advanced gastric cancer: Exploratory analysis of RAINBOW and REGARD phase III trials. Eur J Cancer. 2019;107:115–23.
25. Vaughn DJ, Bellmunt J, Fradet Y, Lee JL, Fong L, Vogelzang NJ, Climent MA, Petrylak DP, Choueiri TK, Necchi A, et al. Health-related quality-of-life analysis from KEYNOTE-045: a phase III study of pembrolizumab versus chemotherapy for previously treated advanced urothelial cancer. J Clin Oncol. 2018;36(16):1579–87.
26. Powles T, Duran I, van der Heijden MS, Loriot Y, Vogelzang NJ, De Giorgi U, Oudard S, Retz MM, Castellano D, Bamias A, et al. Atezolizumab versus chemotherapy in patients with platinum-treated locally advanced or metastatic urothelial carcinoma (IMvigor211): a multicentre, open-label, phase 3 randomised controlled trial. Lancet. 2018;391(10122):748–57.
27. Atkins MB, Rini BI, Motzer RJ, Powles T, McDermott DF, Suarez C, Bracarda S, Stadler WM, Donskov F, Gurney H, et al. Patient-reported outcomes from the phase III Randomized IMmotion151 Trial: Atezolizumab + Bevacizumab versus sunitinib in treatment-naive metastatic renal cell carcinoma. Clin Cancer Res. 2020;26:2506.
28. Unger JM, Griffin K, Donaldson GW, Baranowski KM, Good MJ, Reburiano E, Hussain M, Monk PJ, Van Veldhuizen PJ, Carducci MA, et al. Patient-reported outcomes for patients with metastatic castration-resistant prostate cancer receiving docetaxel and Atrasentan versus docetaxel and placebo in a randomized phase III clinical trial (SWOG S0421). J Patient Rep Outcomes. 2017;2:27.
29. EORTC. Quality of Life. Questionnairres. https://qol.eortc.org/questionnaires/. Accessed 7th May 2020.
30. Mason SJ, Catto JWF, Downing A, Bottomley SE, Glaser AW, Wright P. Evaluating patient-reported outcome measures (PROMs) for bladder cancer: a systematic review using the COnsensus-based Standards for the selection of health Measurement INstruments (COSMIN) checklist. BJU Int. 2018;122(5):760–73.
31. Health USDo, Human Services FDACfDE, Research, Health USDo, Human Services FDACfBE, Research, Health USDo, Human Services FDACfD, Radiological H. Guidance for industry: patient-reported outcome measures: use in medical product development to support labeling claims: draft guidance. Health Qual Life Outcomes. 2006;4:79.
32. Basch E, Deal AM, Kris MG, Scher HI, Hudis CA, Sabbatini P, Rogak L, Bennett AV, Dueck AC, Atkinson TM, et al. Symptom monitoring with patient-reported outcomes during routine cancer treatment: a randomized controlled trial. J Clin Oncol. 2016;34(6):557–65.
33. Loriot Y, Necchi A, Park SH, Garcia-Donas J, Huddart R, Burgess E, Fleming M, Rezazadeh A, Mellado B, Varlamov S, et al. Erdafitinib in locally advanced or metastatic urothelial carcinoma. N Engl J Med. 2019;381(4):338–48.

34. Powles T, Park SH, Voog E, Caserta C, Valderamma BP, H G: Maintenance avelumab + best supportive care (BSC) versus BSC alone after platinum-based first-line (1L) chemotherapy in advanced urothelial carcinoma (UC): JAVELIN Bladder 100 phase III interim analysis. *J Clin Oncol 38: 2020 (suppl; abstr LBA1)* 2020.
35. Rosenberg JE, O'Donnell PH, Balar AV, McGregor BA, Heath EI, Yu EY, Galsky MD, Hahn NM, Gartner EM, Pinelli JM, et al. Pivotal trial of enfortumab vedotin in urothelial carcinoma after platinum and anti-programmed death 1/programmed death ligand 1 therapy. J Clin Oncol. 2019;37(29):2592–600.

19

Transurethral seminal vesiculoscopy for intractable hematospermia: Experience from 144 patients

Wei-Kang Chen[1†], Dong-Dong Yu[1†], Zhi-Xia Chen[1], Peng-Fei Li[1], Jian Cai[1], Yu-Peng Liu[2] and Zhi-Gang Wu[1,3*]

Abstract

Purpose: to describe the methodology of transurethral seminal vesiculoscopy and the anatomy of the area of the verumontanum, and to determine the safety of this procedure, especially in terms of postoperative complications.

Methods: This retrospective observational study enrolled 144 patients with intractable hematospermia from May 2011 and August 2019. A 4.5/6.5-Fr vesiculoscope was inserted into the seminal vesicle to deal with the positive findings. The solution of quinolones was used to rinse each seminal vesicle.

Results: In this study, Transurethral seminal vesiculoscopy was successfully performed in 139 patients (96.53%). Hematospermia was alleviated or disappeared in 116 (80.56%) patients by less than half a year after surgery. Common intraoperative manifestations were hemorrhage, stones, utricle polyps and cysts. The surgical approach in our study were categorized into four types, including 24 (16.7%), 73 (50.7%), 42 (29.2%), and 5 (3.5%) cases in Type A (natural opening of the ejaculatory duct), B (trans-duct fenestration), C (trans-utricle fenestration), and D (not founded), respectively. Sexual function change was recorded in 12 patients of 111 patients, all by the method of trans-utricle fenestration, including 8 (7.21%), 3 (2.70%), and 1 (0.90%) patients in shorter intravaginal ejaculatory latency time, worse erection hardness and loss of orgasm, respectively.

Conclusion: Transurethral seminal vesiculoscopy is an effective and safe procedure for the management of hematospermia. The anatomy of the distal seminal tract should be understood more deeply and Wu'method (uncover-curtain method) needs to be promoted to verify its universality and safety. Besides, the complications of the function dysfunction should be discussed in the future in multi-center clinical trials.

Keywords: Hematospermia, Transurethral seminal vesiculoscopy, Therapy

Introduction

Hematospermia is the presence of blood in the semen. There are various etiologies, including inflammation, duct obstruction, cysts, tumors, vascular abnormalities, systemic factors and iatrogenic causes. In the present study, most hematospermia was self-limiting and could resolve with appropriate antimicrobial treatment [1]. Nevertheless, there remain some patients who suffered recurrent hematospermia, for which the conservative management is not effective. This is a condition that causes great anxiety and panic among patients, leading to damaged physical and mental health [2].

Current non-invasive imaging examinations used for the diagnosis of hematospermia include transrectal ultrasonography (TRUS), pelvic computed tomography (CT) and magnetic resonance imaging (MRI). Whereas

*Correspondence: andrologywzg@wmu.edu.cn
†Wei-Kang Chen and Dong-Dong Yu have contributed equally to this work
[1] Department of Andrology, The First Affiliated Hospital of Wenzhou Medical University, Wenzhou 325000, Zhejiang, China
Full list of author information is available at the end of the article

examinations can diagnose, they may miss some small lesions or produce false positives. Transurethral seminal vesiculoscopy (TUSV) can achieve both diagnosis and therapy and more and more operators have successfully performed this operation with good effect [3–5]. Nevertheless, the long-term efficacy and safety have not been reported, especially regarding postoperative complication of sexual dysfunction. Furthermore, the procedure of the TUSV has not been standardized, because of unfamiliarity with the anatomy of the area of the verumontanum.

Here, we summarize our experience from 144 TUSV patients by illustrating detailed surgical methods, treatment outcomes, and intraoperative findings, with a discussion on the postoperative sexual function change and kinds of operative approaches. We supposed that transurethral seminal vesiculoscopy is an effective and safe procedure for the management of hematospermia, but still needs our future researches.

Materials and methods

Study cohort

This study enrolled consecutive patients who had intractable hematospermia and underwent surgery of TUSV between May 2011 and August 2019 in the Department of Urology, The First Affiliated Hospital of Wenzhou Medical University, Wenzhou, Zhejiang Province, China. All patients presented with continuous or episodic hematospermia.

Regarding the diagnosis of hematospermia, we mainly rely on detailed consultation and photos of semen provided after patients' sex life for reference. Then, they would take a series of physical examination, laboratory test (serum PSA, coagulation profile, blood routine, urine routine, liver function test, kidney function test) and imaging examination (TRUS or MRI) to exclude other diseases and confirm the diagnosis (An additional picture file shows this in more detail [see Additional file 1]). In addition, some patients would provide corresponding semen examination reports. These patients who still have obvious symptoms of hematospermia with the naked eye, after taking antibiotics (usually quinolones) regularly for at least 4 weeks, physical therapy and lifestyle improvements for more than 3 months, were diagnosed as continuous or intractable hematospermia. The specific diagnosis and treatment plan was presented in Additional file 2. Finally, patients who asking for further treatment, and then they were admitted to be treated by TUSV after comprehensive doctor–patient communication, who are enrolled in this study.

Approval for this study was granted by the Ethics Committee of The First Affiliated Hospital of Wenzhou Medical University, Wenzhou, Zhejiang Province, China and written informed consent was obtained from all patients before administering treatment. All methods were carried out in accordance with relevant guidelines and regulations.

Surgical procedures

Each patient was placed in the lithotomy position and received general anesthesia. A small-diameter rigid vesiculoscope (4.5/6.5-Fr, Wolf, Germany) was inserted into the normal anatomic path of the urethra. After passing through two bends of urethra, the verumontanum was shown in the prostatic urethra. The anatomy of the distal seminal tract and its surroundings are noted in Fig. 1 and the subsequent procedure is illustrated in Additional file 3.

There are three ways to enter the seminal vesicle in our study (Fig. 2). In some patients, the opening of the ejaculatory duct was easily found at a position lateral to the verumontanum using a hand-controlled irrigation pressure change, but it usually was found covered with white membranous tissues. The type A way is to through the founded natural opening of the ejaculatory duct. When the path to the ejaculatory duct was not be distinguished on the preface of verumontanum (Type B, C, D), a surgical approach was established. First, a small-diameter rigid vesiculoscope was inserted into the utricle orifice and then the full view of the utricle was shown on the endoscopic monitor. Second, the vesiculoscope was turned back to the opening of utricle, and tentative scratch was made on the bilateral inner wall of the entrance of utricle, approximately in the 5 o'clock and 7 o'clock position. The ejaculatory duct is just beneath the thin layer tissues and the vesiculoscope could be inserted into the ejaculatory duct gently (trans-duct fenestration, Type B); in other patients, the hidden ejaculatory duct could not be found. In Type C patients, the vesiculoscope should be inserted into the utricle. Then, the monitor should focus on the lateroposterior aspect of the utricle wall trying to find the membranous junction between the prostate utricle and the seminal vesicle. In few patients, there was a blue translucent membrane, while in most patients the junction could not be found easily. The trick for identifying the junction is to rhythmically control saline irrigation and watch carefully. The membranous junction often appeared in a periodic motion of sinking and bulging under the change of water pressure. Finally, a fenestration could be made by puncturing using a guidewire (Straight Tip, stiff shaft guidewire, NGCV0557, BARD, NICORE, U.S.A.) through seminal vesicle (trans-utricle fenestration). The typical appearance of the seminal vesicle (SV) is similar to honeycomb. However, in some patients, these pathways could not be found (Type D), and the operation through the seminal vesicle failed.

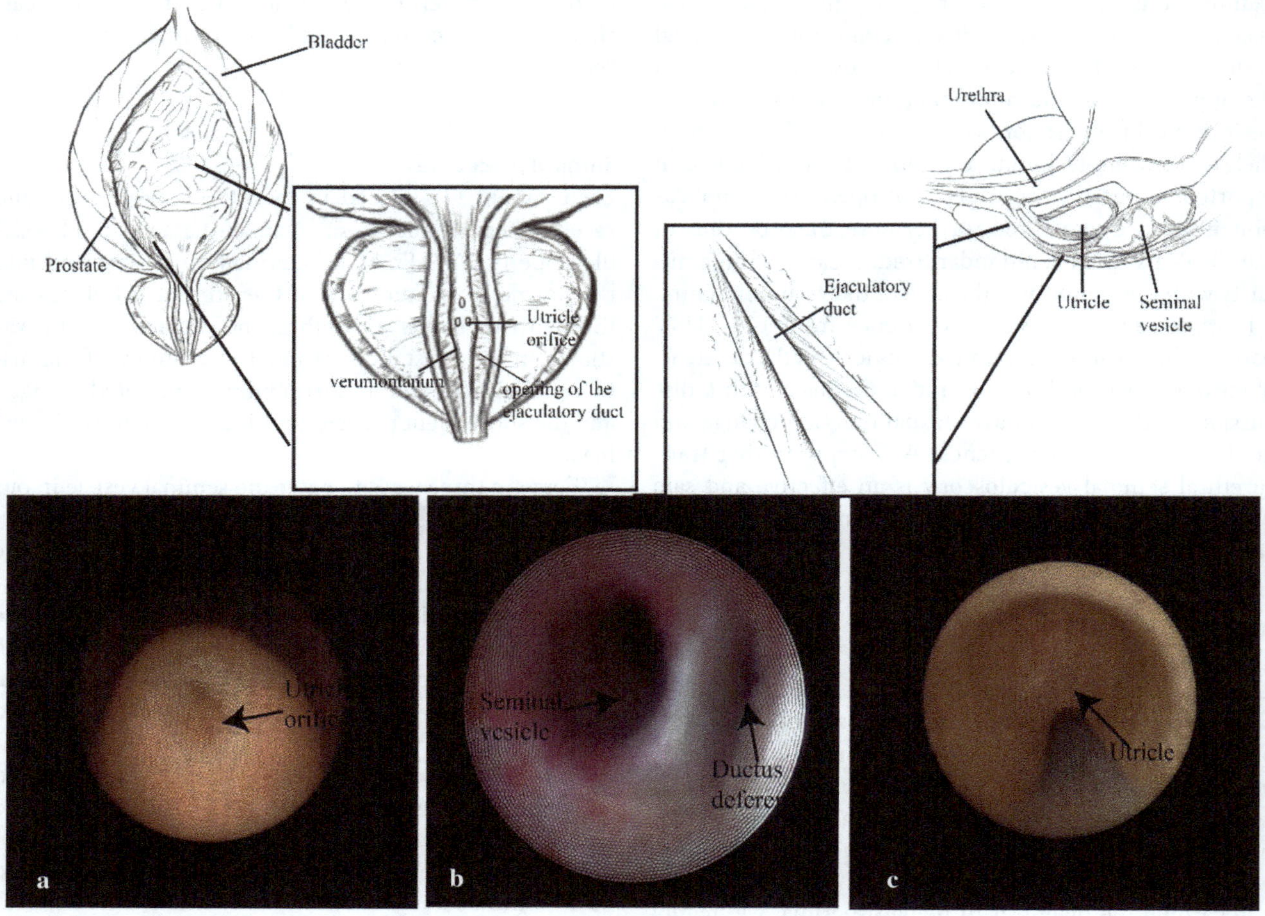

Fig. 1 Anatomy of the verumontanum, utricle and ejaculatory duct

Finally, regardless of pathway to the SV, the surgeon needed to go through every small cavity in the SV. Then, kinds of treatments were performed according to the endoscopic findings of the seminal vesicle. For patients who had large SV stones that could not easily be washed out using continuous saline irrigation but keeping the pressure of SV as low as possible, holmium laser lithotripsy was performed. After this procedure, small crushed stones could be flushed out. When old or new hemorrhage was found in the SV, the subsequent step was to wash it out. Until no stone and hemorrhage could be found in SV, 250 ml solution of quinolones (typically 250 mL of saline solution with 400 mg of Mosifloxacin) would be used to rinse each SV. Meanwhile, the same method was performed for cleaning up utricle. Finally, in patients who underwent trans-utricle fenestration, the surgical path between the prostatic utricle and seminal vesicle was expanded using the scope body or a holmium laser incision to prevent possible stenosis and recurrence, while patients who underwent trans-duct fenestration accepted expanding for new paths by the scope body. After the operation, a 14-Fr Foley catheter was retained for 24 h. Besides, within 48 h after surgery, patients still were infused with intravenous antibiotics (always 250 mL of saline solution with 400 mg of Mosifloxacin) once a day. Before leaving hospital, some patients had MRI to ensure that the operation was successful (large stones or blood clots disappeared compared with pre-operative MRI).

Data collection and statistical methods

We retrospectively recorded demographic and operation data, including age, disease duration, and basic disease history. Therapeutic outcomes were recorded. Patients whose semen turned back to milky white or presented no red blood cells under the microscope were regarded as cured or disappeared; Patients whose semen changed from dark brown or bright red to light red or milky white but presented some red blood cells under the microscope were regarded as reduced. We followed up three times at 3 months, 6 months and 12 months after surgery. We asked the patient's situation of hematospermia

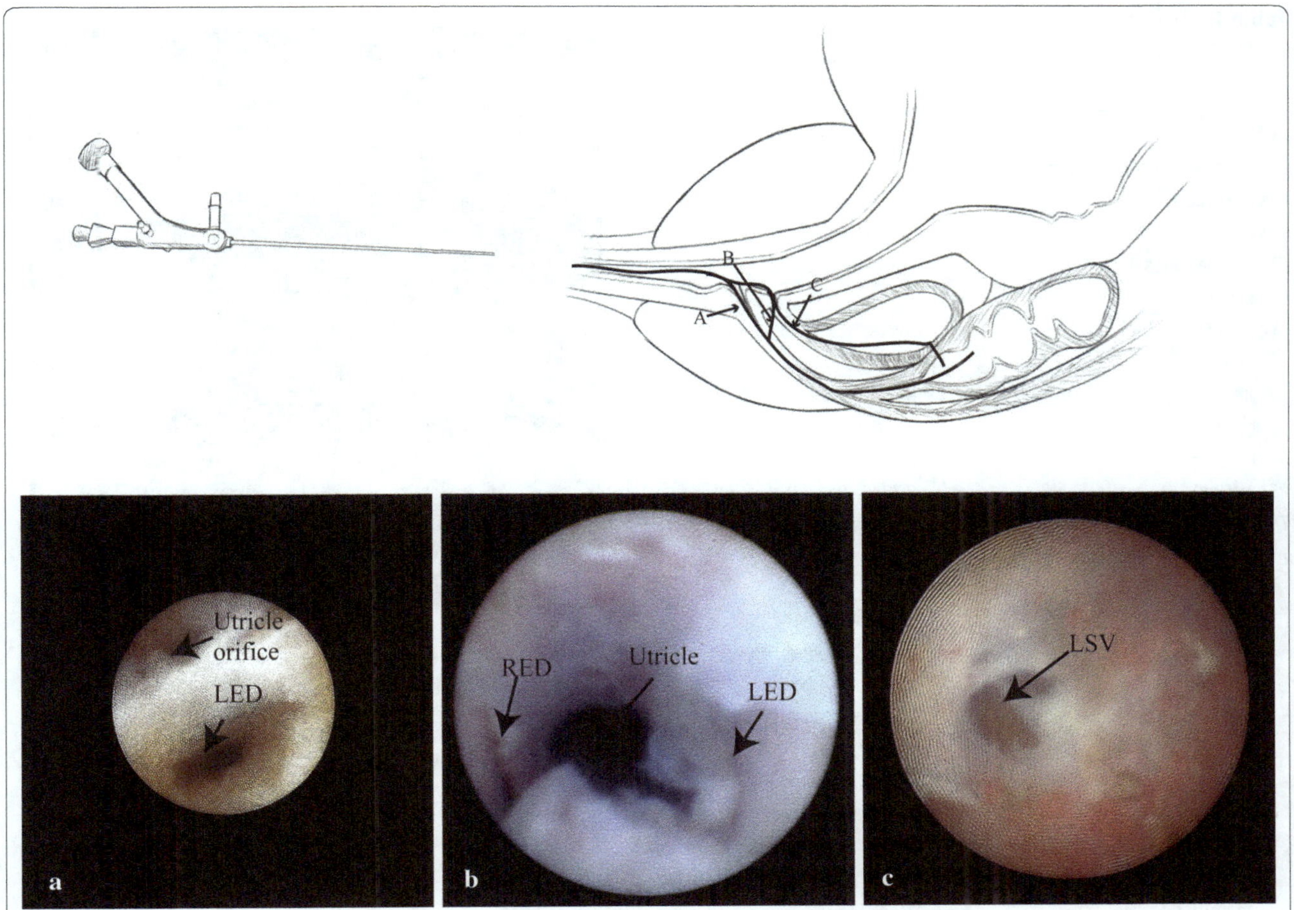

Fig. 2 Approach through seminal vesicle. Arrow A, approach through the opening of ejaculatory duct. Arrow B, approach through the bilateral inner wall of the entrance of utricle. Arrow C, approach through the lateroposterior aspect of the utricle wall. LED, left ejaculatory duct. RED, right ejaculatory duct. LSV, left seminal vesicle

(disappeared or present) and sexual function (i.e. intravaginal ejaculatory latency time and erection hardness scale) at every follow-up interview by call. Continuous variables such as age were presented as mean (Std.), except follow-up period expressed as median (range). Categorical variables such as hypertension were expressed as counts and percentages. The comparison of efficient of TUSV in two kind of patients were used by Chi-square test. All analyses were conducted using Stata 13.0 (Stata Corp, College Station, TX, USA).

Results

Preoperative data and treatment outcomes

A total of 199 patients presented to the urology and andrology department for recurrent hematospermia between 2011 and 2019; however, only 144 patients were enrolled in this study. The specific include/exclude process could be seen in (Additional file 4. The characteristics are shown in Table 1. The effect of TUSV was not immediate. Hematospermia disappeared or reduced in 98 (68.06%) and 18 (12.50%), respectively, by no more than 3 months after surgery (most symptoms disappear within a month). Six of 98 patients experienced recurrence by 12 months after surgery. Symptoms persisted and aggravated in 22 (15.28%) and 6 (4.17%) patients, respectively. The treatments for patients who were dissatisfied with the outcome were always antibiotics and lifestyle improvement; nevertheless the effectiveness remained inadequate. The results of MRI all showed that blood clots or stones disappeared in the seminal vesicles and utricle.

Surgical approach and intraoperative findings

The surgical approaches in our study were categorized into four types, including 24 (16.67%), 73 (50.69%), 42 (29.17%) and 5 (3.47%) patients in Type A, B, C, and D, respectively. Normally, there are nothing in SV, utricle or ED; however, in patients who underwent this surgery, hemorrhage, stones and cyst in the vision (SV, utricle, or

Table 1 Characteristics of patients

	Patient with hemospermia (n = 144)
Age (years)	42 (30.73–52.25)
Duration of hemospermia (months)	12 (12–24)
Hypertension	24/144 (16.67%)
DM	2/144 (1.39%)
Chronic hepatitis B	7/144 (4.86%)
Urine routine	
Microscopic hematuria	39/141 (27.46%)
Pyuria	3/141 (2.11%)
Proteinuria	6/141 (4.23%)
Sugaruria	1/141 (0.70%)
Not tested	n = 3
PSA(ng/ml)	0.72 (0.49–1.13)
TRUS/MRI fingding	
Dilatation or enlargement of SV	70/141 (49.65%)
Hemorrhage	20/141 (14.18%)
Inflammation of SV	25/141 (17.73%)
Overall cyst	52/141 (36.88%)
Prostate	22/141 (15.60%)
Mullerian duct	26/141 (18.44%)
Seminal vesicle	3/141 (2.13%)
Ejaculatory duct	4/141 (2.84%)
Prostate	74/141 (52.48%)
Hyperplasia	42/141 (26.95%)
Enlargement	25/141 (15.60%)
Inflammation	7/141 (3.55%)
Stone	5/141 (1.42%)
Nodular	2/141 (0.71%)
Normal	10/141 (7.09%)
Not tested	n = 3
Successful TUSV	139/144 (96.53%)
Follow-up period (days)	1021.5 (72–2626)

Continuous variables expressed as median (interquartile range), except follow-up period expressed as median (range)

both areas) were presented in 75 (52.08%), 72 (50.00%) and 53 (36.81%) patients, respectively. Utricle polyp was observed in only one patient. Nothing positive occurred in 24 (16.67%) patients (Fig. 3).

The rate of hematospermia disappeared and reduced in patients with different intraoperative findings.

The rate of hematospermia disappeared and reduced in patients whose intraoperative findings were only hemorrhage was 88.00% (22/25), while in patients whose intraoperative findings were both hemorrhage and stones was 73.17% (30/41) ($p > 0.05$).

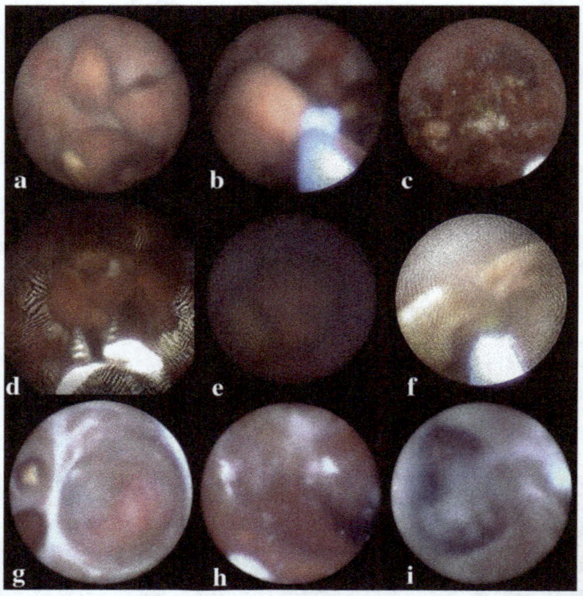

Fig. 3 Perioperative findings in transurethral seminal vesiculoscopy. **a** Stones in the utricle; **b** thulium fiber laser applied to crush stones in the utricle; **c** crushed stones; **d** grasping forceps applied for removal of stones in the utricle; **e** big stones in the seminal vesicle; **f** thulium fiber laser applied to crush stones in the seminal vesicle; **g** small stone in the seminal vesicle; **h** old hemorrhage in the seminal vesicle; **i** seminal plasma in the seminal vesicle

Complications

Complications were as follows: Subjective semen volume decreased in two patients without semen analysis, both of whom underwent TUSV by inserting into the ejaculatory duct opening and refused to have a further medical examination. Every patient was asked about the sexual function before and after operation; however, only 111 patients accepted and answered this question. Of 111 patients, sexual function change was presented in 12 (10.81%), including 8 (7.21%), 3 (2.70%) and 1 (0.90%) patients who reported shorter sexual time, worse erection hardness and loss of orgasm, respectively (Table 2). Of eight patients, five complained of shorter postoperatively self-estimated intravaginal ejaculatory latency time

Table 2 Sexual function change of patients before and after TUSV

	Preoperation	Postoperation	Patients (n = 144)
Intravaginal ejaculatory latency time (minutes)	> 5	> 5	5
	> 5	< 2	2
	< 2	< 2	1
Erection hardness scale	IV	III	3
Frequency of orgasm	HIGH	Low	1

(IELT); however, all their IELT before and after operation was longer than five minutes. However, two patients indicated their IELT changed from longer than 5 min to shorter than 2 min after surgery, which may accord with the clinical standard of premature ejaculation (PE). One patient represented that his IELT was worse, while his IELT had been shorter than 2 min before surgery. Of three patients, all reported their erection hardness scale (EHS) changed from IV to III. All 12 patients denied a history of taking testosterone modulating medications. The remaining 99 patients reported no change in their sexual function. As for other complications, only one patient with postoperative epididymitis was treated with a week of intravenous quinolone antibiotics. No retrograde ejaculation, urinary reflux into the ejaculatory duct, fistula, or other severe complications were observed.

Discussion

Since the first application of endoscopy for examining the interior of the seminal vesicle ex vivo by Shimada et al. [6] in 1996, this new method for observing SV directly had attracted the attention of the andrologists and urologists. Nowadays, the vesiculoscope has been used in some large hospitals. However, there remain many surgeons beginning to operate this procedure, for whom transurethral seminal vesiculoscopy (TUSV) is an advanced but challenging procedure. The present study reported some tricks and details devoting to how to use TUSV, but it is not sufficient enough. Therefore, we focused on sharing our experience and putting forward some views after at least 10 years' application of TUSV.

Transurethral seminal vesiculoscopy has been recommended as the first-line diagnostic modality [7] in hematospermia patients because of its real-time images and low cost. Besides, TUSV is also helpful for therapy.

Xing et al. [8] concluded that TUSV was superior to TRUS for diagnosis, especially for lesions with stones and obstruction. It can also be used to treat recurrent hematospermia and ejaculatory duct obstruction [9] caused by stones or cysts by facilitating removal of calculi, elimination of obstruction and drainage of infection. Liu et al. [3] reported that the hematospermia symptom in 94.4% patients was completely treated and alleviated. Liu et al. [10] reported that hematospermia was alleviated in 89% patients. During the long history of application, it was confirmed to be an effective procedure for both diagnosis and treatment, without severe complications.

In the current study, the improvement rate of hematospermia was 80.56% and the recurrence rate was 6.12%, comparable to similar studies reported in the literature [4, 5]. The reason why our improvement rate of hematospermia was relatively lower than other studies may be the relatively longer duration of hematospermia in enrolled patients. In the meantime, to our knowledge, our median follow-up period of 3.38 years was the longest. For this reason, we are surprised that there were no long-term complications. Our findings provide more powerful evidence supporting the safety and efficiency of TUSV.

We would like to highlight two additional points:

First, we want to name one of approaches of TUSV (*Wu' method*) to capture the attention of surgeons and to promote application of this method (An additional movie file shows this in more detail [see Additional file 5]). In the present articles all over the world, we find four ways to treat hematospermia surgically, including a method of transurethral resection of the ejaculatory duct (TURED) and three methods of TUSV. In our concept, we don't divide TURED into TUSV, due to differences of surgical instrument of vesiculoscope (usually 24-Fr vs. 4.5/6.5-Fr; combine with an electrocautery loop vs. only a scope) and surgical procedure (resection vs. only blunt operation) [11].

We are trying to describe four methods of treating hematospermia as follows: when the opening of the ejaculatory duct is observed from the urethra, inserting into this natural orifice (the first way) is the first choice; whereas in other patients, when the opening is not identified clearly, there are two methods.

First, some surgeons applied TURED (the second way) to observe the covered ejaculatory duct openings. The probable complications of retrograde ejaculation and urinary reflux limited the widely application of this method. At present, surgeons hardly use TURED to locate the opening of the ejaculatory duct exclusively, while some surgeons try to treat patients with Mullerian duct cyst [12]. In addition, surgeons can insert into the verumontanum orifice and establish a surgical path through the ejaculatory duct (the third way) or SV (the fourth way) directly. The only difference between these two approaches is the puncture site (the inner wall of the utricle entrance or the laterposterior aspect of the utricle wall). Anyway, the most important factors are safety and efficacy depending on which method should be used firstly.

We can evaluate safety on the basis of anatomical structure. Nguyen et al. [13] reported the ejaculatory duct and SV consist of three similar histological layers, including a columnar epithelium, a collagenous coat and a muscular layer. The most surprising finding was that all these three layers become thin as the duct proceeds distally, especially the almost disappearing muscular layer. It is not difficult to conclude that the more distal area we puncture, the fewer tissues we destroy. Li et al. [14] reported that the opening of the ejaculatory duct was covered by the valves that needs to be protected in order to prevent urinary reflux into the ejaculatory ducts. This finding may explain why TURED causes these complications of retrograde ejaculation and urinary reflux.

After approximately 10 years' application of rigid vesiculoscope, we recommend an approach (*Wu'method*) through the distal ejaculatory duct, not inserting into the opening of the ejaculatory duct, passing the inner wall of the utricle entrance. The key procedure of this method is to tentatively scratch the entrance of the inner wall of the utricle entrance using the former endoscope. Then, the membrane-like tissue is identified under the monitor. After setting up this tissue, the passageway can be detected and used for entering the ejaculatory duct. Because of the process of the creating and setting up the membrane-like tissue, similar to the action of setting up a curtain or quilt, we would like to call this method the *uncover-curtain method*. In our experience, we found that the success rate of this method was high and the outcomes were good. We emphasize this approach by detailed introduction of seminal tracts and try to make a standard for TUSV so as to encourage its use.

Second, the complications of sexual function are important to discuss. To the best of our knowledge, this study is the first research paying attention to sexual dysfunction after this surgery. The follow-up results showed that 12 patients seemed to suffer sexual dysfunction, including the tendency of premature ejaculation and erectile dysfunction. After we investigated the specific surgical approaches of these 12 patients, we surprisingly discovered that all of them had been treated by puncturing using a guidewire through the SV. This fact triggers our thinking to one guess whether this approach would cause more sexual function influence than other two approaches. Sexuality, as an inherent need for human beings [15], attracts the attention of both patients and doctors. For this reason, we should concentrate on researching the potential relationship between the operation by puncturing using a guidewire through SV and sexual dysfunction. In case this kind of operation can cause sexual dysfunction, we should identify the specific mechanism and countermeasures to prevent these complications by abandoning or improving this method of TUSV. Therefore, our next purpose is to prepare a study to investigate this potential relationship.

There are some limitations in this study. First, its retrospective design invites recall bias. The results of the post-operative outcome are judged by the view of the patients solely. Besides, most patients lacked semen analyses both before and after surgery, due to most patients (always have one or more kids) without the desire to fertile and the expensive price of semen related tests. However, we will collect some younger patients and acquire their semen analyses before and after surgery in the future, because of its effect to verify validity of TUSV. Second, the situation of sexual dysfunction lacks of evaluation of some scales and other examinations, including IIEF-5 or penile Doppler USG investigation. Third, hematospermia is usually a self-limiting disease and the natural course might interfere with the complete remission and improvement rates. However, in this study, patient who have a long history of hematospermia and have been ineffective after long-term treatment were enrolled. In addition, of 16 patients who refused surgery (10 patients before 2011 and 6 patients in this study), only 1 patient recovered within 3 years after a long-term follow-up. Although the probability of natural recovery of our patients is low, it cannot be ruled out that a small number of patients were cured by themselves. Fourthly, we found that the performing of TUSV in patients with single intraoperative finding (only hemorrhage) was more effective than performing in patients with various intraoperative findings (both hemorrhage and stones), which perfectly meet clinical prognosis. However, $p > 0.05$, because of the few number of total cases. Therefore, further verification is needed.

Conclusions

TUSV may be an effective and safe procedure for treating recurrent hematospermia by blocking the vicious cycle of stasis, stones and seminal vesiculitis. The anatomy of the distal seminal tract should be understood more deeply and *Wu'method* (*uncover-curtain method*) needs to be promoted to verify its universality and safety. Besides, the complications of the function dysfunction should be discussed in the future in multi-center clinical trials.

Abbreviations

TRUS: Transrectal ultrasonography; CT: Pelvic computed tomography; MRI: Magnetic resonance imaging; TUSV: Transurethral seminal vesiculoscopy; SV: Seminal vesicle; PE: Premature ejaculation; IELT: Intravaginal ejaculatory latency time; EHS: Erection hardness scale.

Acknowledgements

We thank Pengfei Yan and Prof. Chengdi Li for his valuable proposals to our manuscript.

Authors' contributions

CWK and YDD drafted the manuscript. CZX, LPF and CJ collected data and performed the statistical analysis. WZG conceived of the study, and participated in its design and coordination and helped to draft the manuscript. All authors read and approved the final manuscript.

Competing interests

The authors have no relevant financial or non-financial interests to disclose.

Author details

[1] Department of Andrology, The First Affiliated Hospital of Wenzhou Medical University, Wenzhou 325000, Zhejiang, China. [2] School of Public Administration and Health, Wenzhou Medical University, Wenzhou 325000, Zhejiang, China. [3] Reproductive Health Research Center, Health Assessment Center of Wenzhou Medical University, Wenzhou 325000, Zhejiang, China.

References

1. Ahmad I, Krishna NS. Hematospermia. J Urol. 2007;177:1613.
2. Information from your family doctor. Hematospermia: blood in the semen. Am Fam Physician. 2009; 80: 1428.
3. Liu ZY, Sun YH, Xu CL, Hou JG, Gao X, Lu X, et al. Transurethral seminal vesiculoscopy in the diagnosis and treatment of persistent or recurrent hematospermia: a single-institution experience. Asian J Androl. 2009;11:566.
4. Chen R, Wang L, Sheng X, Piao SG, Nian XW, Cheng X, et al. Transurethral seminal vesiculoscopy for recurrent hematospermia: experience from 419 cases. Asian J Androl. 2018;20:438.
5. Hu JC, Chen CS. Transurethral seminal vesiculoscopy acts as a therapeutic investigation for intractable hematospermia: step-by-step illustrations and single-surgeon experience. Int J Urol. 2018;25:589.
6. Shimada M, Yoshida H. Ex vivo ultrathin endoscopy of the seminal vesicles. J Urol. 1996;156:1388.
7. Hosseinzadeh K, Oto A, Allen BC, Coakley FV, Friedman B, et al. ACR appropriateness criteria hematospermia. J Am Coll Radiol. 2017;14:S154–9.
8. Xing C, Zhou X, Xin L, Hu H, Li L, Fang J, et al. Prospective trial comparing transrectal ultrasonography and transurethral seminal vesiculoscopy for persistent hematospermia. Int J Urol. 2012;19:437.
9. Liao LG, Li YF, Zhang Y, Li K, Zhu T, Li BJ, et al. Etiology of 305 cases of refractory hematospermia and therapeutic options by emerging endoscopic technology. Sci Rep. 2019;9:5018.
10. Liu B, Li J, Li P, Zhang J, Song N, Wang Z, et al. Transurethral seminal vesiculoscopy in the diagnosis and treatment of intractable seminal vesiculitis. J Int Med Res. 2014;42:236.
11. Avellino GJ, Lipshultz LI, Sigman M, Hwang K. Transurethral resection of the ejaculatory ducts: etiology of obstruction and surgical treatment options. Fertil Steril. 2019;111:427–43.
12. Miao C, Liu S, Zhao K, Zhu J, Tian Y, Wang Y, et al. Treatment of Mullerian duct cyst by combination of transurethral resection and seminal vesiculoscopy: an initial experience. Exp Ther Med. 2019;17:2194.
13. Nguyen HT, Etzell J, Turek PJ. Normal human ejaculatory duct anatomy: a study of cadawric and surgical specimens. J Urol. 1996;155:1639.
14. Li ZY, Xu Y, Liu C, Xiao ZM, Luo BH, Xu GW, et al. Anatomical study of the seminal vesicle system for transurethral seminal vesiculoscopy. Clin Anat. 2019;32:244.
15. Montejo AL. Sexuality and mental health: the need for mutual development and research. J Clin Med. 2019;8:1794.

20

Impact of radiation on the incidence and management of ureteroenteric strictures: A contemporary single center analysis

Clinton T. Yeaman[1*], Andrew Winkelman[2], Kimberly Maciolek[1], Mei Tuong[1], Perri Nelson[1], Chandler Morris[1], Stephen Culp[1,2], Sumit Isharwal[1,2] and Tracey L. Krupski[1]

Abstract

Background: Ureteroenteric stricture incidence has been reported as high as 20% after urinary diversion. Many patients have undergone prior radiotherapy for prostate, urothelial, colorectal, or gynecologic malignancy. We sought to evaluate the differences between ureteroenteric stricture occurrence between patients who had radiation prior to urinary diversion and those who did not.

Methods: An IRB-approved cystectomy database was utilized to identify ureteroenteric strictures among 215 patients who underwent urinary diversion at a single academic center between 2016 and 2020. Chart abstraction was conducted to determine the presence of confirmed stricture in these patients, defined as endoscopic diagnosis or definitive imaging findings. Strictures due to malignant ureteral recurrence were excluded (3 patients). Statistical analysis was performed using chi squared test, t-test, and Wilcoxon Rank-Sum Test, logistic regression, and Kaplan–Meier analysis of stricture by cancer type.

Results: 65 patients had radiation prior to urinary diversion; 150 patients did not have a history of radiation therapy. Benign ureteroenteric stricture rate was 5.3% (8/150) in the non-radiated cohort and 23% (15/65) in the radiated cohort ($p = < 0.001$). Initial management of stricture was percutaneous nephrostomy (PCN) in 78% (18/23) and the remaining 22% (5/23) were managed with primary retrograde ureteral stent placement. Long term management included ureteral reimplantation in 30.4% (7/23).

Conclusions: Our study demonstrates a significant increase in rate of ureteroenteric strictures in radiated patients as compared to non-radiated patients. The insult of radiation on the ureteral microvascular supply is likely implicated in the cause of these strictures. Further study is needed to optimize surgical approach such as utilization of fluorescence angiography for open and robotic approaches.

Keywords: Stricture, Ureteroenteric, Radiation, Urinary diversion

Background

Ureteroenteric anastomotic stricture is a well-known complication of urinary diversion which occurs in 4–20% of patients [1–3]. Patients with strictures present clinically with flank pain, decreased renal function, pyelonephritis, or may be asymptomatic and diagnosed incidentally with progressive hydronephrosis and renal impairment. Strictures are a cause of significant morbidity and health care expenditure, as treatment necessitates procedural intervention and often sev-

*Correspondence: Cy5eb@virginia.edu
[1] Department of Urology, UVA Medical Center, Fontaine Research Park, 500 Ray C. Hunt Drive, Charlottesville, VA 22908, USA
Full list of author information is available at the end of the article

eral repeat admissions. Numerous studies have sought to identify risk factors for development of ureteroenteric strictures, as well as opportunities for technical approaches to reduce stricture risk. Stricture is traditionally more common on the left side, in patients with elevated BMI, longer operative time, and those with Clavien-Dindo ≥ 3 complication, however these studies have not identified radiation therapy as a significant risk factor [3–6]. Increased stricture risk of the left side has been attributed to the need for greater ureteral mobilization in order to transpose it to the right side for anastomosis. This extended dissection is likely to compromise distal ureteral vasculature. Operative time and high-grade complications are associated with stricture development likely in part due to fluid shifts, hypoperfusion of the ureteroenteric anastomosis. These as well as increased risk with elevated BMI are suggestive of the risks seen with difficult urinary diversion surgeries.

Ischemia of the anastomosis related to the tenuous ureteral blood supply is implicated in the formation of ureteroenteric stricture [7]. Basic science and animal data have established the detrimental impact of radiation therapy on microvasculature [8]. Radiation-induced ureteral ischemia, in conjunction with periureteral fibrosis, make the preservation of distal ureteral blood supply during urinary diversion tenuous. This is of concern in patients requiring pelvic exenteration for colorectal or gynecological malignancy, which may necessitate radiation therapy prior to surgical intervention [9–11]. Radiation history is also an important contributor commonly in patients undergoing benign diversion for radiation cystitis or fistulas. Radiation has been demonstrated to be an independent risk factor for development of ureteral strictures, with a 2% ureteral stricture rate from radiation therapy alone [11]. One institutional review examined 25 ureteral strictures and found urolithiasis was the most common cause (60%) while 28% were due to radiation, 4% endometriosis, 4% iatrogenic (without stone), and 4% unknown or other causes [12]. These findings were demonstrated in a cohort of patients with intact urinary tracts and have not been reproduced in a cohort undergoing urinary diversion. Recent work by Beller et al. demonstrated that patients with ureteral stricture following radiation therapy for gynecologic malignancy underwent a mean of 25 procedures per patient, highlighting the significant morbidity and cost associated with ureteral stricture [13].

Radiation therapy continues to improve targeting techniques that spare adjacent organs and urologists have more precision with robotic assisted techniques. With these new innovations, it is possible radiation is less of a risk factor than previously thought. We sought to determine if radiation continues to adversely affect ureteroenteric anastomotic stricture rates in a contemporary series and identify other contributing risk factors.

Methods

An IRB-approved prospectively maintained cystectomy database was utilized to identify ureteroenteric strictures amongst patients who underwent urinary diversion at a single academic center between 2016 and 2020. The cohort of interest was any patient who underwent a urinary diversion whether it was for a benign and malignant etiology. Particular interest was in those with prior radiotherapy for colorectal, gynecologic or urologic malignancy. There were no exclusions in terms of surgeon, operative technique, or type of diversion. Even for robotic extirpation, the diversion was performed in open fashion. For robotic-assisted cases, the ureteral dissection was completed robotically. All ureteroenteric anastomoses were completed using the Bricker technique with interrupted absorbable monofilament. The most common suture used in anastomosis was 4–0 monocryl. Postoperative care was conducted per surgeon preference, including length of stent duration. Procedurally, care was taken to limit ureteral mobilization and manipulation and preserve periureteral tissue.

The outcome of interest was ureteroenteric anastomotic stricture. Chart abstraction was necessary to evaluate imaging reports and clinical presentation to confirm the presence of a clinically relevant stricture. We defined a stricture as endoscopic diagnosis or definitive imaging findings. Endoscopic diagnosis was defined as visualization of focal narrowing at the anastomosis on ureteroscopy, and definitive imaging findings were defined on Computed Tomography (CT) reports indicating focal narrowing at the anastomoses with related hydronephrosis. In the latter case, patients were excluded from the confirmed stricture cohort if their ureteral stricture was suspected to be a result of malignant recurrence; such findings would be indicated by the presence of focal enhancement at the site of ureteral obstruction/stricture and/or biopsy pathology with proven malignancy. Radiation dose delivered was extrapolated based upon current cancer guideline-based protocols. Statistical analysis performed using chi squared test, Student's T-test, Wilcoxon Rank-Sum Test, and logistic regression where appropriate using $\alpha = 0.05$. Given the heterogeneity of the cohort, subset analysis was performed comparing stricture rates between the highest volume surgeon and the remaining surgeons for both radiated and non-radiated patient populations using chi square test. A Kaplan–Meier survival curve was used to compare UES rates between radiation treated cancers.

Results

Over the four year period ending Feb 2020, 215 patients with urinary diversions performed by six surgeons were identified. Figure 1 shows the total cohort broken down by benign versus malignant etiology and for those with malignancy, the number with a non-urologic malignancy. 196 patients underwent construction of ileal conduit, while the other 19 had continent diversions, all of which had refluxing Bricker ureteroenteric anastomoses. 65 patients underwent radiation prior to urinary diversion; 150 patients did not undergo preoperative radiation. The demographics of the cohort comparing the radiated to non-radiated patients are shown in Table 1, including operative intervention and chosen urinary diversion. Patients who underwent pelvic exenteration and supratrigonal cystectomy were more likely to have had radiation, while patients who had radical cystectomy and urinary diversion (RCUD) were less likely to have had radiation ($p < 0.0001$). Patients who underwent radiation therapy were more likely to undergo ileal conduit rather than continent diversion ($p = 0.013$). There was no significant difference between age, sex, Body Mass Index (BMI), Charlson Comorbidity Index, or robotic-assisted surgical approach. The length of stent duration postoperatively was a median of 6 days for the non-radiated group and 7.5 days for the radiated group ($p = 0.08$). The median stent duration postoperatively for patients who would go on to develop stricture was 5.5 days in the non-radiated group and 5 days in the radiated group. In the non-radiated cohort, 7 patients did not have surgical excision of their primary pathology, but did undergo urinary diversion. In the radiated cohort, 10 patients did not have surgical excision of their primary pathology. There was no association between primary pathologic resection and ureteroenteric stricture development.

The overall benign ureteroenteric stricture rate was 10.6% (23/215). Ureteroenteric stricture rate was 5.3% (8/150) in the non-radiated cohort and 23% (15/65) in the radiated cohort ($p < 0.0001$). Stricture diagnosis was made on average 10.3 months after urinary diversion. Logistic regression was used to adjust for BMI as a risk factor. Radiation was found to be a significant predictor of ureteroenteric stricture ($p = 0.0005$) while BMI was not significant ($p = 0.75$). The odds ratio for radiation was 5.2. Diagnosis was made on average 12.7 months postoperatively in radiated patients and 5.7 months postoperatively

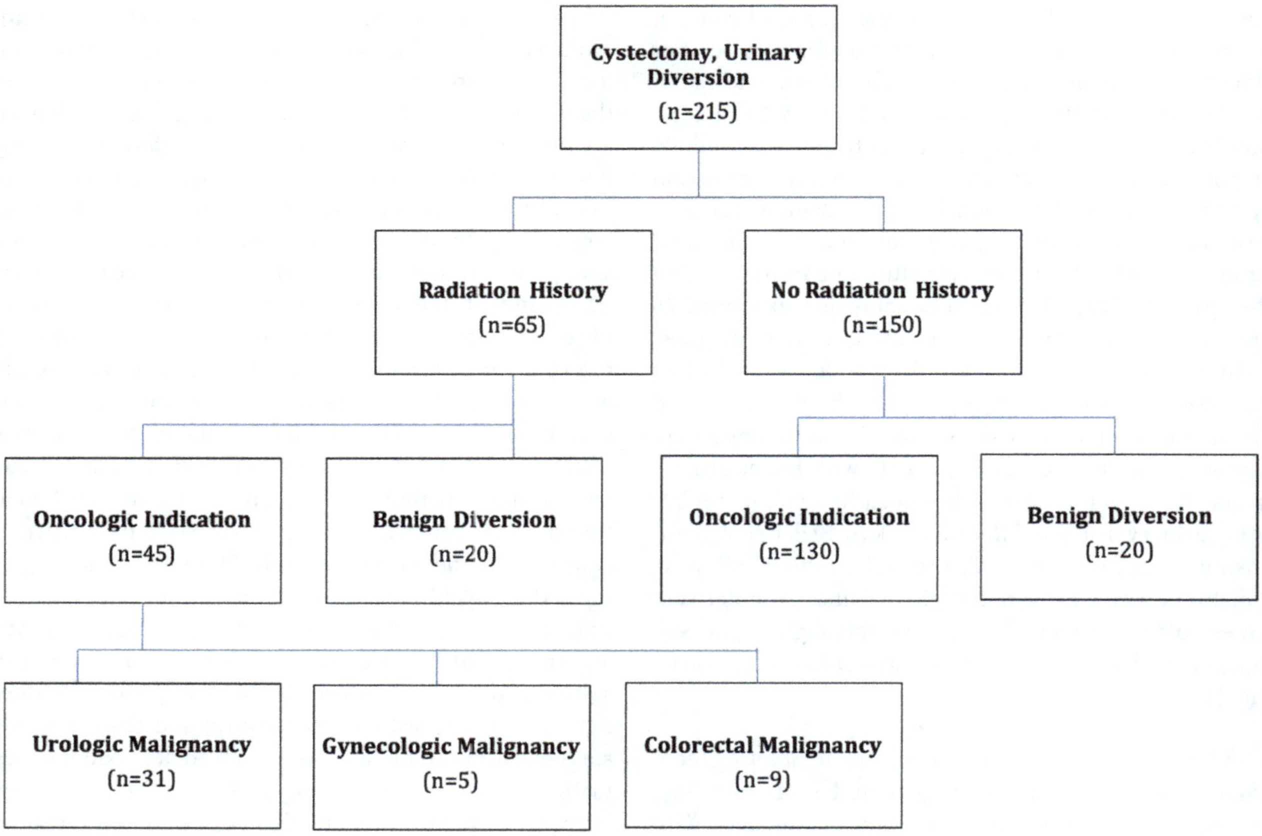

Fig. 1 Breakdown of patient cohorts, radiation status, and indication for urinary diversion

Table 1 Demographic and surgical information

	Overall cohort (n = 215) N (%)	Non-radiated (n = 150) N (%)	Radiated (n = 65) N (%)	*p*
Age	66.5	65.3	67	0.2
BMI (kg/m^2)	27.57	28.93	26.98	0.06
Female	70 (32.5)	44 (29.3)	26 (40.0)	0.12
CCI	3.9	3.6	4.1	0.1
Pelvic exenteration	15 (7)	0	15 (23.1)	< 0.0001
				< 0.0001
Radical cystectomy/urinary diversion	160 (74.4)	130 (86.6)	30 (46.2)	0.002
Supratrigonal cystectomy/urinary diversion	40 (18.6)	20 (13.3)	20 (30.8)	
Ileal conduit	196 (91)	132 (88)	64 (98.5)	0.01
Orthotopic neobladder	7 (3)	7 (4.7)	0	
Indiana pouch	12 (6)	11 (7.3)	1 (15.3)	
Robotic-assisted	22 (11)	18 (12)	4 (6.2)	0.19
Open approach	193 (89)	132 (88)	61 (93.8)	

BMI, body mass index; CCI, Charlson comorbidity index

in non-radiated patients, however this difference was not significant ($p = 0.06$). Of those with prior radiation, 10 were left-sided, 4 were right-sided, and 1 was bilateral. In the non-radiated group, 5 were right-sided and 3 were left-sided. Initial management of stricture was percutaneous nephrostomy (PCN) in 78% (18/23) and the other 22% (5/23) were managed with primary ureteral stent. 30.4% (7/23) patients went on to have open reimplantation, 52.2% (12/23) continued to have stent exchanges, and 17.4% (4/23) live with percutaneous nephrostomy tubes. 3 of the 7 patients who had open reconstruction had prior radiation and 4 were non-radiated.

There was no significant difference between rates of 90-day readmission. To account for variability in stricture rates between surgeons, we analyzed rates of stricture between the single surgeon who performed 127 of the included cases in comparison with the 5 surgeons who performed the remaining 88 cases. There was no difference in stricture risk by surgeon for those with radiation ($p = 0.2$) or those without radiation ($p = 0.07$). Clinical presentation of each of the ureteroenteric strictures was determined. Each of these clinical factors was not mutually exclusive. Pyelonephritis was the most common presenting symptom of stricture. 6 non-radiated and 8 radiated patients presented with pyelonephritis. 2 non-radiated patients and 8 radiated patients presented with renal impairment. 1 non-radiated patient and 3 radiated patients experienced flank pain. 3 radiated patients were clinically asymptomatic and diagnosed on imaging. Of the 3 patients who were diagnosed primarily with hydronephrosis noted on imaging, 2 had renal impairment noted on concurrent laboratory evaluation as well. Of note, nine patients would go on to have ureteroscopy confirming stricture presence, however each of the diagnosed strictures was first evaluated with cross-sectional imaging, which demonstrated the presence of ureteroenteric stricture. Six patients had a Mag-3 renal lasix scan performed as a component of their work-up for stricture.

Within the radiated cohort, we examined patients by indication for radiation therapy. 7 patients underwent radiation for cervical cancer (target dose 85 Gy) and 4 patients (57%) experienced ureteroenteric stricture. 11 patients had radiation for colorectal malignancy (target dose 50 Gy) and 3 patients (27%) developed strictures. 40 patients had radiation therapy for urologic malignancy (target dose 45–50 Gy pelvis), with 7 patients (18%) developing ureteroenteric stricture. An additional 7 patients had radiation therapy for other non-cervical gynecologic malignancies (45–50 Gy) and 1 patient experienced ureteroenteric stricture. Kaplan–Meier estimation demonstrated radiation treated cervical cancer had a statistically significant higher probability of developing UES compared with other radiation treated cancers ($p = 0.046$), which is shown in Fig. 2.

Discussion

Our study demonstrates evidence that a contemporary series of patients with a history of prior radiation therapy had higher rates of ureteroenteric stricture following urinary diversion while other covariates were similar with an odds ratio of 5.2. This is in spite of our knowledge of radiation as a risk factor and utilizing known strategies for mitigation such as extensive spatulation, mucosal eversion and no-touch technique. It is also the practice

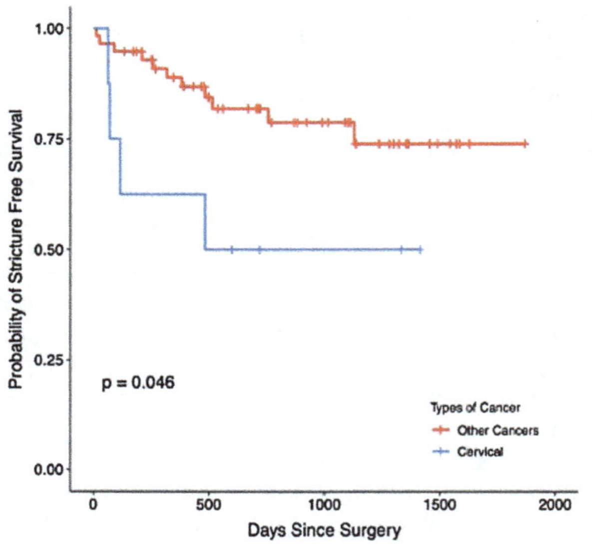

Fig. 2 Ureteroenteric stricture free survival by radiation treated cancers

of our surgeons, including the highest volume surgeon, to emphasize only mobilization and manipulation of the ureters to the degree surgically necessary and preservation of ureteral vasculature is paramount. Though previous studies have identified BMI as a risk factor for stricture, we did not find this to be significant in our series. Ureteroenteric stricture remains a well-known complication of urinary diversion, yet little progress has been made in reduction of stricture rates, either by means of surgical technique or postoperative management [5, 6, 14–17]. Demonstrating that radiation is a risk factor for ureteroenteric stricture is important in preoperative counseling, particularly for exenteration, continent or incontinent diversion selection, and possibly post-operative imaging follow up. It is well demonstrated that radiation therapy affects tissue causing fibrosis and impairment of microvascular tissue perfusion. Ischemia to the distal ureter due to compromise of the microvascular blood supply is implicated in the formation of ureteroenteric strictures [7].

Several groups have tested whether varied surgical methods may offer risk reduction. Surgical anastomotic approach has not significantly impacted ureteroenteric stricture rate [5, 14–16]. However, a more recent study suggests that intracorporeal diversion confers a higher risk of ureteroenteric stricture [14]. This is counterintuitive as robotics is advertised as more precise with better visualization. Later work has suggested that this increased risk noted with intracorporeal diversion diminishes after a surgeon performs 75 diversions on the learning curve [18]. A study of 47 robotic assisted urinary diversions by Ahmadi et al. demonstrated intraoperative use of indocyanine green had a lower ureteroenteric stricture rate [19]. Recent work by Shen et al. has demonstrated potential for the use of intraoperative fluorescent angiography during open urinary diversion in reduction of ureteroenteric stricture rates. In a series of 47 patients, no ureteroenteric strictures were detected in the experimental group [20]. These studies show promise for widespread reduction in ureteroenteric stricture rates by assessing ureteral perfusion prior to making ureteroenteric anastomosis, as the technique will not be limited to robotic only approach. The gold standard for treatment of ureteroenteric stricture is open repair with ureteral reimplantation. These are challenging surgeries and are most successful when redundancy in the conduit allows the bowel to be moved to the non-diseased ureter. Patients must be counseled on the risk of nephrectomy or continued stricture if reimplantation fails. Open surgical repair has a success rate of 92–100%, while endoscopic management has a success rate of 30–50% [21–23].

We found that patients who underwent pelvic exenteration and supratrigonal cystectomy were more likely to have had radiation. The difference within the pelvic exenteration population is attributable to the standard of care for gynecologic and colorectal malignancy consisting of neoadjuvant radiation therapy protocols [9–11]. Obtaining exact radiation dosing information by chart abstraction proved difficult as many patients undergo radiation therapy in the community outside of our institution. We did note a high incidence of ureteroenteric stricture in those who had radiation for cervical cancer, however this study was not powered to evaluate differences on the basis of malignancy type. Cervical cancer has a high radiation dose (85 Gy) delivered in close proximity to the distal ureters [9]. Additionally, there exists the risk of iatrogenic ureteral devascularization in those patients with masses abutting or invading the ureters. This is of particular interest in the radiated gynecologic malignancy patient, where radiation may impair the development of collateral blood supply in the setting of iatrogenic ureteral vascular compromise. For some patients who underwent supratrigonal cystectomy, the indication was radiation cystitis or fistula, which contributes to that demographic difference. We found that while the stricture rate was higher within the radiation cohort, the 90-day readmission rate was not significantly higher. While cystectomy and urinary diversion remains a complex surgery that carries high risk of readmission, lowering rates of ureteroenteric stricture would alleviate the morbidity associated with repeated procedural intervention as well as readmission beyond 90 days. With mean time to stricture diagnosis of 10.3 months postoperatively, reduction in readmission in the early postoperative period may not be seen, but reduction in late readmission and concomitant costs may be realized. Ureteroenteric stricture and related complications and readmissions also confer significant healthcare cost and remain one of the most costly per day reasons for readmission following urinary diversion [24]. Treatment of a stricture with prolonged stent placement also obviates a risk factor for the rare but catastrophic ureteroiliac fistula.

A factor that makes study and minimization of ureteroenteric stricture difficult is the lack of consensus on stricture definition and proper diagnosis. We defined stricture as endoscopic diagnosis or definitive imaging findings. Endoscopic diagnosis consisting of visualization of focal narrowing at the anastomosis on ureteroscopy, and definitive imaging findings on CT indicating focal narrowing at the anastomoses with related hydronephrosis without concern for malignant recurrence. This is consistent with work by other groups [24]. However, others have defined ureteroenteric stricture by the need for future procedures [25]. Further, urologists have different protocols for postoperative surveillance imaging which may detect asymptomatic/subclinical ureteroenteric strictures. The varied utilization of cross-sectional imaging, loopogram, antegrade/retrograde fluoroscopy, Mag-3 renal lasix scan, and ureteroscopy in the diagnosis of ureteroenteric stricture offers opportunity for standardization of the clinical workup. With the workforce shortage in urology, we often have no local urologists to perform follow-up testing. It is possible our surveillance is closer, leading to detection bias. Our colorectal and gynecologic surgeons prefer to perform total pelvic exenterations in an open fashion as opposed to robotic assisted. Further, our institution serves a predominately rural population and patients often presents with advances disease at initial presentation, which necessitates a larger number of open cystectomies.

Ureteroenteric stricture minimization remains an area of need for continued research. The use of fluorescent angiography or indocyanine green and firefly technology gives surgeons the ability to assess ureteral perfusion and have demonstrated significant improvement in ureteroenteric stricture rates in single institution series [19, 20]. Further work is merited to validate these findings and incorporate them into standard practice.

Conclusion

Our study demonstrates a significant increase ureteroenteric strictures rate in radiated patients as compared to non-radiated patients. The insult of radiation on the ureteral microvascular supply is likely implicated in the cause of these strictures. Further study is needed to optimize surgical approach such as utilization of indocyanine green fluorescence angiography or fluorescein angiography.

Authors' contributions

CTY: Protocol/project development, Data analysis, Manuscript writing/editing. AJW: Data collection or management. KAM: Data analysis. MT: Data analysis, manuscript writing/editing. PFN: Data collection or management. CM: Data collection or management. STC: Manuscript writing/editing. SI: Manuscript writing/editing. TLK: Protocol/project development, Manuscript writing/editing. Authorship confirmation statement: All authors meet criteria for definitions of authorship as defined by ICMJE.

Competing interests

The author(s) declare(s) that they have no competing interests.Author disclosure statement: No disclosures.

Author details

[1]Department of Urology, UVA Medical Center, Fontaine Research Park, 500 Ray C. Hunt Drive, Charlottesville, VA 22908, USA. [2]University of Virginia School of Medicine, Charlottesville, VA, USA.

References

1. Katherine A A, Emily A V, Gillian S, et al. Predictors of benign ureteroenteric anastomotic strictures after radical cystectomy and urinary diversion [published online ahead of print, 2018 Jun 29]. *Urology*. 2018;S0090–4295(18)30613–7.
2. Shimko MS, Tollefson MK, Umbreit EC, Farmer SA, Blute ML, Frank I. Long-term complications of conduit urinary diversion. J Urol. 2011;185(2):562–7.
3. Anderson CB, McKiernan JM. Surgical complications of urinary diversion. Urol Clin North Am. 2018;45(1):79–90.
4. Yang DY, Boorjian SA, Westerman MB, Tarrell RF, Thapa P, Viers BR. Persistent, long-term risk for ureteroenteric anastomotic stricture formation: the case for long term follow-up. Transl Androl Urol. 2020;9(1):142–50.
5. Richards KA, Cohn JA, Large MC, Bales GT, Smith ND, Steinberg GD. The effect of length of ureteral resection on benign ureterointestinal stricture rate in ileal conduit or ileal neobladder urinary diversion following radical cystectomy. Urol Oncol. 2015;33(2):65.e1-65.e658.
6. Ahmed YE, Hussein AA, May PR, et al. Natural history, predictors and management of ureteroenteric strictures after robot assisted radical cystectomy. J Urol. 2017;198(3):567–74.
7. Lobo N, Dupré S, Sahai A, Thurairaja R, Khan MS. Getting out of a tight spot: an overview of ureteroenteric anastomotic strictures. Nat Rev Urol. 2016;13(8):447–55.
8. Baker DG, Krochak RJ. The response of the microvascular system to radiation: a review. Cancer Invest. 1989;7(3):287–94.
9. NCCN Guidelines: Cervical Cancer. Version 1.2021. Cerv-7.
10. NCCN Guidelines: Colon Cancer.Version 4.2020. Col-2.
11. Fokdal L, Tanderup K, Pötter R, Sturdza A, Kirchheiner K, Chargari C, Jürgenliemk-Schulz IM, Segedin B, Tan LT, Hoskin P, Mahantshetty U, Bruheim K, Rai B, Kirisits C, Lindegaard JC; EMBRACE Collaborative Group. Risk Factors for Ureteral Stricture After Radiochemotherapy Including Image Guided Adaptive Brachytherapy in Cervical Cancer: Results From the EMBRACE Studies. Int J Radiat Oncol Biol Phys. 2019 Mar 15;103(4):887–894.
12. Tran H, Arsovska O, Paterson RF, Chew BH. Evaluation of risk factors and treatment options in patients with ureteral stricture disease at a single institution. Can Urol Assoc J. 2015 Nov-Dec;9(11–12):E921–4.
13. Beller HL, Rapp DE, Zillioux J, Abdalla B, Duska LR, Showalter TN, Krupski TL, Cisu T, Congleton JY, Schenkman NS. Urologic complications requiring intervention following high-dose pelvic radiation for cervical cancer. Urology. 2020;S0090–4295(20):31153–5.
14. Baten E, Akand M, Floyd MS Jr, et al. Evaluation of conservative approach in the management of ureteroenteric strictures following radical cystectomy with Bricker ileal conduit: a single-center experience. Scand J Urol. 2016;50(6):439–44.
15. Large MC, Cohn JA, Kiriluk KJ, et al. The impact of running versus interrupted anastomosis on ureterointestinal stricture rate after radical cystectomy. J Urol. 2013;190(3):923–7.

16. Ficarra V, Giannarini G, Crestani A, et al. Retrosigmoid versus traditional Ileal conduit for urinary diversion after radical cystectomy. Eur Urol. 2019;75(2):294–9.
17. Beano H, He J, Hensel C, Worrilow W, Townsend W, Gaston K, Clark PE, Riggs S. Safety of decreasing ureteral stent duration following radical cystectomy. World J Urol. 2020 Apr.
18. Ericson KJ, Thomas LJ, Zhang JH, Knorr JM, Khanna A, Crane A, Zampini AM, Murthy PB, Berglund RK, Pascal-Haber G, Lee BHL. Uretero-enteric anastomotic stricture following radical cystectomy: a comparison of open, robotic extracorporeal, and robotic intracorporeal approaches. Urology. 2020;144:130–5. https://doi.org/10.1016/j.urology.2020.06.047.
19. Ahmadi N, Ashrafi AN, Hartman N, Shakir A, Cacciamani GE, Freitas D, Rajarubendra N, Fay C, Berger A, Desai MM, Gill IS, Aron M. Use of indocyanine green to minimise uretero-enteric strictures after robotic radical cystectomy. BJU Int. 2019;124(2):302–7.
20. Shen JK, Jamnagerwalla J, Yuh BE, Bassett MR, Chenam A, Warner JN, Zhumkhawala A, Yamzon JL, Whelan C, Ruel NH, Lau CS, Chan KG. Real-time indocyanine green angiography with the SPY fluorescence imaging platform decreases benign ureteroenteric strictures in urinary diversions performed during radical cystectomy. Ther Adv Urol. 2019;4(11):1756287219839631.
21. DiMarco DS, LeRoy AJ, Thieling S, Bergstralh EJ, Segura JW. Long-term results of treatment for ureteroenteric strictures. Urology. 2001;58(6):909–13.
22. Gin GE, Ruel NH, Parihar JS, et al. Ureteroenteric anastomotic revision as initial management of stricture after urinary diversion. Int J Urol. 2017;24(5):390–5.
23. Fransen van de Putte EE, de Wall LL, van Werkhoven E, et al. Endo-Urological Techniques for Benign Uretero-Ileal Strictures Have Poor Efficacy and Affect Renal Function. *Urol Int*. 2018;100(1):18–24.
24. Wittig K, Ruel N, Barlog J, Crocitto L, Chan K, Lau C, Wilson T, Yuh B. Critical analysis of hospital readmission and cost burden after robot-assisted radical cystectomy. J Endourol. 2016;30(1):83–91.
25. Goh AC, Belarmino A, Patel NA, Sun T, Sedrakyan A, Bochner BH, Hu JC. A population-based study of ureteroenteric strictures after open and robot-assisted radical cystectomy. Urology. 2020;135:57–65.

21

Newly designed solid coupling medium for reducing trapped air pockets during extracorporeal shock wave lithotripsy

Chien-Sheng Wang[1], Ching-Chia Li[1], Wen-Jeng Wu[1], Wen-Chin Liou[2], Yusen Eason Lin[3,4] and Wei-Chuan Chen[1,2*]

Abstract

Introduction: Air pockets between the lithotripter head and body surface are almost inevitably generated when applying a handful of gel onto the contact portion of the treatment head and that on the patient's skin during coupling procedure. These air pockets can compromise the transmission of acoustic energy of shock wave and may significantly affect efficacy of stone disintegration. Comparing to conventional gel, this study aims to investigate efficacy of stone disintegration by using a proprietary isolation-coupling pad ("icPad") as the coupling medium to reduce trapped air pockets during ESWL procedure.

Method: In this phantom study, Dornier lithotripter (Delta-2 RC, Dornier MedTech Europe GmbH Co., Germany) was used with a proprietary gel pads (icPad, Diameter = 150 mm, Thickness = 4 mm and 8 mm). The lithotripter was equipped with inline camera to observe the trapped air pockets between the contact surface of the lithotripter head. A testing and measuring device were used to observe experimental stone disintegration using icPad and semi-liquid gel. The conventional semi-liquid gel was used as control for result comparison.

Results: The stone disintegration rate of icPad 4 mm and 8 mm after 200 shocks of energy at level 2 were significantly higher than that of the semi-liquid gel (disintegration rate 92.3%, 85.0% vs. 45.5%, respectively, $p < 0.001$). The number of shocks for complete stone disintegration by icPad of 4 mm and 8 mm at the same energy level 2 were significantly lower than that of the semi-liquid gel (the number of shocks 242.0 ± 13.8, 248.7 ± 6.3 vs. 351.0 ± 54.6, respectively, $p = 0.011$). Furthermore, quantitative comparison of observed air pockets under Optical Coupling Control (OCC) system showed that the area of air pockets in semi-liquid group was significantly larger than that of the group using icPad (8 mm) and that of the group using icPad (8 mm) after sliding (332.7 ± 91.2 vs. 50.3 ± 31.9, 120.3 ± 21.5, respectively, $p < 0.05$).

Conclusion: The advantages of icPad includes: (1) reduced the numbers of shock wave and increased stone disintegration rate due to icPad's superior efficacy; (2) significantly reduce trapped air pockets in ESWL coupling. Due to the study limitation, more data are needed to confirm our observations before human trials.

*Correspondence: coupe055@ms28.hinet.net
[1] Department of Urology, School of Medicine, College of Medicine, Kaohsiung Medical University Hospital, No.100, Shiquan 1st Rd., Sanmin Dist., Kaohsiung City 807, Taiwan
Full list of author information is available at the end of the article

Keywords: Coupling, Air pockets, Extracorporeal shock wave lithotripter

Introduction

There has been a marked development of lithotripsy techniques in the late 1990s or the early 2000, including precise localization (in-line navigation systems) with automatic ultrasound robotic arm, monitoring and stone fixation, implementation of different focal sizes with new acoustic lenses, coupling control, slower pulse rates, and ramping strategies [1–4]. Modern lithotripters are dry-head devices in which the treatment head is shifted into contact with the patient. The typical protocol for coupling is to apply a handful of gel onto the contact portion of the treatment head, and to the contact area on the patient's skin. However, quality of coupling is usually not concerned by operators during ESWL procedure [5]. Entrapped air pockets can get caught at the coupling interface and impair the transmission of shock waves [6, 7]. Neucks et al. has conducted an in vitro study and discovered that air pockets covering 1.5–19% of coupling area result in a reduction in shock wave (SW) amplitude of 20%, and even 2% air coverage could decrease stone breakage rate by 20–40% [8]. Good quality of coupling, with minimal or no air trapped between the two contact surfaces, is the key factor to prevent transmission of acoustic energy loss and to improved efficacy of stone disintegration for ESWL.

Several strategies have been proposed to minimize air pockets in the coupling area. Coupling technique by applying a larger amount of semi-liquid gel to the lithotripter head leads to better coupling [8]. Bergsdorf et al. invented a coupling membrane and demonstrated better efficacy over semi-liquid gel, but not being widely adopted [9]. Lithotripter equipped with optical coupling control (OCC) system was invented. Under visual surveillance, the physician can halt and re-apply gels to treatment head if the air pockets are observed [10]. However, the high cost might hinder its widespread adoption. Thus, we conducted an observational study on the use of a single-use, proprietary isolation-coupling pad ("icPad") (Taiwan patent, utility model patent, M480354) as coupling medium to reduce trapped air pockets and increase efficacy of stone disintegration during ESWL procedure.

Materials and methods

Test medium

The medium tested are proprietary gel pads (icPad) (Diameter = 150 mm, Thickness = 4 mm and 8 mm) consisting of chemical-gel, mainly polyacrylamide, (Fig. 1) and standard semi-liquid gel (Sonogel®), which is widely used in clinical practice, as control. We used a clinical lithotripter (Delta-2 RC, Dornier MedTech Europe GmbH Co., Germany) equipped with an inline video camera with OCC (Optical Coupling Control) system for coupling monitoring. In the study group, we applied the icPad on the treatment head similar to the

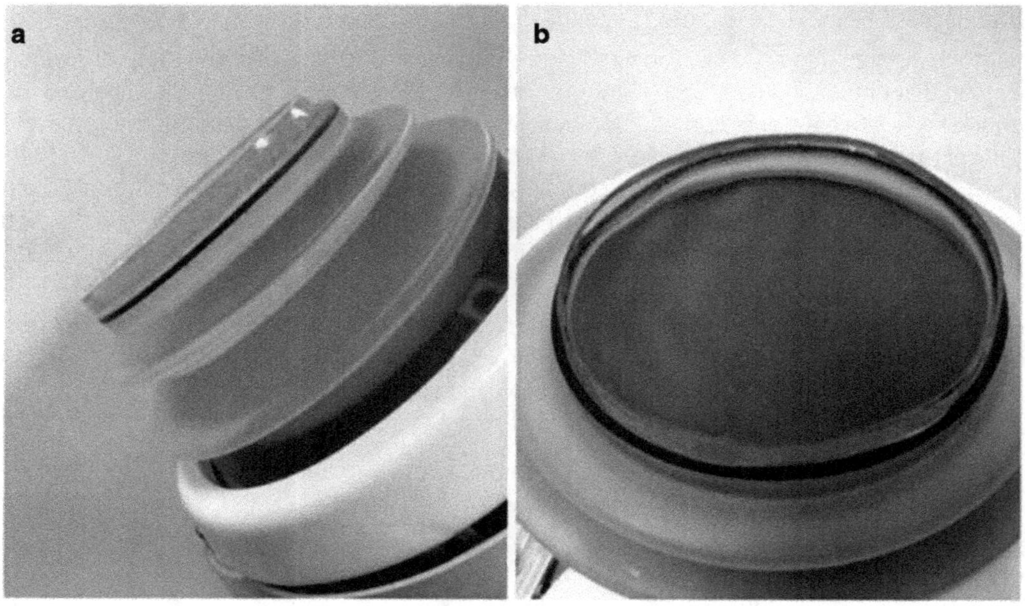

Fig. 1 A proprietary icPad (light green color) sticking on the treatment head. **a** side view and **b** bottom view

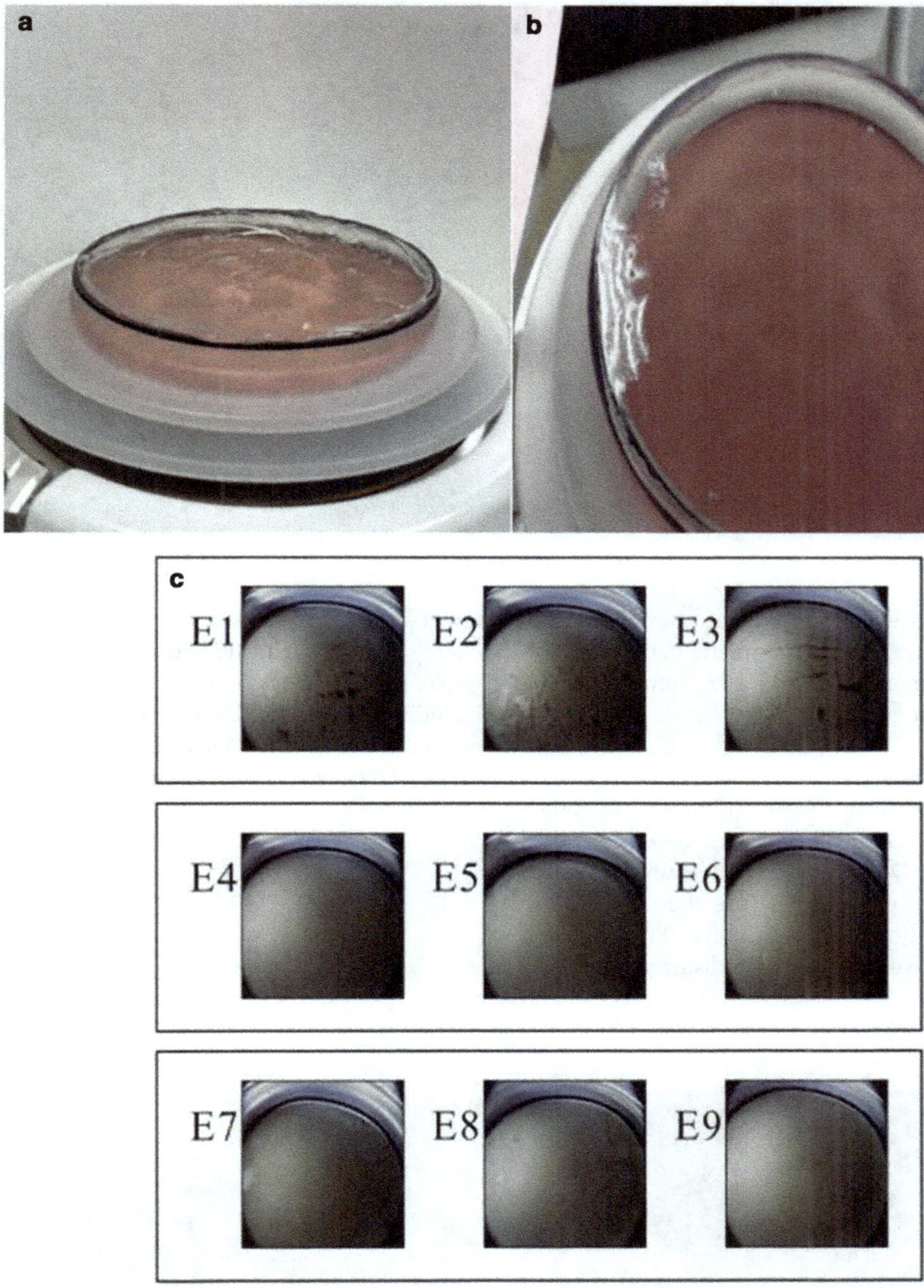

Fig. 2 **a** Uneven surface and **b** smooth surface using semi-liquid gel and icPad on treatment head. **c** Comparisons of trapped air pockets between icPad and semi-liquid gel. Apparent air pockets were seen on experiments (E) using semi-liquid gel (E1–E3). No obvious air pockets were observed in the experiments using icPad (E4–E6) and remained almost air-free after sliding the icPad (E7–E9)

method we apply thin-film screen protector to a smart phone. The other side of icPad then was sprayed with specified liquid lubricant and attached to the water tank of the testing device in which the model stone was immersed. In the control group, we applied abundant amount of semi-liquid gel to the lithotripter head as Neucks et al. described to decrease the air pockets trapped shown on Fig. 2a, b [8]. If air pockets still existed under OCC system in both groups, we would reapply up to 3 times in our study protocol. Then, experiments were triplicated for each group. The procedure of sliding test was also performed to observe

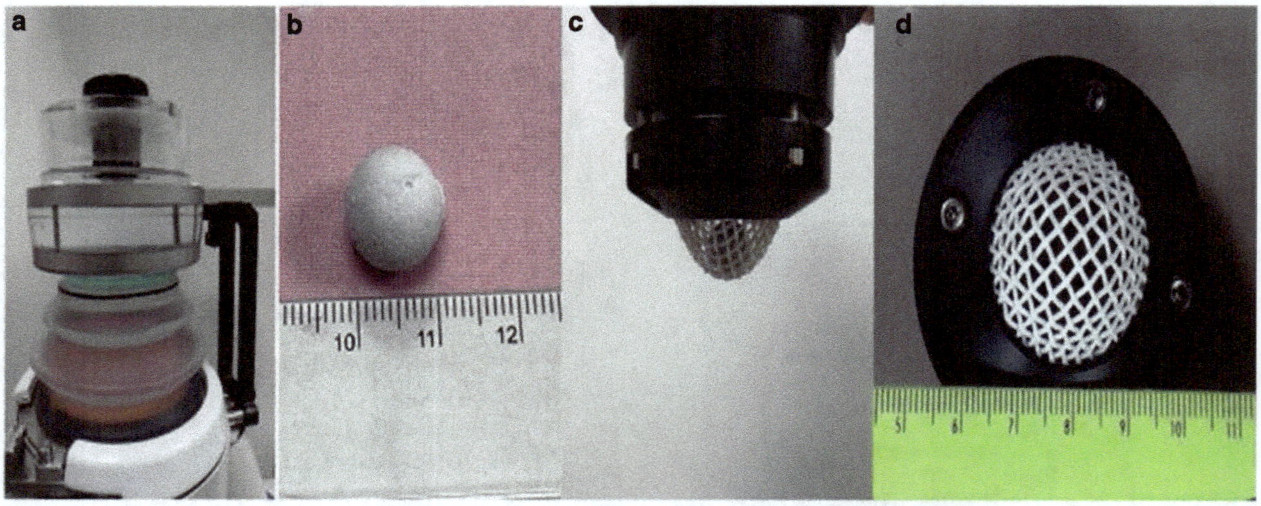

Fig. 3 **a** A testing and measuring device containing **b** a model stone placed in the **c** basket with the **d** sieve size of 2 mm. The icPad (green part) placed between treatment head and water tank in which a model stone immersed shown on (**a**)

whether air pockets would be present after sliding the icPad. This procedure aimed to simulate patient's involuntary body movement during localization of targeted stone and ESWL procedure.

Experimental procedure

A testing and measuring device (Dornier MedTech Europe GmbH Co., Germany) and standardized model stones (K0742691, Dornier MedTech Europe GmbH Co., Germany) were used to measure the performance of stone disintegration of lithotripters (Fig. 3). Each model stone was weighted before disintegration and underwent 200 shocks at energy level 2(corresponding energy = 20 mJ, acoustic pressure range 50–90 MPa) at rate of pulse of shock of 80 per minutes. Two parameters, including disintegrated stone rate and number of shocks needed for complete stone disintegration, were measured for the efficacy of stone disintegration. First, fragments

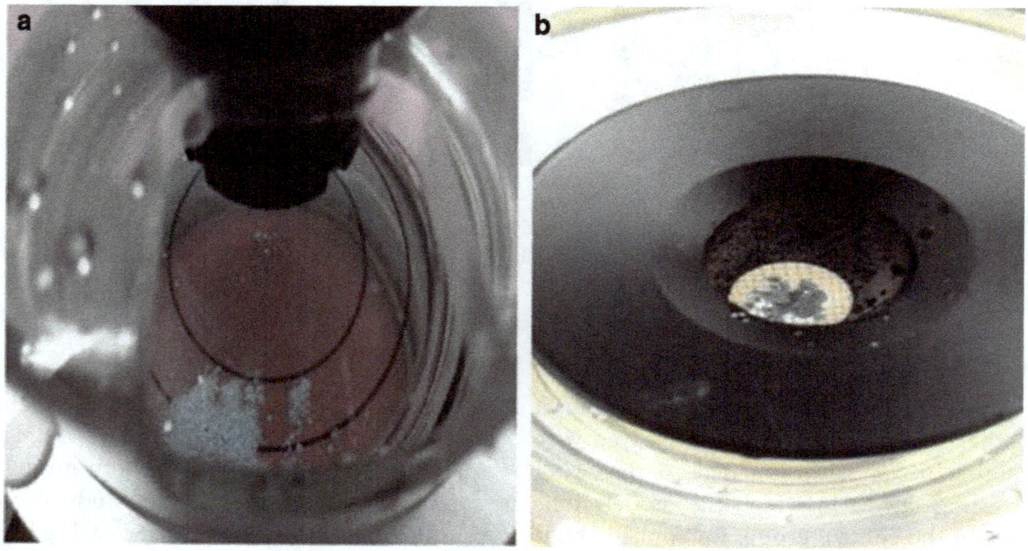

Fig. 4 **a** Disintegrated stone fragments passed through the sieve after shock wave. **b** The fragments remained on the sieve

passed through the sieve and those which remained on the sieve (sieve size = 2 mm) were collected as residual portion after shock wave (Fig. 4). The residual fragments were later weighed after desiccation. Stone disintegration rate then was defined as the following formula:

$$\text{Stone disintegration rate} = \frac{\text{Weight of model stone} - \text{Weight of residual stone}}{\text{Weight of model stone}}$$

Second, the number of shocks needed for complete stone disintegration was recorded when no visible residual stone fragments on the sieve during the test.

Quantitative comparison of observed air pockets between the contract surface and the lithotripter head was performed using icPad (8 mm) and semi-liquid gel. We calculated the irregular area covered by air pockets using imaging recognition (@5 × 5 pixel grid, Photoshop CS6) (Additional file 1: Figure S1).

Statistical analysis

One-way ANOVA with post-hoc pairwise two-group comparisons were used for numerical variables. Statistical significance was set at $p < 0.05$. IBM SPSS 26.0 (IBM Corp., Armonk, NY) was used for all statistical analyses.

Results

Stone disintegration

The post hoc comparison showed that icPad 4 mm and 8 mm have significantly higher stone disintegration rate (icPad 4 mm 93.5%, icPad 8 mm 85.0%) than semi-liquid gel group (45.5%) ($p < 0.001$). The number of shocks needed for complete stone disintegration also revealed similar results: icPad 4 mm and 8 mm have significantly lower number needed for complete stone disintegration (icPad 4 mm 242.0, icPad 8 mm 248.7) than semi-liquid group (351.0) ($p < 0.05$), more than 20% faster than semi-liquid gel (Table 1).

Air pockets observation

The amount of air pockets observed from OCC in icPad and semi-liquid gel were shown on Fig. 2c. Despite the attempt to reduce trapped air pockets under OCC system, there were still noticeable amount of air pockets (in dark-gray or bright color) observed from the camera in the group using semi-liguid gel (E1–E3). Almost air-free on the central area and few marginal air pockets were observed using icPad (E4–E6). The procedure of icPad sliding was performed on the testing device to simulate the patient's body movement for localization of target stone during ESWL and the trapped air pockets remain the same (E7-E9).

The area of air pockets in semi-liquid (Fig. 2c E1–E3) is significantly larger that of the group using icPad (8 mm) (Fig. 2c E4–E6) and that of the group after sliding (Fig. 2c E7–E9)(332.7 ± 91.2, 50.3 ± 31.9, 120.3 ± 21.5, respectively, $p < 0.05$) (Table 2).

Table 1 The results of disintegration rate after 200 shocks and number of shocks for complete stone disintegration for different test groups using icPad and semi-liquid gel

	Group	Mean ± SD	F value	Post-hoc Scheffé results
Stone disintegration rate (%) after 200 shocks	icPad 4 mm	92.3 ± 2.1	79.166***	Semi-liquid gel < icPad 4 mm and 8 mm
	icPad 8 mm	85.0 ± 7.5		
	Semi-liquid gel	45.5 ± 3.6		
Number of shocks for complete disintegration	icPad 4 mm	242.0 ± 13.8	10.446*	Semi-liquid gel > icPad 4 mm and 8 mm
	icPad 8 mm	248.7 ± 6.3		
	Semi-liquid gel	351.0 ± 54.6		

*$p < 0.05$; **$p < 0.01$; ***$p < 0.001$

Table 2 The results of quantitative comparison of observed air pockets between the icPad (8 mm) and semi-liquid gel

	Group	Mean ± SD	F Value	Post-hoc Scheffé results
Area of air pockets (pixel grid)	icPad 8 mm	50.3 ± 31.9 (0.38%)	16.051**	Semi-liquid gel > icPad 8 mm and 8 mm after sliding
	icPad 8 mm after sliding	120.3 ± 21.5 (0.92%)		
	Semi-liquid gel	332.7 ± 91.2 (2.55%)		

*$p < 0.05$; **$p < 0.01$; ***$p < 0.001$

Discussion

Since the first procedure performed in 1980, ESWL has revolutionized the management of urolithiasis [11]. Ever since, several techniques of ESWL including shock wave generation, localization system, larger focal zone, ramping strategy, lower pulse rate, stone localization, and adequate coupling in lithotripter design have evolved to achieve better stone disintegration over the past four decades [12–14]. In this study, we proposed a new strategy to reduce the trapped air pockets during ESWL coupling by using a new acoustic, proprietary isolation-coupling pad (icPad). icPad exhibits higher efficacy and faster stone disintegration (Table 1). For example, under the same condition of 200 shocks, icPad group showed significant better efficacy than the semi-liquid gel (92.3% and 85.0% vs. 45.5%). Under the inline camera attached to the lithotripter, the trapped air pockets observed is only 0.38% in icPad groups over the treatment head, which is significantly lower than that of semi-liquid gel group (2.55%). Even sliding occurred, the air pockets only increased as little as 0.54%. Thus, icPad demonstrated better stone disintegration efficacy and lower air pockets in comparison with semi-liquid gel. In addition, our data support Neucks et al. and Jain et al. that the air pocket coverage over 1.5% could compromise the ESWL efficacy [6, 8]. In our study, icPad can maintain air pocket coverage rate below 1% and exhibits better ESWL efficacy.

When using icPad, three advantages are worth considering: coupling, adhesion and isolation. First, the transmission coefficient for an acoustic wave moving from water to air is only 0.1%, which means 99.9% of the wave will be reflected [15]. In our study, OCC system showed that we can achieve minimal air pockets (< 0.5%) at the coupling area when using icPad. Even after sliding, the air pockets only increased as little as 0.54%, comparing to the air pockets as much as 2.55% when using semi-liquid gel. This may enhance the transmission of shock-wave and improve ESWL efficacy. Second, icPad is a solid polyacrylamide gel which can firmly attach to the receiving object to ensure minimal air pockets in the coupling area. Third, from the practical infection control point of view, icPad provides a good isolation between lithotripter treatment head and the receiving object. However, this feature requires further experimental data under case-control clinical study design to support our hypothesis.

The limitation of this study is that we only demonstrate the correlation between ESWL efficacy and the presence of air pockets. In addition, we are unable to differentiate whether better ESWL efficacy is due to low air pockets or the nature of the solid coupling medium. Therefore, more data are needed to confirm our observations before human trials.

To our knowledge, this is the first evidence-based observational study showing that a solid gel pad (icPad) can minimize the trapped air pockets during ESWL, utilizing an inline camera for quantitative evaluation. The experimental results show that icPad has advantages in better efficacy in stone disintegration and lower air pockets.

Authors' contributions

CSW, WCC: Project development, Data Collection, Data analysis, Manuscript writing. CCL, WJW, WCL, YEL: Project development. All authors read and approved the final manuscript.

Competing interests

The authors declare that they have competing interests.

Author details

[1]Department of Urology, School of Medicine, College of Medicine, Kaohsiung Medical University Hospital, No.100, Shiquan 1st Rd., Sanmin Dist., Kaohsiung City 807, Taiwan. [2]Department of Surgery, St. Joseph Hospital, Kaohsiung City, Taiwan. [3]Graduate Institute of Human Resource and Knowledge Management, National Kaohsiung Normal University, Kaohsiung City, Taiwan. [4]CleanWave Medical Co., LTD, Kaohsiung City, Taiwan.

References

1. Duryea AP, Roberts WW, Cain CA, Tamaddoni HA, Hall TL. Acoustic bubble removal to enhance SWL efficacy at high shock rate: an in vitro study. J Endourol. 2014;28(1):90–5.
2. Rassweiler J, Rassweiler M-C, Frede T, Alken P. Extracorporeal shock wave lithotripsy: an opinion on its future. Indian J Urol IJU J Urol Soc India. 2014;30(1):73.
3. Elmansy H, Lingeman J. Recent advances in lithotripsy technology and treatment strategies: a systematic review update. Int J Surg. 2016;36:676–80.
4. Pereira-Arias J, Gamarra-Quintanilla M, Urdaneta-Salegui L, Mora-Christian J, Sanchez-Vazquez A, Astobieta-Odriozola A, et al. Current status of extracorporeal shock wave lithotripsy in urinary lithiasis. Arch Esp Urol. 2017;70(2):263–87.
5. Lingeman JE, McAteer JA, Gnessin E, Evan, AP. Shock wave lithotripsy: advances in technology and technique. Nat Rev Urol. 2009;6(12):660–70.
6. Jain A, Shah TK. Effect of air bubbles in the coupling medium on efficacy of extracorporeal shock wave lithotripsy. Eur Urol. 2007;51(6):1680–7.
7. Lawler AC, Ghiraldi EM, Tong C, Friedlander JI. Extracorporeal shock wave therapy: current perspectives and future directions. Curr Urol Rep. 2017;18(4):25.
8. Neucks JS, Pishchalnikov YA, Zancanaro AJ, VonDerHaar JN, Williams JC, McAteer JA. Improved acoustic coupling for shock wave lithotripsy. Urol Res. 2008;36(1):61–6.
9. Bergsdorf T, Chaussy C, Thueroff S. 1815 Coupling gel viscosity—a relevant factor for efficient shock wave coupling in SWL. J Urol. 2010;183(4S):e704–e704.
10. Tailly GG, Tailly-Cusse MM. Optical coupling control: an important step toward better shockwave lithotripsy. J Endourol. 2014;28(11):1368–73.
11. Wess OJ. Physics and technique of shock wave lithotripsy (SWL). In: Talati J, Tiselius HG, Albala D, YE Z. editors. Urolithiasis. London: Springer; 2012.
12. Chaussy C, Brendel W, Schmiedt E. Extracorporeally induced destruction of kidney stones by shock waves. Lancet. 1980;316(8207):1265–8.
13. Basulto-Martínez M, Klein I, Gutiérrez-Aceves JJ. The role of extracorporeal shock wave lithotripsy in the future of stone management. Curr Opin Urol. 2019;29(2):96–102.
14. Talso M, Tefik T, Mantica G, Rodriguez MS, Kartalas IG, Somani BK, et al. Extracorporeal shockwave lithotripsy: current knowledge and future perspectives. Minerva urologica e nefrologica Ital J Urol Nephrol. 2019;71(4):365–72.
15. Cleveland, RO.; McAteer, JA. Smith's textbook on endourology. In: Smith AD, et al., editors. B. C. Decker, Inc; Hamilton: 2007. p. 317–32.

22

Presepsin as a predictor of septic shock in patients with urinary tract infection

Yoshitaka Sekine[1*], Kazuhiko Kotani[2], Daisuke Oka[1], Hiroshi Nakayama[1], Yoshiyuki Miyazawa[1], Takahiro Syuto[1], Seiji Arai[1], Masashi Nomura[1], Hidekazu Koike[1], Hiroshi Matsui[1], Yasuhiro Shibata[1], Masami Murakami[3] and Kazuhiro Suzuki[1]

Abstract

Background: Recently, presepsin has been reported to be a useful biomarker for early diagnosis of sepsis and evaluation of prognosis in septic patients. However, few reports have evaluated its usefulness in patients with urinary tract infections (UTI). This study aimed to evaluate whether presepsin could be a valuable marker for detecting severe sepsis, and whether it could predict the therapeutic course in patients with UTI compared with markers already used: procalcitonin (PCT) and C-reactive protein (CRP).

Methods: From April 2014 to December 2016, a total of 50 patients with urinary tract infections admitted to Gunma university hospital were enrolled in this study. Vital signs, presepsin, PCT, CRP, white blood cell (WBC) count, causative agents of urinary-tract infections, and other data were evaluated on the enrollment, third, and fifth days. The patients were divided into two groups: with (n = 11) or without (n = 39) septic shock on the enrollment day, and with (n = 7) or without (n = 43) sepsis on the fifth day, respectively. Presepsin was evaluated as a biomarker for systemic inflammatory response syndrome (SIRS) or septic shock.

Results: Regarding the enrollment day, there was no significant difference of presepsin between the SIRS and non-SIRS groups ($p = 0.276$). The median value of presepsin (pg/mL) was significantly higher in the septic shock group ($p < 0.001$). Multivariate logistic regression analysis showed that presepsin (≥ 500 pg/ml) was an independent risk factor for septic shock ($p = 0.007$). ROC curve for diagnosing septic shock indicated an area under the curve (AUC) of 0.881 for presepsin (vs. 0.690, 0.583, and 0.527 for PCT, CRP and WBC, respectively). Regarding the 5th day after admission, the median presepsin value on the enrollment day was significantly higher in the SIRS groups than in the non-SIRS groups ($p = 0.006$). On the other hand, PCT (≥ 2 ng/ml) on the enrollment day was an independent risk factor for SIRS. ROC curve for diagnosing sepsis on the fifth day indicated an AUC of 0.837 for PCT (vs. 0.817, 0.811, and 0.802 for presepsin, CRP, and WBC, respectively).

Conclusions: This study showed that presepsin may be a good marker for diagnosing septic shock based on admission data in patients with UTI.

Keywords: Bacterial infections, Biomarkers, C-reactive protein, Cytokines, Endotoxins, Flank pain, Presepsin, Urinary tract infection, Sepsis; procalcitonin

Background

Urinary tract infections (UTI) are common, and sometimes progress to sepsis or septic shock, which can be lethal. Mortality rate due to severe sepsis and septic shock has been reported to be between 20 and 50% [1, 2],

*Correspondence: ysekine@gunma-u.ac.jp
[1] Department of Urology, Gunma University Graduate School of Medicine, 3-39-22 Showa-Machi, Maebashi 371-8511, Japan
Full list of author information is available at the end of the article

and 9–31% of all cases of severe sepsis and septic shock has been reported to arise from UTI [2]. Therefore, diagnosis and evaluation of severity of sepsis or septic shock are important at the beginning of treatment of UTI.

Clinically, C-reactive protein (CRP) and procalcitonin (PCT) are used as markers for disease severity in patients with UTI. However, both CRP and PCT have some limitations. The response time to bacterial infections is delayed (CRP, 6 h; PCT, 2–3 h), production triggers might not be living bacteria (CRP, cytokine; PCT, endotoxin and cytokine), and serum half-time is long (CRP, 4–6 h; PCT, 20–24 h) [3, 4]. Therefore, a novel biomarker for bacterial infection, which reflects clinical condition at the time of measurement, is required.

Presepsin is a 13KDa N-terminal fragment of soluble CD14 [5]. Granulated leukocytes phagocytose both bacteria and CD14 and expel presepsin into the blood after enzymatic digestion of bacteria within two hours [5, 6]. Recently, presepsin has been reported to have a high sensitivity in detecting sepsis and be a biomarker for early diagnosis of sepsis [7]. Moreover, elevated presepsin levels on day one might evaluate prognosis of patients with sepsis in intensive-care units [8, 9]. However, there are a few reports on the use of presepsin as a biomarker in patients with UTI.

This study aimed to evaluate whether presepsin could be a useful marker for detecting sepsis or severe sepsis, and whether it could predict therapeutic courses in patients with UTI compared with other markers, such as PCT or CRP.

Methods

Patients

We performed a prospective observational study. From April 2014 to December 2016, a total of 57 patients with UTI, who were admitted into Gunma university hospital, were enrolled in this study. Seven patients were excluded from this study due to data unavailability. The urologist diagnosed UTI based on urinary sediment (≥ 5 leucocytes/high power field) and symptoms (fever and/or micturition pain and/or flank pain). Data of patient age, sex, medical history, oral medicine, blood pressure, body temperature, heart rate, respiratory rate, urine and blood culture results, surgical procedure for UTI after admission, causative agents of UTI, presepsin, PCT, CRP, white blood cell (WBC), Aspartate transaminase (ALT), Alanine transaminase (AST), γ-glutamyl transpeptidase (γGPT), and Creatinine (Cr) were collected. Vital signs and blood test results were evaluated at enrollment, and on the 3rd and 5th day after admission. The written informed consent was obtained from all of the enrolled patients. This study was approved by the Institutional Review Board of Gunma University Hospital (No.1650).

Assessment of systemic inflammatory response syndrome (SIRS) and septic shock

Diagnosis of SIRS and septic shock were established according to the criteria set by the American College of Chest Physicians/Society of Critical Care Medicine (ACCP/SCCM) [10].

Outcomes

Three outcome variables: SIRS and septic shock on the enrollment day and SIRS on the 5th day after admission were evaluated by dividing the participants into two groups for each of these variables; with (n = 39) or without (n = 11) SIRS on the enrollment day, with (n = 11) or without (n = 39) septic shock on the enrollment day, and with (n = 7) or without (n = 43) SIRS on the 5th day after admission, respectively.

Statistical analysis

Mann–Whitney U-test was used for continuous variables (age, CRP, presepsin, PCT, ALT, AST, γGPT, and Cr). We estimated independence using the chi-squared test or Fisher`s exact test for categorical variables (sex, placement of urinary catheter, urological cancer, urinary calculi, diabetes mellitus, and internal use of steroids). Independent predictors were evaluated using logistic regression analysis. The predictive accuracy of presepsin, PCT, CRP and WBC for septic shock or SIRS was evaluated by the area under the curve (AUC) of receiver operating characteristics (ROC) analysis. The Youden's index (sensitivity + specificity—1) was used to calculate optimal cutoff values for presepsin. *P* values ≤ 0.05 were considered statistically significant. SPSS Statistics Ver. 25 (IBM Corp. IL, USA) was used for statistical analyses.

Results

Patients characteristic

Table 1 shows the clinical characteristics of the 50 patients. On the enrollment day, septic shock was detected in 22% (n = 11) and SIRS in 78% (n = 39) of the patients. The mean age was 66.5 years, and 33 patients (66%) were men and 17 (34%) were women. Urine and blood cultures were positive and revealed bacterial growth in in 90% (n = 45) and 48% (n = 24) of samples, respectively. Forty-eight% (n = 24), 30% (n = 15), 24% (n = 12), 18% (n = 9), 56% (n = 28), and 18% (n = 9) were with placement of urinary catheter, urological cancer, urinary calculi, diabetes mellitus, surgical procedure after admission, and internal use of steroids, respectively.

Table 1 Characteristics of Patients with or without septic shock on the enrollment day

Variable	Total N=50	Septic shock group N=11	Non-septic shock group N=39	*p* value
Age (years)	66.5 [60.3–75.5]]	64 [49–70]	68 [61–78]	0.055
White blood cell (/mm^3)	13,600 [10,375–18,000]	13,600 [9900–25600]	13,600 [10400–16600]	0.788
C-reactive protein (mg/L)	10.45 [4.26–23.06]	11.47 [6.41–25.63]	10.2 [4.21–22.37]	0.406
Presepsin (pg/mL)	483 [277–1130]	1380 [924–5219]	399 [254–707]	<0.001
Procalcitonin (ng/mL)	0.87 [0.20–17.1]	25.06 [0.42–103.73]	0.66 [0.14–2.06]	0.056
Aspartate transaminase (U/L)	24.5 [19.8–35.3]	44 [24–133]	24 [18–29]	0.003
Alanine transaminase (U/L)	17 [11.8–30.0]	19 [15–52]	17 [11–24]	0.049
γ-glutamyl transpeptidase (U/L)	31 [21.0–53.3]	70 [43–74]	26 [20–43]	0.002
Creatinine (mg/dL)	1.24 [0.87–1.99]	1.85 [1.19–3.86]	1.05 [0.85–1.84]	0.020
sex (male/female)	33/17	8/3	25/14	0.440
placement of urinary catheter (Y/N)	24/26	6/5	18/21	0.623
urological cancer (Y/N)	15/35	1/10	14/25	0.085
urinary calculi (Y/N)	12/38	4/7	8/31	0.240
DM (Y/N)	9/41	3/8	6/33	0.308
internal use of steroid (Y/N)	9/41	3/8	6/33	0.308

Values are expressed as number or median [interquartile range, IQR]

DM diabetes mellitus, *Y* yes, *N* No

Prediction of SIRS on the enrollment day

The overall median baseline presepsin, PCT, and CRP levels were 483 pg/mL, 0.87 ng/mL, and 10.45 mg/L, respectively, with no significant difference between the SIRS and non-SIRS groups (Additional file 1: Table S1)."

Prediction of septic shock on the enrollment day

The median presepsin level (pg/mL) was significantly higher in the septic shock group (1380 vs. 399, $p<0.001$). The PCT and CRP levels were not significantly different between the septic shock and non-septic shock groups. Other blood test results that were significantly higher in the septic group included: AST ($p=0.003$), ALT ($p=0.049$), γGTP ($p=0.002$ and Cr ($p=0.02$), respectively (Table 1). Logistic regression analysis for evaluating factors associated with septic shock on the enrollment day is shown in Table 2. The factors associated with septic shock on univariate analysis included presepsin (≥500 pg/mL), PCT (≥2 ng/ml), AST (≥34 U/L) and γGTP (≥47 U/L). Only presepsin level retained a significant value after adjusting for confounders using multivariate logistic regression analysis (Table 2). ROC curve for diagnosing septic shock indicated an AUC of 0.881 for presepsin, which was greater than these for other markers (Fig. 1). The Cutoff level of presepsin with the optimum diagnostic efficiency by the ROC curves was 492 ng/ml, which was broadly similar to the clinical cut off value (500 pg/mL).

Prediction of SIRS on the 5th day after admission

The median presepsin level (pg/mL) was significantly higher in the SIRS group on the 5th day after admission (day1; 1167 vs. 419, $p<0.001$, day3; 633 vs. 311, $p=0.027$). The PCT (day1: 73.1 vs. 0.55, $p=0.003$; day3: 20.34 vs. 1.35, $p=0.005$)) and CRP (day1: 25.63 vs. 8.23, $p=0.007$; day3: 25.58 vs. 10.71, $p<0.001$) levels were also significantly different between the SIRS and non-SIRS groups on the 5th day after admission. Other blood test results that were significantly higher in the SIRS group on the 5th day after admission included: day1/AST (34 vs. 24, $P=0.013$); day1/Cr (2.3 vs. 1.05, $p=0.007$); day1/WBC (18,200 vs. 13,600, $p=0.009$); and day3/WBC (11,900 vs. 8400, $p=0.021$) (Table 3). The ratio of positive blood culture (86% vs. 42%, $p=0.039$) and urinary calculi (57% vs. 19%, $p=0.048$) significantly differed between the SIRS and non-SIRS groups on the 5th day after admission. Logistic regression analysis to evaluate factors associated with SIRS on the 5th day after admission is shown in Table 4. These factors included day1/presepsin (≥500 pg/mL), day1/PCT (≥2 ng/ml) and urinary calculi. Only day1/PCT level retained statistical significance after adjusting for confounders using multivariate logistic regression analysis (Table 4). ROC curve in patients with definitive diagnosis of SIRS on the 5th day after admission indicated an AUC of 0.837 for PCT, which is larger than these for other markers (Fig. 1). Regarding presepsin, the cutoff level with the optimum diagnostic efficiency using the

Table 2 Prediction of septic shock on the enrollment day by logistic regression analysis

Variable	Univariate analysis			Multivariable analysis		
	P value	HR	95% CI	*P* value	HR	95% CI
Sex (male vs female)	0.595					
WBC (4000–12,000 vs other)	0.497					
CRP (≥ 0.5 vs < 0.5)	0.360					
CRP (≥ 10 vs < 10)	0.848					
Presepsin (≥ 500 vs < 500)	0.007	20.000	2.305–173.553	0.029	12.157	1.298–113.892
PCT (≥ 0.05 vs < 0.05)	0.630					
PCT (≥ 2 vs < 2)	0.025	5.075	1.223–21.065	0.673		
AST (≥ 34 vs < 34)	0.006	8.000	1.829–34.996	0.375		
ALT (≥ 28 vs < 28)	0.105					
γGPT (≥ 47 vs < 47)	0.005	8.889	1.941–40.711	0.081		
Cr (male; ≥ 1.07 vs < 1.07, female; ≥ 0.79 vs < 0.79)	0.095					
placement of urinary catheter (Y vs N)	0.624					
urological cancer (Y vs N)	0.118					
urinary calculi (Y vs N)	0.284					
DM (Y vs N)	0.371					
internal use of steroid (Y vs N)	0.371					

WBC white blood cell, *CRP* C-reactive protein, *PCT* procalcitonin, *AST* aspartate transaminase, *ALT* Alanine transaminase, *γGTP* γ-glutamyl transpeptidase, *Cr* creatinine, *DM* diabetes mellitus, *Y* yes, *N* no

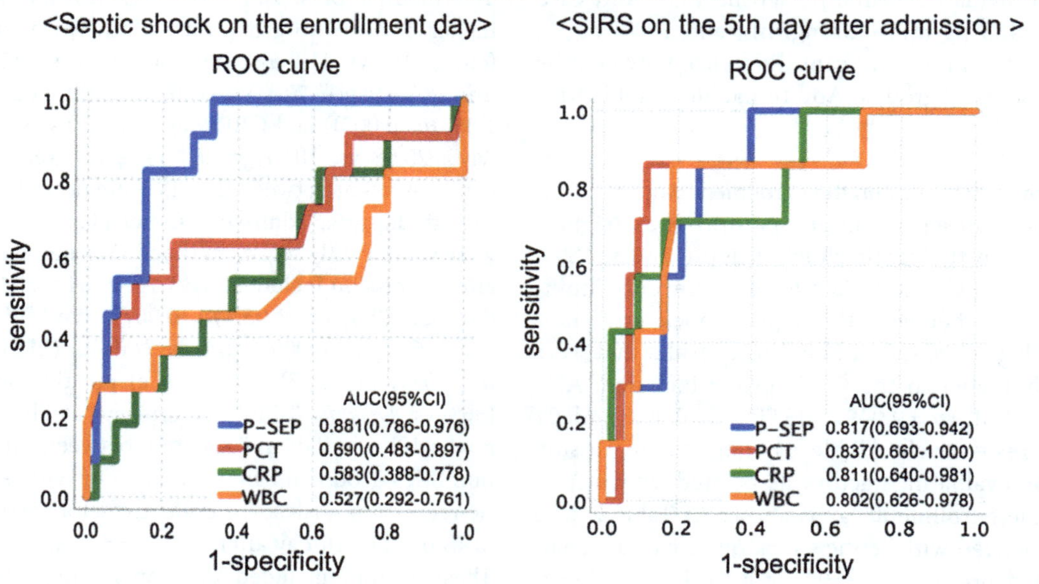

Fig. 1 ROC curve for presepsin, procalcitonin, CRP, and WBC in patients with definitive diagnosis of septic shock on the enrollment day and SIRS on the 5th day after admission. Abbreviations: P-SEP; presepsin, PCT; procalcitonin, CRP; C-reactive protein, WBC; white blood cell

ROC curves was 492 ng/ml, which was broadly similar to the clinical cut off value (500 pg/mL).

Discussion

In this study, elevated presepsin level on admission was an independent risk factor for septic shock, while elevated PCT on admission was independently associated with SIRS on the 5th day after admission in patients with UTI. Presepsin and PCT originate from different sources [3–5]. These results support our hypothesis that presepsin could be a useful marker for detecting severe sepsis in patients with UTI. On the other hand, PCT could predict therapeutic courses in patients with UTI better than did presepsin.

Table 3 Characteristics of Patients with or without SIRS on the 5th day

Variable	SIRS group N = 7	Non-SIRS group N = 43	*p*-value
Age (years)	64 [54–68]	68 [61–77]	0.126
Day1/White blood cell (/mm^3)	18,200 [17,200–24900]	13,600 [9900–16,000]	0.009
Day1/C-reactive protein (mg/L)	25.63 [9.58–31.38]	8.23 [4.1–16.6]	0.007
Day1/Presepsin (pg/mL)	1167 [878–5129]	419 [277–922]	0.006
Day1/Procalcitonin (ng/mL)	73.1 [25.06–103.73]	0.55 [0.14–2.06]	0.003
Day1/Aspartate transaminase (U/L)	34 [28–126]	24 [18–33]	0.013
Day1/Alanine transaminase (U/L)	23 [18–52]	16 [11–25]	0.056
Day1/γ-glutamyl transpeptidase (U/L)	48 [38–72]	28 [21–51]	0.133
Day1/Creatinine (mg/dL)	2.30 [1.72–2.71]	1.05 [0.85–1.84]	0.007
Day3/White blood cell (/mm^3)	11,900 [9400–20,100]	8400 [5900–10,400]	0.021
Day3/C-reactive protein (mg/L)	25.58 [16.47–34.54]	10.71 [6.55–15.40]	< 0.001
Day3/Presepsin (pg/mL)	633 [464–1360]	311 [196–695]	0.027
Day3/Procalcitonin (ng/mL)	20.34 [14.23–32.27]	1.35 [0.30–15.09]	0.005
Sex (male/female)	4/3	29/14	0.446
Urinary culture (P/N)	7/0	38/5	0.454
Blood culture (P/N)	6/1	18/25	0.039
Placement of urinary catheter (Y/N)	2/5	22/21	0.244
Urological cancer (Y/N)	1/6	14/29	0.311
Urinary calculi (Y/N)	4/3	8/35	0.048
DM (Y/N)	1/6	8/35	0.630
Surgical procedure (Y/N)	6/1	22/21	0.095
Internal use of steroid(Y/N)	2/5	7/36	0.370

Values are expressed as number or median [interquartile range, IQR]

DM diabetes mellitus, *P* positive, *N* no, *Y* yes

Presepsin is one of the biomarkers that increase after bacterial infections [11]. Its levels are increased in acute pyelonephritis patients with bacteremia [12]. Moreover, elevation of presepsin levels before initiating treatment might predict the development of sepsis in patients with obstructive acute pyelonephritis [13]. In this study, we evaluated the patients who needed hospitalization due to not only pyelonephritis, but also prostatitis. Additionally, elevation of presepsin levels on the enrollment day was a predictor of septic shock. Therefore, presepsin might be a useful for detecting severe urosepsis that needs vasopressor therapy.

Sever sepsis and septic shock can be fatal, with mortality rates: 28.3% in the United States and 41.1% in Europe [2]. Clinically, it is very useful to predict septic shock on admission. Therefore, it is essential that biomarkers increase immediately after infections and have high sensitivity for sepsis to be reliable. Presepsin levels have been shown to increase within 2 h together with blood bacterial counts, and peak at 3 h after infection [6]. On the other hand, elevated PCT and CRP levels are detected within 3–6 and 6 h, and peak at 6–8 and 36–50 h, respectively [14, 15]. It has also been reported that patients with severe sepsis had significantly higher presepsin levels than did those with sepsis, local infection, or SIRS [16]. In this study, elevation of presepsin levels on the enrollment day was a predictor of septic shock, not of SIRS. These results suggest that presepsin may be used to identify patients at increased risk of more severe infections at early stages.

One important characteristic of biomarkers is their prognostic values. Presepsin levels on day 1 were reported to be correlated with 60-day in-hospital mortality in patients with sepsis, severe sepsis, or septic shock [17]; a longer intensive-care unit stay; and a lower degree of resolution of primary infection [8, 9]. Mortality is one of the prognostic variables. Since there were no mortalities in this current study, we used presence or absence of SIRS on day 5 for prognosis. In this study, the levels of presepsin were significantly higher in the SIRS group than in the non-SIRS group on day 5 after admission. However, the levels of PCT on day1 were only identified as a predictor of SIRS on day5 using multivariate logistic regression analysis. Regarding PCT, the AUC for PCT to predict 30-day mortality in patients with febrile UTI was reported to be 0.71 (95% CI: 0.56–0.85) [18]. There

Table 4 Prediction of SIRS on the 5th day by logistic regression analysis

Variable	Univariate analysis			Multivariable analysis		
	P-value	HR	95% CI	*P*-value	HR	95% CI
Day1/WBC (4000–12,000 or other)	0.19					
Day1/CRP (≥ 10 or < 10)	0.280					
Day1/Presepsin (≥ 500 or < 500)	0.049	9.176	1.013–83.108	0.366		
Day1/PCT (≥ 2 or < 2)	0.012	17.455	1.886–161.528	0.012	17.455	1.886–161.528
Day1/AST (≥ 34 or < 34)	0.079					
Day1/ALT (≥ 28 or < 28)	0.283					
Day1/γGPT (≥ 47 or < 47)	0.177					
Day1/Cr (male; ≥ 1.07 or < 1.07, female; ≥ 0.79 or < 0.79)	0.998					
Day3/WBC (4000–12,000 or other)	0.120					
Day3/CRP (≥ 10 or < 10)	0.998					
Day3/Presepsin (≥ 500 or < 500)	0.067					
Day3/PCT (≥ 2 or < 2)	0.998					
Sex (male or female)	0.596					
Urinary culture (P vs N)	0.999					
Blood culture (P vs N)	0.059					
Placement of urinary catheter (Y vs N)	0.280					
Urological cancer (Y vs N)	0.346					
Urinary calculi (Y vs N)	0.040	5.833	1.084–31.377	0.182		
DM (Y vs N)	0.783					
Surgical procedure (Y vs N)	0.120					
Internal use ofsteroid (Y vs N)	0.439					

WBC white blood cell, *CRP* C-reactive protein, *PCT* procalcitonin, *AST* aspartate transaminase, *ALT* alanine transaminase, *γGTP* γ-glutamyl transpeptidase, *Cr* creatinine, *DM* diabetes mellitus, *P* positive, *N* no, *Y* yes

are a few reports that compared between presepsin and PCT for evaluating their prognostic values in patients with UTI. Further research that includes a large sample size of patients with severe urosepsis than does this study is needed to evaluate the reliability of each of these biomarkers for predicting treatment outcomes.

This study has several limitations. First, since 2016, sepsis has been defined according to the Sequential (Sepsis-Related) Organ Failure Assessment (SOFA) [19]. This study began in 2014, and we did not assess the level of consciousness, which is a requirement for the SOFA scoring. Therefore, instead of the SOFA, SIRS criteria [10] were used for defining sepsis and septic shock. Second, this study might have been limited by its single-center design and small sample size. Third, we did not consider renal function in setting the reference values of presepsin and PCT. The levels of presepsin and PCT have been previously reported to be affected by renal function [20, 21]. It would have been ideal to set the reference values depending on assessment of renal function. However, these adjustments are yet to be clarified. Fourth, all patients were discharged from our hospital alive in this study. However, it has been reported that severe sepsis and septic shock could be fatal, with mortality rate of 28.3%-41.1% [2]. Regarding 11 patients with septic shock on the enrollment day, seven patients were without SIRS on the fifth day. Six patients underwent surgical procedures out of these seven patients, and it seems that the combination of antibiotics and surgical procedures might have been quite effective. There is a possibility that these patients might have not needed any vasopressors infusion in the course of treatments. Moreover, the number of patients was not enough to evaluate presepsin for detecting severe sepsis and predicting the therapeutic course in comparison with PCT and CRP. Further research with a larger number of patients is needed.

Conclusions

This study showed that, in patients with UTI, presepsin may be a good marker for diagnosis of septic shock based on the data of admission.

Abbreviations

ALT: Aspartate transaminase; AST: Alanine transaminase; AUC: The area under the curve; Cr: Creatinine; CRP: C-reactive protein; γGPT: γ-Glutamyl transpeptidase; PCT: Procalcitonin; ROC: A receiver operating characteristics; SIRS: Systemic inflammatory response syndrome; SOFA: The Sequential Organ Failure Assessment UTI: Urinary tract infections; WBC: White blood cell.

Acknowledgements

We thank Ms. Atsuko Oyama, and Ms. Rie Suzuki for their technical assistance.

Authors' contributions

YSe perfomed project development, data collection, data analysis and manuscript writing. KK contributed to project development and manuscript editing. DO, HN, YM, TS, SA, MN, HK, HM and YSh contributed to data collection. MM contributed to data analysis. KS contributed to project developments. All authors read and approved the final manuscript.

Competing interests

The authors declare no competing interests.

Author details

[1]Department of Urology, Gunma University Graduate School of Medicine, 3-39-22 Showa-Machi, Maebashi 371-8511, Japan. [2]Division of Community and Family Medicine, Department of Clinical Laboratory Medicine, Jichi Medical University, Shimotsuke, Japan. [3]Department of Clinical Laboratory Medicine, Gunma University Graduate School of Medicine, Maebashi, Japan.

References

1. Angus DC, Linde-Zwirble WT, Lidicker J, Clermont G, Carcillo J, Pinsky MR. Epidemiology of severe sepsis in the United States: analysis of incidence, outcome, and associated costs of care. Crit Care Med. 2001;29:1303–10.
2. Levy MM, Artigas A, Phillips GS, Rhodes A, Beale R, Osborn T, et al. Outcomes of the surviving sepsis campaign in intensive care units in the USA and Europe: a prospective cohort study. Lancet Infect Dis. 2012;12:919–24.
3. Brunkhorst FM, Heinz U, Forycki ZF. Kinetics of procalcitonin in iatrogenic sepsis. Intensive Care Med. 1998;24:888–9.
4. Dandona P, Nix D, Wilson MF, Aljada A, Love J, Assicot M, et al. Procalcitonin increase after endotoxin injection in normal subjects. J Clin Endocrinol Metab. 1994;79:1605–8.
5. Yaegashi Y, Shirakawa K, Sato N, Suzuki Y, Kojika M, Imai S, et al. Evaluation of a newly identified soluble CD14 subtype as a marker for sepsis. J Infect Chemother. 2005;11:234–8.
6. Nakamura M, Takeuchi T, Naito K, Shirakawa K, Hosaka Y, Yamasaki F, et al. Early elevation of plasma soluble CD14 subtype, a novel biomarker for sepsis, in a rabbit cecal ligation and puncture model. Crit Care. 2008;12(Suppl 2):194.
7. Zou Q, Wen W, Zhang XC. Presepsin as a novel sepsis biomarker. World J Emerg Med. 2014;5:16–9.
8. Masson S, Caironi P, Fanizza C, Thomae R, Bernasconi R, Noto A, et al. Circulating presepsin (soluble CD14 subtype) as a marker of host response in patients with severe sepsis or septic shock: data from the multicenter, randomized ALBIOS trial. Intensive Care Med. 2015;41:12–20.
9. Kim H, Hur M, Moon HW, Yun YM, Di Somma S. Multi-marker approach using procalcitonin, presepsin, galectin-3, and soluble suppression of tumorigenicity 2 for the prediction of mortality in sepsis. Ann Intensive Care. 2017;7:27.
10. Bone RC, Balk RA, Cerra FB, Dellinger RP, Fein AM, Knaus WA, et al. Definitions for sepsis and organ failure and guidelines for the use of innovative therapies in sepsis. The ACCP/SCCM Consensus Conference Committee. American College of Chest Physicians/Society of Critical Care Medicine. Chest. 1992;101:1644–55.
11. Memar MY, Baghi HB. Presepsin: a promising biomarker for the detection of bacterial infections. Biomed Pharmacother. 2019;111:649–56.
12. Claessens Y-E, Trabattoni E, Grabar S, Quinguis L, Sahakian G, Anselmo M, et al. Plasmatic presepsin (sCD14-ST) concentrations in acute pyelonephritis in adult patients. Clin Chim Acta. 2017;464:182–8.
13. Tambo M, Taguchi S, Nakamura Y, Okegawa T, Fukuhara H. Presepsin and procalcitonin as predictors of sepsis based on the new sepsis-3 definitions in obstructive acute pyelonephritis. BMC Urol. 2020;20:23.
14. Maruna P, Nedelníková K, Gürlich R. Physiology and genetics of procalcitonin. Physiol Res. 2000;49(Suppl 1):57–61.
15. Lelubre C, Anselin S, Boudjeltia KZ, Biston P, Piagnerelli M. Interpretation of C-reactive protein concentrations in critically ill patients. Biomed Res Int. 2013;2013:124021.
16. Shozushima T, Takahashi G, Matsumoto N, Kojika M, Okamura Y, Endo S. Usefulness of presepsin (sCD14-ST) measurements as a marker for the diagnosis and severity of sepsis that satisfied diagnostic criteria of systemic inflammatory response syndrome. J Infect Chemother. 2011;17:764–9.
17. Ulla M, Pizzolato E, Lucchiari M, Loiacono M, Soardo F, Forno D, et al. Diagnostic and prognostic value of presepsin in the management of sepsis in the emergency department: a multicenter prospective study. Crit Care. 2013;17:R168.
18. Starre WE, Zunder SM, Vollaard AM, Nieuwkoop CV, Stalenhoef JE, Delfos NM, et al. Prognostic value of pro-adrenomedullin, procalcitonin and C-reactive protein in predicting outcome of febrile urinary tract infection. Clin Microbiol Infect. 2014;20:1048–54.
19. Singer M, Deutschman CS, Seymour CW, Shankar-Hari M, Annane D, Bauer M, et al. The third international consensus definitions for sepsis and septic shock (sepsis-3). JAMA. 2016;315:801–10.
20. Nakamura Y, Ishikura H, Nishida T, Kawano Y, Yuge R, Ichiki R, et al. Usefulness of presepsin in the diagnosis of sepsis in patients with or without acute kidney injury. BMC Anesthesiol. 2014;14:88.
21. Amour J, Birenbaum A, Langeron O, Le Manach Y, Bertrand M, Coriat P, et al. Influence of renal dysfunction on the accuracy of procalcitonin for the diagnosis of postoperative infection after vascular surgery. Crit Care Med. 2008;36:1147–54.

23

Incidental para-ureteral aggressive angiomyxoma: A rare case report and literature review

Ming Liu[1†], Ting-Shuai Zhai[2†], Xiao-Feng Zhao[1], Li-Jin Feng[3], Xin-Sheng Lyu[4], Lan-Ting Hu[1], Zheng-Xin Wang[1], Wei-Guo Ma[1], Jian Zhang[2], Xiao Chen[1], Bin-Jie Su[1], Xu-Dong Yao[2], Jing-Yi Lu[1] and Lin Ye[1,2*]

Abstract

Background: Aggressive angiomyxoma (AA) is a rare tumor that typically occurs in the pelvis and perineum, most commonly in women of reproductive age. However, no para-ureteral AA has been reported according to the literature.

Case presentation

We herein describe the first case of para-ureteral AA. A 62-year-old male presented to our institute in March 2017 with a para-ureteral mass that was 15 mm in diameter incidentally. No symptom was observed and laboratory analysis was unremarkable. Magnetic resonance and computed tomography imaging showed a non-enhancing mass abutting the left ureter without causing obstruction. Laparoscopic resection of the mass was performed without injury to the ureter. Pathologic and immunohistochemical results were consistent with AA. Till now, no recurrence was noticed.

Conclusions: We reported a rare case of para-ureteral AA, along with a literature review. Early diagnosis, proper surgical plan and long-term close follow-up is recommended for its high risk of recurrence and malignant potential.

Keywords: Angiomyxoma, Ureter, Case management

Background

Aggressive angiomyxoma (AA), synonymously referred to deep angiomyxoma (DAM), is a very rare mesenchymal tumor characterized by local aggressiveness and high risk of recurrence [1]. AA preferentially grows in pelvis and perineum of females aged 30 to 60, with a female-to-male ratio approximately 6:1 [2]. In 1983 Steeper and Rosai first described this disease and named it "aggressive angiomyxoma" [3]. According to the latest WHO classification AA was classified as "tumors of uncertain differentiation". Pre-operative diagnosis is difficult due to its rarity and lack of typical presenting signs and symptoms. Wide surgical excision is the curative and foremost treatment method for AA [4]. Local recurrence is common even after complete excision. So long-term close follow-up is recommended [5]. However, no para-ureteral AA has been reported. A case of para-ureteral AA of a 62-year-old male is presented herein. To the best of our knowledge, this is the first reported case of para-ureteral AA.

Case presentation

A 62-year-old male was hospitalized in March 2017 with a para-ureteral mass that was 15 mm in diameter found through a routine check-up incidentally. There was no symptom. On physical examination no abnormality was

*Correspondence: ericyelin@163.com
†Ming Liu and Ting-Shuai Zhai have contributed equally to this work
[2] Department of Urology, Shanghai Tenth People's Hospital, Tongji University School of Medicine, No.301, Middle Yan-Chang Rd., Jing-An District, Shanghai 200072, China
Full list of author information is available at the end of the a'ticle

detected. Laboratory tests (blood routine test, urine routine test, biochemical tests) including tumor markers (β-HCG, CA125, CA242, CA15-3, CA199, CEA, AFP, NSE, CYK-19, SCC, t-PSA, f-PSA) were unremarkable. CT imaging showed an irregular-shaped non-enhancing mass abutting the left ureter was 15 mm in diameter, with unclear boundaries to the ureter, hypodense relative to muscle (Fig. 1). MRI appearances of the tumor demonstrated hyperintensity on T2-weighted images (Fig. 2). And No hydronephrosis was observed in the imaging.

Laparoscopic resection of the tumor was performed. The intraoperative situs revealed a well-defined and gelatinous cystic mass with a smooth surface abutting the upper left ureter, 2.3 × 2.0 × 1.0 cm in size (Fig. 3). Histopathological analysis revealed spindle-shaped cells in loose myxoid stroma with variable calibre blood vessels (Fig. 4), consistent with AA. Mitotic figures were absent. Immunohistochemically the tumor cells were positive for Vimetin, Ki-67(weakly, 0–2%) and S-100(focally), while negative for Desmin, SMA, CD34, EMA and CK(AE1/AE3). The postoperative period was uneventful. After 30-month follow-up, no evidence of recurrence was noted. The patient has been informed to keep the follow-up because of the high risk of recurrence.

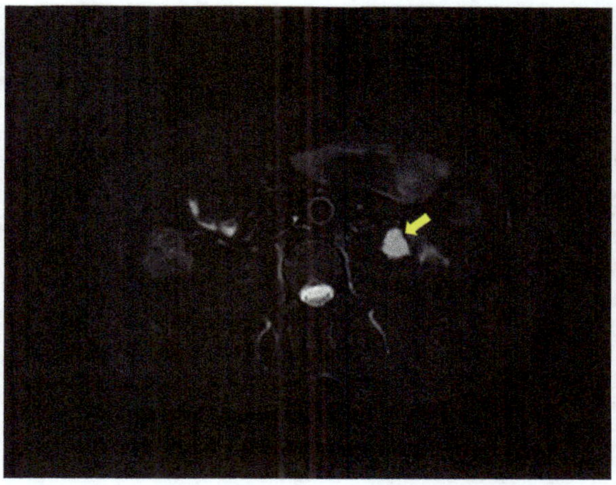

Fig. 2 MRI appearances of the tumor demonstrated hyperintensity on T2-weighted images

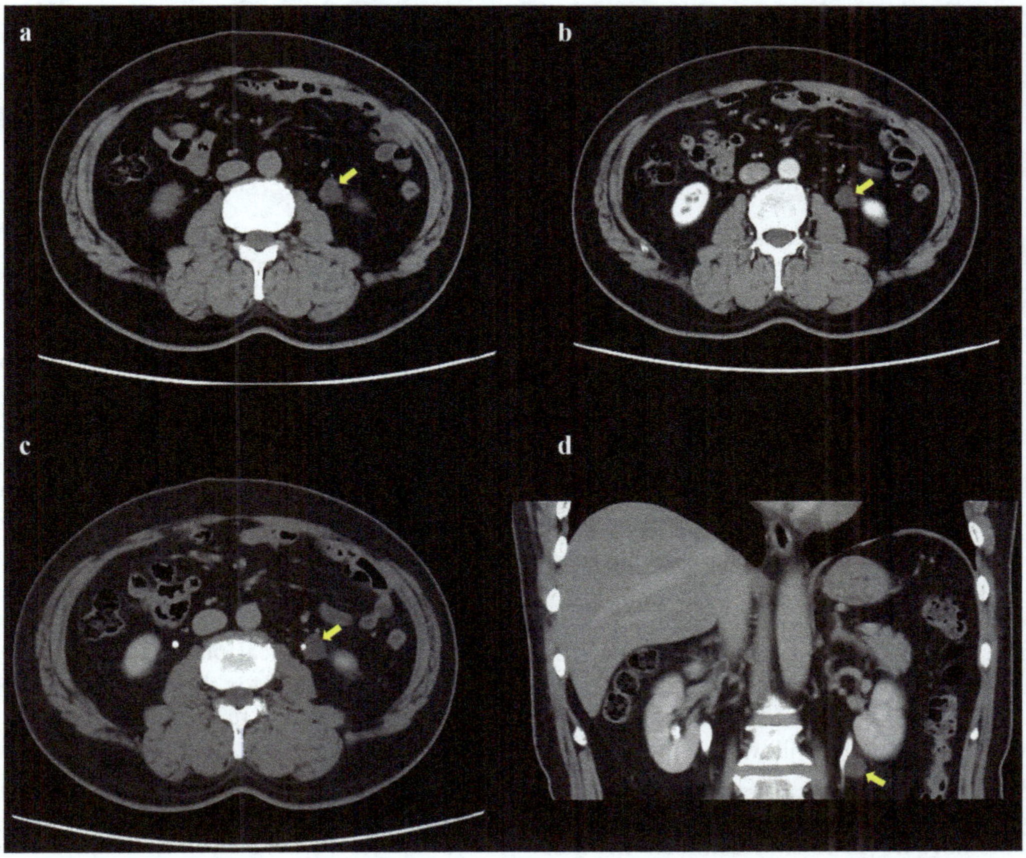

Fig. 1 Axial (**a**–**c**) and coronal (**d**) contrast-enhanced CT of the abdomen. CT imaging showed the mass abutting the left ureter was 15 mm in diameter without causing obstruction (**a**, **b**), which could been obviously seen in the excretory phase (**c**). The mass was located between the left ureter and the lower pole of the left kidney (**d**)

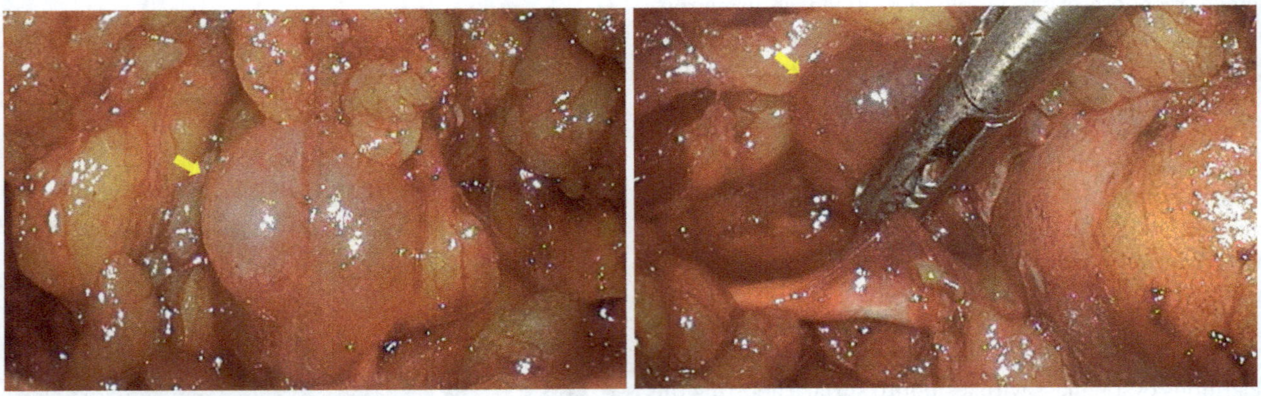

Fig. 3 Surgical photograph. A well-defined and gelatincus cystic mass, 2.3 × 2.0 × 1.0 cm in size, with a smooth surface was observed abutting the upper left ureter with a stent inside

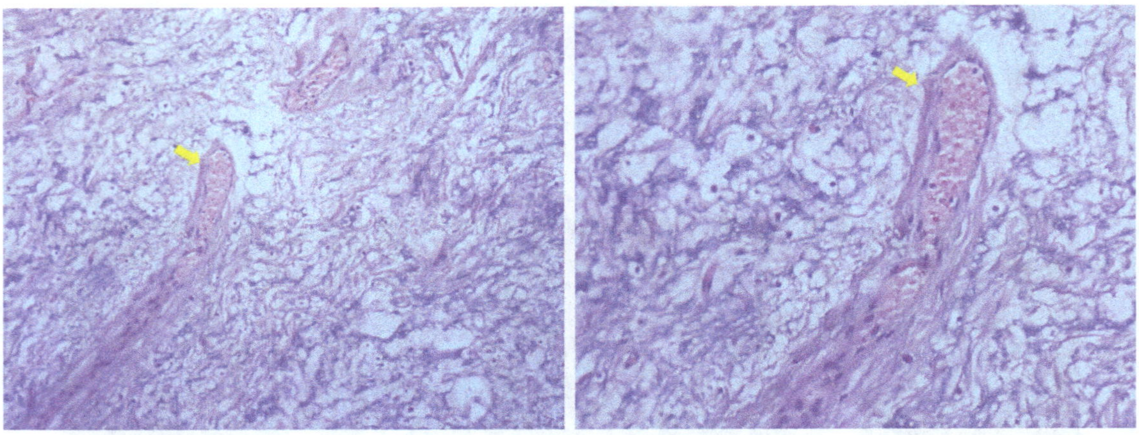

Fig. 4 Pathological photos. Histopathological analysis revealed spindle-shaped cells in loose myxoid stroma with variable calibre blood vessels

Discussion and conclusions

Aggressive Angiomyxoma, as a rare soft-tissue neoplasm, seldom occurs in urinary system especially in ureter. We reviewed the latest 100 AA patients published, analyzed the localization and found no paraureteral AA (Additional file 1: Fig. 1). "Aggressive" refers to the nature of its local infiltration and recurrence [6]. Because of its rarity, the preoperative misdiagnosis rate of AA is rather high and the pathogenesis is poorly understood. Both of proper management and prognosis have not been investigated very well. In the present case, the patient benefited from early detection, proper treatment and regular follow-up. The literature review focused on the clinical characteristics, pathological feature and the treating effect.

Most patients have no obvious discomfort. The mass often grows at the perineal or pelvic region [1]. If the tumor is large enough, compressive symptoms may occur. Imageological examinations of AA have low specificity. Color doppler ultrasound usually indicates a hypoechoic or cystic mass [7]. CT often shows a well-defined mass, hypodense to muscle [9]. MRI revealed T1 hypointensity and T2 hyperintensity and a characteristic "swirled" appearance inside the mass can be observed [8]. Furthermore, MRI can identify the infiltrating borders and relationship between the tumor and surrounding organs, which could help surgeons make optimal surgical plan. Pathological examination is the gold standard for the diagnosis of AA. On gross examination, the soft tumors are white and have a rubbery consistency with a gelantinous, translucent and glistening cut surface [7]. Microscopically, stellate to spindle-shaped tumor cells with ill-defined cytoplasmic borders, fibromyxoid stroma and hyalinized thin-to-thick wall vessels can always observed. Mitotic figures are always absent [8, 9]. Immunohistochemically the tumor has no specific marker, showing diffuse positivity for Vimentin, SMA, Desmin, CD-34, estrogen receptor and progesterone receptors. While, S-100, cytokeratins and CD68 are usually negative [1, 7].

At present surgical resection of the tumor with wide free margin is the most effective treatment [8]. However, surgical plan differs in different patients. For the small and superficial well-defined tumors, wide local excision is suitable. For the large and deep tumors but with clear borders to the adjacent tissue, efforts should be made to perform complete excision. While, for those extensively and deeply invading the surrounding vital organs, if complete excision is infeasible or severe surgical injuries may happen, incomplete resection combined with adjuvant therapy are recommended [10]. Zugail et al. reported a 35-mm AA mimicking an upper tract urothelial carcinoma (UTUC) of the right pelvic ureter treated with nephroureterectomy [11]. In our case, the tumor was small and well-defined, so wide local excision was performed successfully. If the tumor grew larger and invaded the ureter, it would not be easy to perform complete excision. Hormonal treatment, including raloxifene, tamoxifen, and gonadotropin-releasing hormone analogs, is sometimes used to shrink the tumor before surgery. Moreover, hormonal treatment is necessary especially for the residual or recurrent tumors [10]. However, chemotherapy, radiation and embolization are generally considered to be of limited use due to the tumor's low mitotic activity and numerous feeding vessels [8].

Because AA has a high recurrence rate (36–72%) [2, 12], postoperative surveillance is necessary. MRI is considered as a useful tool to detect recurrence. The factors affecting risk of recurrence remain unclear. Some researchers hold that incomplete surgical resection increases the risk of recurrence [2] but remains unproven. According to the literature, most of patients have had a relatively favorable prognosis, despite local multiple recurrences and infiltration to adjacent organs and tissues. However, two metastasizing cases were reported, ending in death [13, 14], which highlight the need to consider it as potentially malignant in a small percentage of cases.

From our perspective, diagnosis mainly depends on CTU and MRI. Complete resection of tumor should be performed and partial pelvis or ureter should also be resected if necessary. During follow-up, US can be used to detect hydronephrosis and MRI can be used to detect recurrence. To conclude, we reported a rare case of para-ureteral AA, along with a literature review. CT or MRI is helpful to detect early stage para-ureteral AA, which can be removed intactly and safely by laparoscopy. Thus, it can help increase the cure rate and decrease the recurrence rate and mortality. Early diagnosis, proper surgical plan and long-term close follow-up is recommended for its high risk of recurrence and malignant potential.

Abbreviations

AA: Aggressive angiomyxoma; DAM: Deep angiomyxoma; CT: Computerized tomography; MRI: Magnetic resonance imaging.

Acknowledgements

We would like to thank Dr. Min Zhu and Dr. Guo-Qing Guo (Department of pathology, Karamay Central Hospital) for pathological suggestions to our study.

Authors' contributions

ML, TSZ: manuscript writing; LJF, LTH, ZW: data collection; WGM: image analysis; LY, ML, XFZ, XC, BJS: patient treatment; XDY, JYL, LY, XSL: manuscript revision. All authors read and approved the final manuscript.

Competing interests

The authors declare that they have no competing interests.

Author details

[1] Department of Urology, Karamay Central Hospital, Karamay 834000, Xinjiang, China. [2] Department of Urology, Shanghai Tenth People's Hospital, Tongji University School of Medicine, No.301, Middle Yan-Chang Rd., Jing-An District, Shanghai 200072, China. [3] Department of Pathology, Shanghai Tenth People's Hospital, Tongji University School of Medicine, Shanghai 200072, China. [4] Department of Radiology, Karamay Central Hospital, Karamay 834000, Xinjiang, China.

References

1. Sutton BJ, Laudadio J. Aggressive angiomyxoma. Arch Pathol Lab Med. 2012;136(2):217.
2. Chan YM, Hon E, Ngai SW, Ng TY, Wong LC. Aggressive angiomyxoma in females: is radical resection the only option? Acta Obstet Gynecol Scand. 2000;79:216–20.
3. Steeper TA, Rosai J. Aggressive angiomyxoma of the female pelvis and perineum. Report of nine cases of a distinctive type of gynecologic soft-tissue neoplasm. Am J Surg Pathol. 1983;7(5):463.
4. Simo M, Zapata C, Esquius J, Domingo J. Aggressive angiomyxoma of the female pelvis and perineum: report of two cases and review of the literature. Br J Obstet Gynaecol. 1992;99:925–7.
5. Morag R, Fridman E, Mor Y. Aggressive angiomyxoma of the scrotum mimicking huge hydrocele: a case report and literature review. J Case Rep Med. 2009;15:7624.
6. Elchalal U, Lifschitz-Mercer B, Dgani R, Zalel Y. Aggressive angiomyxoma of the vulva. Gynecol Oncol. 1992;47:260–2.
7. Haldar K, Martinek IE, Kehoe S. Aggressive angiomyxoma: a case series and literature review. Eur J Surg Oncol. 2010;36(4):335–9.
8. Lee KA, Seo JW, Yoon NR, Lee JW, Bae DS. Aggressive angiomyxoma of the vulva: a case report. Obstet Gynecol Sci. 2014;57(2):164.
9. Schoolmeester JK, Fritchie KJ. Genital soft tissue tumors. J Cutan Pathol. 2015;42(7):441–51.
10. Bai HM, Yang JX, Huang HF, Cao DY, Chen J, Yang N, et al. Individualized managing strategies of aggressive angiomyxoma of female genital tract and pelvis. Eur J Surg Oncol. 2013;39(10):1101–8.
11. Zugail AS, Baowaidan F, Comperat EM, Guillonneau B, Colau A. Angiomyxoma of the ureter imitating an upper tract urothelial carcinoma: a case report. Int J Surg Case Rep. 2018;53:39–42.
12. Giraudmaillet T, Mokrane FZ, Delchier-Bellec MC, Motton S, Cron C, Rousseau H. Aggressive angiomyxoma of the pelvis with inferior vena cava involvement: MR imaging features. Diagn Interv Imaging. 2015;96(1):111–4.
13. Siassi RM, Papadopoulos T, Matzel KE. Metastasizing aggressive angiomyxoma. N Engl J Med. 1999;341(23):1772.
14. Blandamura S, Cruz J, Faure VL, Machado PI, Ninfo V. Aggressive angiomyxoma: a second case of metastasis with patient's death. Hum Pathol. 2003;34(10):1072–4.

24

The utilization of perfused cadaver simulation in urologic training

Daniel McClelland[1], Luke P. O'Connor[1*], John Barnard[1], Ali Hajiran[1], Chad Crigger[1], Tyler Trump[1], Emma Bacharach[1], Amr Elbakry[1], Zach Werner[1], Chad Morley[1], Daniel Grabo[2] and Adam Luchey[1]

Abstract

Background: We sought to determine if participating in a surgical training session using perfused fresh human cadavers (PFHC) had a positive effect on urology residents' confidence in performing open and endoscopic procedures.

Methods: Urology residents at our institution participated in a surgical training session in the West Virginia University Fresh Tissue Training Program, which utilized fresh cadavers with vascular perfusion. The session consisted of performing different urologic procedures (open and endoscopic) on the perfused fresh human cadavers (PFHC). Residents were given a survey to rate their confidence in different urologic procedures before, after, and 6 months after the session. Each procedure on the survey had 3–6 questions associated with it, with scores ranging from 0 (no confidence) to 4 (great confidence). Scores for each procedure before and after the session were compared.

Results: Six residents participated in the session. There was an increase in the score for every procedure performed after the session. Scores at 6 month follow up remained higher than the pre-session scores.

Conclusion: PFHCs offer an excellent opportunity to teach a wide variety of urologic procedures to residents. Incorporation of PFHCs may be very useful in urologic training, and further studies on its use are warranted.

Keyword: Education, Resident, Training, Cadaver, Simulation

Background

With new technologies and surgical techniques being incorporated into the practice of urology, today's residents are tasked with learning a broader skillset than ever before. This has led to some concern that residents are not prepared for practice after completion of a 5-year surgical residency program. In fact, one study found that 23% of PGY-5 general surgery residents across 55 programs did not believe that a 5-year residency fully prepared them to practice independently [1]. In this constant-changing world of surgery, it is crucial that residency programs adapt and incorporate new methods of training to maximize residents' readiness to practice on their own. It has been well documented that cadaver training is an effective method to enhance surgical skills by helping residents become more familiar with the anatomy and steps of surgical procedures in a low-risk setting [2–4]. In the realm of urology, studies have shown that residents believe cadaver simulation training helped them learn the steps of an operation, boosted their confidence for many procedures, and improved their surgical skills in the operating room [5]. In 2018, the West Virginia University Fresh Tissue Training Program (FTTP) was established as part of the WVU Critical Care and Trauma Institute and in partnership with the Department of Pathology, Anatomy, and Lab Medicine. The FTTP utilizes fresh, never-frozen cadavers with vascular perfusion in surgical skills training. Educational sessions

*Correspondence: loconnor419@gmail.com; luke.oconnor@hsc.wvu.edu
[1] Department of Urology, West Virginia University, 1 Medical Center Drive, PO Box 9251, Morgantown, WV 26506-9251, USA
Full list of author information is available at the end of the article

take place in the FTTP lab, which includes a training room with standard operating room equipment and are moderated by surgical faculty. A case-based approach is used in surgical and procedural skills training for all levels. In this pilot study, we aim to determine if utilization of perfused fresh human cadavers (PFHC) for surgical simulation improves residents' confidence in open/laparoscopic urologic procedures. The use of PFHCs allows residents to experience urologic procedures on full-size models where realistic adverse events, such as bleeding, can be recreated with our perfusion technology. To date, this is the first documented use of PFHCs in urology.

Methods

Cadaver preparation

Fresh human cadavers were obtained from the West Virginia University Human Gift Registry. All practices regarding fresh human cadaver procurement, storage, usage and removal were in accordance with the protocols and policies of the WVU Human Gift Registry and Fresh Tissue Training Program.

Fresh human cadavers used in this FTTP session were prepared in the same fashion as those previously described in the literature [2–4]. Cadavers were fresh, non-embalmed, and never frozen. They were stored in coolers maintained at 4 °C and allowed to warm at ambient temperature (20 °C) prior to scheduled training sessions. They were perfused via exposure and cannulation of the femoral vessels with Simms connectors (Fig. 1A). A centrifugal pump was used to achieve perfusate flow (Fig. 1B). Red, non-toxic paint with water was used as a blood substitute. Clamping and unclamping of the blood tubing allowed regulation of vascular perfusion [2, 3].

Setting/participants

Urology residents at West Virginia University participated in a surgical skills training session in the FTTP. Residents of all levels (PGY 1 through PGY 5) participated. Prior to the start of the session, residents completed a survey that assessed confidence levels in several different urologic procedures. Each procedure on the survey had 4–6 associated questions/statements, with responses ranging from 0 (no confidence) to 4 (great confidence). For example, the section for partial nephrectomy consisted of four questions or statements (i.e. "my confidence in gaining exposure for partial nephrectomy..."), so the highest score possible for this section was 20 (as seen in Fig. 2). These procedures were then carried out in the training session under faculty supervision. Procedures performed on the PFHC model included: exploratory laparotomy, partial/radical nephrectomy,

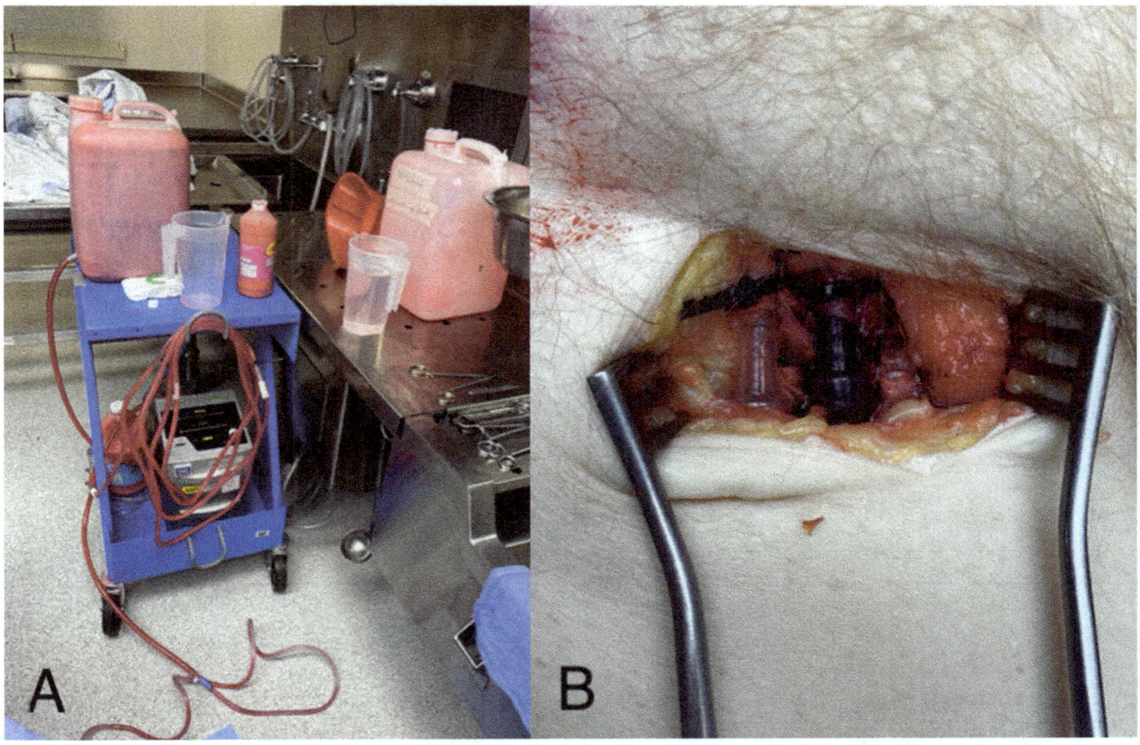

Fig. 1 **A** Centrifugal pump set up. **B** Cannulation of femoral vessels

Urology Training Confidence Assessment

1. Partial Nephrectomy/Radical Nephrectomy

My confidence in exposure for partial/radical nephrectomy ....

No Confidence	0	1	2	3	4	Great Confidence

My confidence in control of the renal hilum ....

No Confidence	0	1	2	3	4	Great Confidence

My confidence in repair of the collecting system ...

No Confidence	0	1	2	3	4	Great Confidence

My confidence in renorrhahy

No Confidence	0	1	2	3	4	Great Confidence

2. Transurethral Resection of the Prostate

My confidence in selecting the appropriate equipment (i.e. scope, loop, irrigation, etc) ....

No Confidence	0	1	2	3	4	Great Confidence

My confidence in resecting the median lobe ....

No Confidence	0	1	2	3	4	Great Confidence

My confidence in resecting the lateral lobes ...

No Confidence	0	1	2	3	4	Great Confidence

My confidence in controlling bleeding ...

No Confidence	0	1	2	3	4	Great Confidence

My confidence in identifying prostatic capsule ...

No Confidence	0	1	2	3	4	Great Confidence

My confidence in identifying the veru and resecting apical tissue ...

No Confidence	0	1	2	3	4	Great Confidence

Fig. 2 Survey questions for partial/radical nephrectomy and TURP

repair of ureteral/bladder injury, RPLND, groin dissection, TURBT/TURP, ureteroscopy, difficult foley catheter placement, and orchiectomy/orchiopexy. Comparisons of ureteroscopy and TURP in a live patient to a PFHC can be seen in Fig. 3. Residents then filled out the same survey immediately following the session, and again

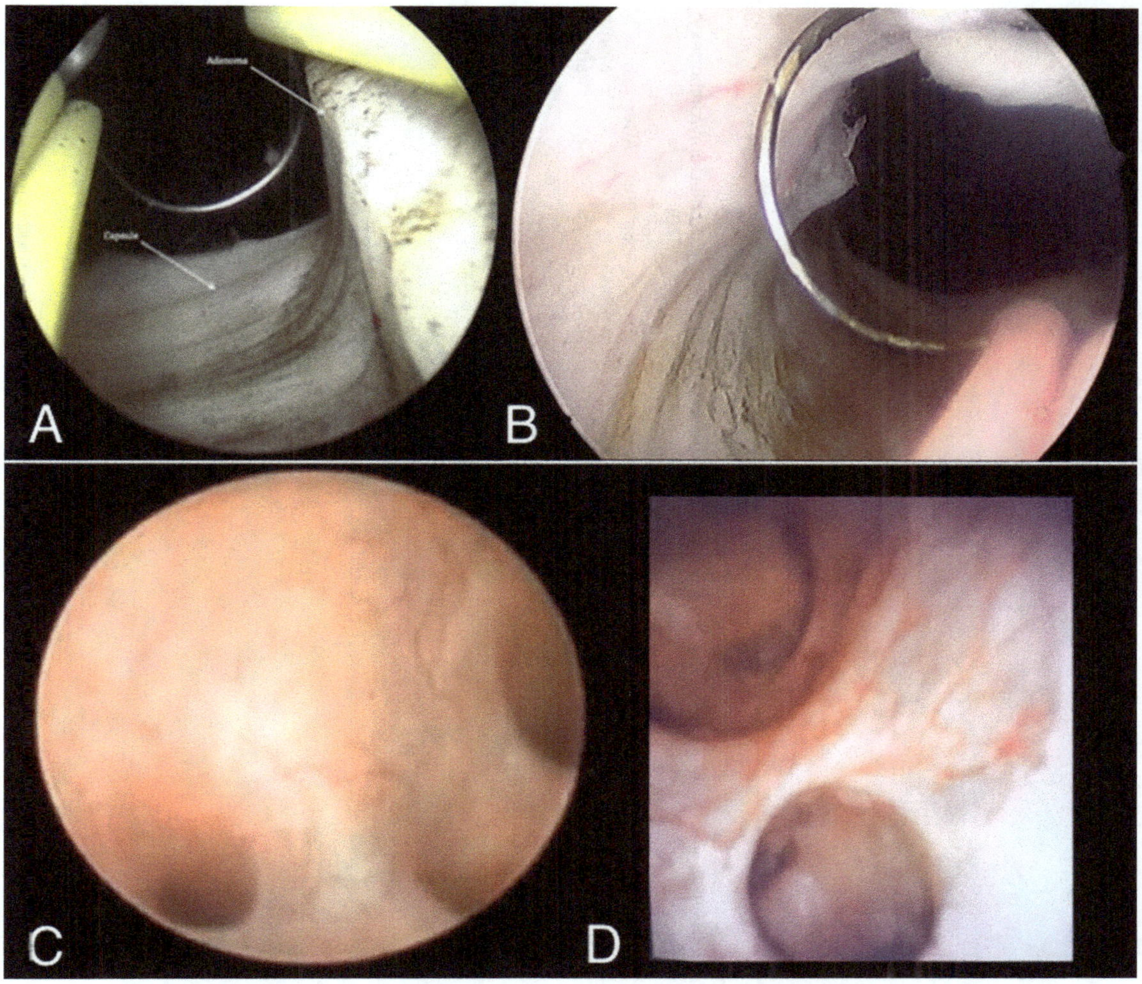

Fig. 3 **A** TURP in a live patient. **B** TURP in a PFHC. **C** Ureteroscopy in a live patient. **D** Ureteroscopy in a PFHC

6 months later. Residents also completed a questionnaire immediately following the session to assess their perception of the training session.

Results

Six urology residents from our institution participated in this training session. The total scores for each procedure before the session, immediately after the session, and 6 months after the session were compared. We also evaluated the responses on the perception of the training session. When comparing scores before the session and immediately following the session, there was an increase in score for every procedure performed in all residents, with the exception of procedures in which senior residents already had a maximum score prior to the session. With outliers removed (100% confidence or no prior experience with the simulated procedure), we found that senior level residents (PGY 4+5) had a 9% increase in confidence scores from baseline versus 30% increase for junior level residents (PGY 1–3). For open procedures, senior level residents had a 34.1% increase in confidence level from baseline versus 37.7% for junior level residents. At six-month follow-up, scores on the survey remained higher than the pre-session scores, indicating that residents retained at least some of the knowledge and skills from the session. Scores for open and endoscopic procedures can be seen in Tables 1 and 2. Residents believed the session was a true simulation of the conditions of live surgery (100% agree or strongly agree), promoted acquisition of surgical skills (100% agree or strongly agree), and would increase their confident in handling future intra-operative consults (100% agree or strongly agree). They also believed this simulation offered benefits not available in existing training models (100% agree or strongly agree) and would recommend this training method to their colleagues (100% agree or strongly agree).

Table 1 Scores before, immediately following, and 6 months after session for open procedures

	Survey scores (total possible points)																	
	Exploratory laparotomy (16)			**Partial/radical nephrectomy (16)**			**Ureteral/bladder injury repair (16)**			**RPLND (16)**			**Groin dissection (12)**			**Orchiectomy/orchopexy (20)**		
	Before	**After**	**6 Months after**	**Before**	**After**	**6 Months after**	**Before**	**After**	**6 Months after**	**Before**	**After**	**6 Months after**	**Before**	**After**	**6 Months after**	**Before**	**After**	**6 Months after**
PGY-5	13	16	16	12	16	16	15	16	16	2	14	11	8	12	12	19	20	20
PGY-4	5	9	11	4	12	12	9	15	16	1	11	10	5	12	12	20	20	20
PGY-3	1	3	5	0	2	3	1	4	5	0	2	2	2	3	4	13	17	20
PGY-2a	1	3	2	0	6	4	1	6	5	1	2	2	3	6	5	10	12	18
PGY-2b	1	7	5	0	7	4	2	7	4	0	1	8	1	6	6	10	15	16
PGY-1	0	2	1	0	2	1	0	2	1	0	1	0	0	3	3	0	9	5

Table 2 Scores before, immediately following, and 6 months after session for endoscopic procedures

	Survey scores (total possible points)											
	Difficult foley placement (20)			TURBT (16)			TURP (24)			URS (20)		
	Before	After	6 Months after	Before	After	6 Months after	Before	After	6 Months after	Before	After	6 Months after
PGY-5	20	20	20	16	16	16	24	24	24	20	20	20
PGY-4	20	20	20	16	16	16	22	24	24	20	20	20
PGY-3	19	20	20	13	14	16	18	24	24	20	20	20
PGY-2	13	18	19	1	8	3	0	8	10	9	15	14
PGY-2	15	20	18	2	12	11	1	18	17	16	20	20
PGY-1	10	13	14	1	5	2	1	5	3	2	6	5

Discussion

This pilot study shows that that the use of PFHCs in urologic training can be very beneficial in increasing residents' confidence in performing a variety of urologic procedures, both open and endoscopic. Residents of all levels reported an increased score in all procedures performed. It also demonstrates that the skills and confidence gained in these sessions were at least partially retained as scores 6 months after the session remained higher than scores prior to the session. It was noted that some scores at 6 months were higher than they were immediately following the session. This was likely due to more exposure to these procedures in the operating room within the first 6 months of completing the session. With the introduction of laparoscopy, robotics, and new minimally invasive endourologic procedures, urology residents must learn a very broad skillset during their training. Simulations such as this provide residents with extra opportunities to learn and improve their skillset in a low stress environment. Residents that participated believed the session accurately simulated the conditions of live surgery, promoted the acquisition of surgical skills, and increased their confidence of handling future intraoperative consults. Furthermore, they felt that this simulation offered benefits not available in existing training models and would recommend this training model to their colleagues.

One major advantage of PFHC over 3D printing is having the ability to operate on human tissue versus synthetic material. Many educators believe that there is truly no substitute for human tissue when learning surgical techniques [6]. 3D printing also requires highly trained computer scientists/engineers who are experts in 3D-printing. These personnel are not widely available, making it difficult for widespread implementation as there are significant barriers when starting a program as well as for maintenance of machines/software. In addition, there are significant costs to consider with 3D-printing based surgical simulation as some printers can cost > $250,000 (http://www.aniwaa.com/).

In 2012, Lewis et al. reported their experience utilizing fresh frozen cadavers to teach anatomy and operative skills to their general surgery residents [7]. Residents indicated that sessions with the cadavers were useful for learning anatomy, learning the steps of various operations, and improved their confidence in doing an operation on their own. Furthermore, the vast majority of residents expressed interest in participating in additional sessions and stated they would spend their free time in the cadaver laboratory if allowed to do so. Our study varied as we utilized fresh cadavers that never underwent a freeze/thaw cycle. In addition, junior residents were able to participate in all procedures in our simulation, even those deemed to be above their training level such as complex open procedures.

The addition of vascular perfusion further improves the validity of cadaver sessions. By using a red, non-toxic water-based paint, trainees are able to visualize bleeding in real-time during a simulated operation. Carey et al. demonstrated that mean arterial pressures of 80 mm Hg could be established, resulting in microvascular perfusion [3]. This allows for a life-like simulation for residents; bleeding will be encountered, as it would in a real surgical scenario. This type of experience is invaluable when learning how to perform minimally invasive procedures such as TURP as bleeding is one the most common complication of this procedure [8]. Encountering intraoperative bleeding on a cadaver allows residents to experience real-life complications without jeopardizing patient safety. Perfused cadavers have also been used to simulate traumatic injuries in the realm of trauma surgery. In one study, fully trained trauma surgeons participated in a session with perfused cadavers in which various injuries were simulated. Surgeons that participated reported that the perfused cadaver model allowed for an accurate simulation of the challenges faced during operative trauma and helped familiarize them with different techniques and skills [9]. While this study was primarily focused on creating a realistic training simulation, our study assessed the impact of PFHC on trainees' confidence. While having the recreation of a realistic situation is essential, having a positive impact on trainees' skills and confidence level is equally as important with any surgical simulation. To date, this is the first documentation of utilizing PFHCs in urologic training.

There are limitations to this study. One inherent limitation is our small sample size of 6 residents. With this small of a sample size, meaningful statistical analysis was unable to be performed. Further sessions with a larger number of urology residents need to be organized to evaluate the true impact that PFHCs may have on urologic training. Another potential limitation of this method is cost. Carey et al. reported that the average cost per PFHC was $1262.55 [3]. This may limit some training programs from using this resource depending on their funding.

The objective of this study was to introduce a new method of training to our urology residents and assess its impact on our residents' confidence. The increase in survey scores and positive reception by our residents after just one session are very promising, and further investigation into the use of PFHCs in urologic training is warranted.

Conclusion

This study is the first-ever documented use of perfused fresh human cadavers in urologic surgical training. This novel approach to urology training allows residents to experience the wide scope of surgical procedures and associated complications prior to real life scenarios. Further study with a larger cohort of residents is necessary to better understand the impact of perfused fresh human cadavers on urology training.

Authors' contributions

Conception of work: DM, CM, DG, AL. Design of work: DM, CM, DG, AL. Data acquisition/analysis: DM, JB, AH, CC, TT, EB, AE, ZW. Interpretation of data: DM, CM, DG, AL. Manuscript drafting/revising: DM, LO, CM, DG, AL. All authors have read and approved this manuscript.

Competing interests

The authors of this paper certify that they have NO affiliations with or involvement in any organization or entity with any financial interest (such as honoraria; educational grants; participation in speakers' bureaus; membership, employment, consultancies, stock ownership, or other equity interest; and expert testimony or patent-licensing arrangements), or non-financial interest (such as personal or professional relationships, affiliations, knowledge or beliefs) in the subject matter or materials discussed in this manuscript.

Author details

[1]Department of Urology, West Virginia University, 1 Medical Center Drive, PO Box 9251, Morgantown, WV 26506-9251, USA. [2]Department of Surgery, West Virginia University, Morgantown, WV, USA.

References

1. Coleman JJ, Esposito TJ, Rozycki GS, et al. Early subspecialization and perceived competence in surgical training: are residents ready? J Am Coll Surg. 2013;216:764.
2. Grabo D, Bardes J, Sharon M, Borgstrong D. Initial report on the impact of a perfused fresh cadaver training program in general surgery resident trauma education. Am J Surg. 2019. https://doi.org/10.1016/j.amjsurg.2019.10.033.
3. Carey JN, Minneti M, Leland HA, Demetriades D, Talving P. Perfused fresh cadavers: method for application to surgical simulation. Am J Surg. 2015;210(1):179–87.
4. Minneti M, Baker CJ, Sullivan ME. The development of a novel perfused cadaver model with dynamic vital sign regulation and real-world scenarios to teach surgical skills and error management. J Surg Educ. 2018;75(3):820–7.
5. Ahmed K, Aydin A, Dasgupta P, Khan MS, McCabe JE. A novel cadaveric simulation program in urology. J Surg Educ. 2015;72(4):556–65. https://doi.org/10.1016/j.surg.2015.01.005.
6. Crafts TD, Ellsperman SE, Wannemuehler TJ. Three-dimensional printing and its applications in otorhinolaryngology-head and neck surgery. Otolaryngol Head Neck Surg. 2017;156(6):999–1010.
7. Lewis CE, Peacock WJ, Tillou A, Hines OJ, Hiatt JR. A novel cadaver-based educational program in general surgery training. J Surg Educ. 2012;69(6):693–8.
8. Kavanagh LE, Jack GS, Lawrentschuk N. Prevention and management of TURP-related hemorrhage. Nat Rev Urol. 2011;8(9):504–14.
9. Aboud ET, Krisht AF, O'Keeffe TO, et al. Novel simulation for training trauma surgeons. J Trauma. 2011;71(6):1484–90.

25

Sperm parameters and anti-Müllerian hormone remain stable with *Helicobacter pylori* infection

Chun Feng[1†], Ping-Ping Lv[2†], Chang-Chang Huang[1], Song-Qing Yang[1], Qiu-Ping Yao[1], Jin-Ming Shen[3*] and Min Jin[1*]

Abstract

Background and aims: It has been reported that *Helicobacter pylori* (HP) infection was more prevalent in infertile populations. HP infection could lead to decreased sperm parameters, and treating the HP infection could improve the quality of sperm. However, studies investigating the relationship between infertility and HP infection are still limited, and more evidence is required. Therefore, we performed the present study to investigate the impact of HP infection on sperm quality in males and on ovarian reserve in females.

Methods: A total of 16,522 patients who visited the Second Hospital of Zhejiang University from January 2016 to June 2019 due to abdominal discomfort and underwent a $^{13/14}$C-urea breath HP test were included in this retrospective cross-sectional study. Among them, 565 had performed sperm analysis or ovarian reserve tests in the past three months and were involved for further analyses. Sperm parameters were examined with a computer-assisted sperm analysis system, and serum anti-Müllerian hormone (AMH) and sex hormones were tested with an electrochemiluminescence method.

Results: Among 363 patients who underwent the sperm test, 136 (37.47%) had HP infection. Among 202 patients who underwent the AMH test, 55 (27.23%) had HP infection. There was no difference in sperm concentration and motility between the HP+ and HP− groups ($P > 0.05$). Further subgroup analyses stratified into 5-year age groups confirmed that there was no significant difference in sperm parameters ($P > 0.05$). When pooled with previously published data, no significant difference in sperm concentration or motility was found ($P > 0.05$). Meanwhile, this study found that the serum AMH level was similar between the HP+ and HP− groups ($P > 0.05$). Further subgroup analyses confirmed that there was no significant difference in serum AMH level ($P > 0.05$).

Conclusions: There were no differences in sperm parameters and AMH levels based on history of HP infection among Chinese patients.

Keywords: *Helicobacter pylori* (HP), Anti-müllerian hormone (AMH), Sperm parameters, Progressive motility

*Correspondence: shenjinmg@gmail.com; min_jin@zju.edu.cn
†Chun Feng and Ping-Ping Lv contributed equally to this work
[1] Department of Reproductive Medicine, The Second Affiliated Hospital of Zhejiang University School of Medicine, 88 Jiefang Road, Hangzhou 310009, Zhejiang, China
[3] Department of Orthopedics, The First Affiliated Hospital of Zhejiang Chinese Medicine University, 54 Youdian Road, Hangzhou 310006, Zhejiang, China
Full list of author information is available at the end of the article

Background

Currently, it is widely accepted that *Helicobacter pylori* (HP) may be related to a series of extragastric diseases, including cardiovascular, neurologic, respiratory, hematologic, metabolic, dermatologic, obstetric, autoimmune, and kidney diseases [1, 2]. Among them, the impact of HP on fertility has attracted much attention. As early as

20 years ago, a study in Italy suggested that the prevalence of HP infection was significantly higher in an infertile population than in controls, and antibodies against HP could be found in follicular fluids, semen, and vaginal secretions [3]. Ten years ago, a study in Japan found that the seropositive rate of HP in an infertile population with unknown etiology was higher than that in a population with known infertility factors, indicating that HP infection could be the cause of infertility [4]. In a cytotoxin-associated gene A (CagA)-positive population, the incidence of early pregnancy loss (EPL) after assisted reproductive technology increased significantly [5]. Recently, studies about infertility have focused on the impact of HP infection on sperm quality.

The first study from Italy reported a lower sperm quality in HP-infected patients with idiopathic infertility than in HP-uninfected patients. In CagA-positive patients, both sperm motility and fertility index are reduced [6, 7]. It has been suggested that anti-CagA antibodies might block spermatozoa acrosomes and disturb fertilization [8]. Further study found that compared with HP− patients, HP+ patients showed reduced sperm concentration, motility, and fertility index [9]. All the above studies indicate that HP infection may be a deteriorating factor for sperm quality, which deserves further investigation and treatment. However, most studies are from Italy, and additional data from different ethnicities may provide more robust evidence.

In females, there is a possible association between HP infection and polycystic ovarian syndrome (PCOS). A study from Turkey reported that the proportion of HP seropositivity was almost doubled in the PCOS population [10]. It is speculated that HP infection may lead to the release of certain substances or stimulate the immune response of the host, leading to the occurrence of PCOS. PCOS is manifested by increased ovarian reserve, while decreased ovarian reserve is an even worse problem that is difficult to treat. Since anti-Müllerian hormone (AMH) is an excellent indicator of ovarian reserve, we plan to investigate the association between HP infection and AMH.

Overall, there appears to be an association between HP infection and infertility, but available support is not sufficient and thus requires further validation. The purpose of the present study is as follows: (1) to investigate the correlation between HP infection and sperm quality in males and (2) to explore the association between HP infection and ovarian reserve in females.

Methods

Population of study

From January 2016 to June 2019, patients aged 20–50 years who came to the Second Hospital of Zhejiang University School of Medicine due to abdominal discomfort and underwent HP testing were included in this study. Among them, 565 had plans for pregnancy and had performed sperm analysis or ovarian reserve tests in the past three months, who were involved for further analyses (Fig. 1).

Detection of HP infection

The ^{13}C-urea breath test (UBT) or ^{14}C-UBT was used to examine HP infection. Two breath samples were collected before and after ingestion of a ^{13}C-urea (Richen–Force, Beijing, China) or ^{14}C-urea (Xinke, Shanghai, China) reagent dissolved in water. For the ^{13}C-urea breath test, a change over baseline value greater than 4.0 delta over baseline (DOB) was taken as a positive result (HP+). For ^{14}C-UBT, a result greater than 100 DPM was taken as a positive result (HP+).

Detection of sperm parameters

Sperm samples were collected with sterile containers by masturbation after 2–7 days of sexual abstinence. After liquefaction at 37 °C for 30 min, routine parameters including sperm concentration and motility were examined with a computer-assisted sperm analysis (CASA) system (WLJY-9000, Beijing, China) according to World Health Organization guidelines [11]. Sperm morphology was assessed by the Papanicolaou staining modified for spermatozoa according to World Health Organization guidelines [11].

Detection of serum AMH and sex hormones

Serum AMH was tested with the electrochemiluminescence method by an Elecsys ® AMH from Roche Diagnostics on a Roche Cobas e602 analyzer. The total imprecision for the assays was 1.2% at a level of 1.19 ng/mL with a measuring range of 0.01–23 ng/mL. Serum

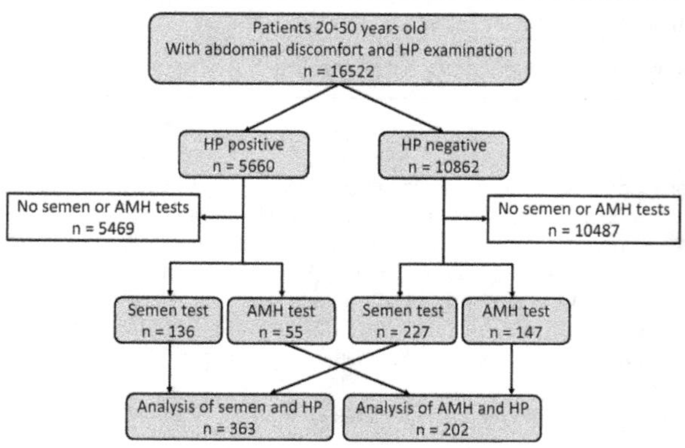

Fig. 1 Flow chart of the present study. HP: *Helicobacter pylori*; AMH: anti-Müllerian hormone

sex hormone levels were detected with the electrochemiluminescence method by kits from Siemens Healthcare Diagnostics Inc.. The total imprecision for the assays was 3.0% at a level of 10,585 pmol/L for estradiol (E_2), 12.6% at a level of 0.37 nmol/L for testosterone (T), 2.7% at a level of 4.2 IU/L for luteinizing hormone (LH), 3.9% at a level of 6.9 IU/L for follicle-stimulating hormone (FSH), 4.8% at a level of 69.9 mIU/L for prolactin (PRL), and 12.7% at a level of 3.8 nmol/L for progesterone (P). The measuring ranges were 43.6–11,010 pmol/L for E_2, 0.24–52.05 nmol/L for T, 0.07–200 IU/L for LH, 0.3–200 IU/L for FSH, 6.4–4240 mIU/L for PRL, and 0.67–190.8 nmol/L for P.

Search strategy and data extraction

To search for studies investigating the correlation between HP and sperm parameters, two reviewers independently searched the studies published in English via three databases, including PubMed, Embase, and Cochrane CENTRAL, until June 30, 2019. Articles were identified through computerized searches using the keywords as follows: ("semen analysis" OR "sperm count" OR "sperm motility") AND ("*Helicobacter pylori*" OR "Campylobacter pylori"). Meanwhile, we hand-searched the references listed in the achieved papers to obtain additional studies.

Two reviewers extracted the common characteristics and outcome parameters of the searched manuscripts independently. The common characteristics included the name of the first author, publication year, country, and number of patients. The clinical outcomes included sperm concentration and progressive motility percentage (PR).

Statistical analysis

Analyses were performed by using the SPSS 19.0 statistics package (SPSS, Chicago, IL, USA). Continuous variables are expressed as the mean values ± standard deviation (SD). Student's t test was used for comparisons between two groups. Pearson correlation analysis was performed to analyze the relationship between two variables. A *P* value of < 0.05 was considered statistically significant.

Data from our hospital and previously published results were pooled and calculated together by Review Manager Software (RevMan Version 5.3). When the mean and SD were not provided in the published article, we used formulas to estimate them [12–14]. The results were presented as the mean difference (MD) and 95% confidence interval (CI), and statistical significance was calculated by the Z test. If there was no serious heterogeneity (P value ≥ 0.1 by the Q test), a fixed-effects model (FEM) was applied for calculation, and if there was serious heterogeneity, a random-effects model (REM) was applied [15].

Results

Baseline characteristics of the involved population.

As shown in Fig. 1, a total of 16,522 patients who underwent the HP test were included in this study. Among these patients, 34.26% (5660) were HP positive. Among the patients with HP infection, 136 underwent the sperm test, and 55 underwent the AMH test. Among the patients without HP infection, 227 underwent the sperm test, and 147 underwent the AMH test. Finally, 363 were involved in the analysis between sperm and HP and 202 between AMH and HP.

As shown in Table 1, the baseline characteristics were similar in both the sperm and AMH analyses. In the analysis of sperm and HP, there was no significant difference in age, weight, height, or body mass index (BMI) between the HP+ and HP− groups ($P > 0.05$). Similarly, in the analysis of AMH and HP, no significant difference was found in age, weight, height, or BMI between the HP+ and HP− groups ($P > 0.05$).

Comparison of sperm parameters between groups with or without HP infection

As shown in Table 1, the mean sperm concentration was 53.00×10^6 Sp/mL and 53.90×10^6 Sp/mL in the HP+ and HP− groups, respectively, with no significant difference ($P > 0.05$). Sperm PR was also similar between the HP+ and HP− groups (39.39% vs. 39.92%), with no significant difference ($P > 0.05$). There was no difference in either normal sperm morphology percentage or sperm head defects ($P > 0.05$).

To further exclude the impact of age, we divided the population into subgroups of 20–24, 25–29, 30–34, 35–39, 40–44, and 45–50 years of age. As shown in Fig. 2a, c, there was no significant difference in sperm concentration or PR between the HP+ and HP− groups for any age group ($P > 0.05$). As shown in Fig. 2b, d, in both the HP+ and HP− groups, there was no significant correlation between sperm concentration and age or between PR and age ($P > 0.05$).

Comparison of AMH and sex hormones between groups with or without HP infection

As shown in Table 1, the mean serum AMH level was 3.49 in the HP+ group and 3.25 in the HP− group, with no significant difference ($P > 0.05$). No difference was found between HP+ and HP− groups in serum E_2, T, LH, FSH, PRL, or P levels ($P > 0.05$).

As shown in Fig. 2e, there was no significant difference in AMH level between the HP+ and HP− groups in every age span ($P > 0.05$). Meanwhile, AMH correlated

Table 1 Characteristics of the present study

Characteristics	Sperm and HP			AMH and HP		
	HP+	HP−	*P*	HP+	HP−	*P*
	n=136	n=227		n=55	n=147	
Age (y)	31.08±4.28	31.19±4.52	0.822	32.89±6.82	34.27±6.83	0.202
Weight (kg)	69.72±10.05	69.58±9.82	0.898	52.91±8.57	52.85±7.01	0.961
Height (m)	1.74±0.06	1.74±0.06	0.838	1.61±0.05	1.61±0.04	0.546
BMI (kg/m^2)	22.98±2.78	22.97±2.78	0.967	20.26±2.72	20.39±2.50	0.757
Conc. (Sp/ml × 10^6)	53.00±42.36	53.90±46.95	0.855	NA	NA	NA
PR (%)	39.39±18.61	39.92±18.81	0.793	NA	NA	NA
Normal (%)	6.73±3.97	6.63±4.43	0.865	NA	NA	NA
Head (%)	86.61±8.71	84.77±13.44	0.248	NA	NA	NA
AMH (ng/ml)	NA	NA	NA	3.49±3.03	3.25±2.82	0.605
E2 (pmol/L)	NA	NA	NA	194.46±78.53	192.56±68.24	0.906
T (nmol/L)	NA	NA	NA	0.94±0.71	1.12±0.78	0.118
LH (IU/L)	NA	NA	NA	6.31±4.32	4.98±3.32	0.106
FSH (IU/L)	NA	NA	NA	8.36±3.84	8.38±3.43	0.978
PRL (mIU/L)	NA	NA	NA	256.19±154.03	234.81±129.36	0.489
P (nmol/L)	NA	NA	NA	1.99±1.03	1.65±0.97	0.128

BMI: body mass index; AMH: anti-Müllerian hormone; NA: not available; Conc.: concentration; PR: progressive motility; Normal: normal sperm morphology percentage; Head: sperm head defects; DFI: sperm DNA fragmentation index; E_2: estradiol; T: testosterone; LH: luteinizing hormone; FSH: follicle-stimulating hormone; PRL: prolactin; P: progesterone

significantly negatively with age (Fig. 2f, for HP−, Pearson correlation coefficient = −0.482, $P=0.000$; for HP+, Pearson correlation coefficient = −0.431, $P=0.001$).

Pooled analysis of the association between sperm parameters and HP infection

Since 2010, six studies investigated the correlation between HP infection and sperm parameters, as listed in Table 2. Most studies found that sperm motility was reduced significantly in CagA+ patients [6, 7, 16, 17]. The latest study found that sperm concentration and PR were reduced in the HP+ population, and in the CagA+ population PR was reduced further than in the CagA− population [9].

Five studies including 703 participants were pooled to compare HP+ and HP− groups, and five studies including 210 participants were pooled to compare CagA+ and CagA− groups. As shown in Fig. 3a, c, FEM analysis showed that there was no significant difference in sperm concentration between the HP+ and HP− groups or between the CagA+ and CagA− groups ($P>0.05$ for both). In the sperm motility analysis between HP+ and HP−, since serious heterogeneity ($P<0.01$) was found, a REM was applied and suggested no significant difference in PR (Fig. 3b, 95% CI −11.44 to 1.87, $P=0.16$). FEM analysis was applied to compare sperm PR between CagA+ and CagA− groups, which suggested that PR was 16.18% lower in the CagA+ group than in the CagA− group (Fig. 3d, 95% CI −18.86 to −13.50, $P<0.01$).

Discussion

In the present study, no difference was found in sperm concentration or sperm motility between HP+ and HP− groups. Further subgroup analyses confirmed that there was no significant difference in sperm parameters between HP+ and HP− groups. Furthermore, we pooled our data and those of previous studies and found no significant difference in sperm concentration or motility, indicating that in the Chinese population, HP infection does not disturb spermatogenesis.

The results of previous studies were not consistent. Some suggested that sperm concentration and motility were reduced in HP+ patients [9] and that treating HP could improve the quality of sperm [18], while some suggested no significant difference in sperm parameters between HP+ and HP− groups [6, 7, 16, 17]. The inconsistent results may be due to different test methods and ethnicities investigated.

This is the first study that used UBT to detect HP infection and to investigate its relationship with sperm quality. In previous studies, HP infection was detected with a serology test by enzyme-linked immunosorbent assay (ELISA) and confirmed with western blotting (WB) [6, 7, 9, 16–18], whereas in the present study, ^{13}C- and ^{14}C-UBT were used to detect HP infection. UBT is the best

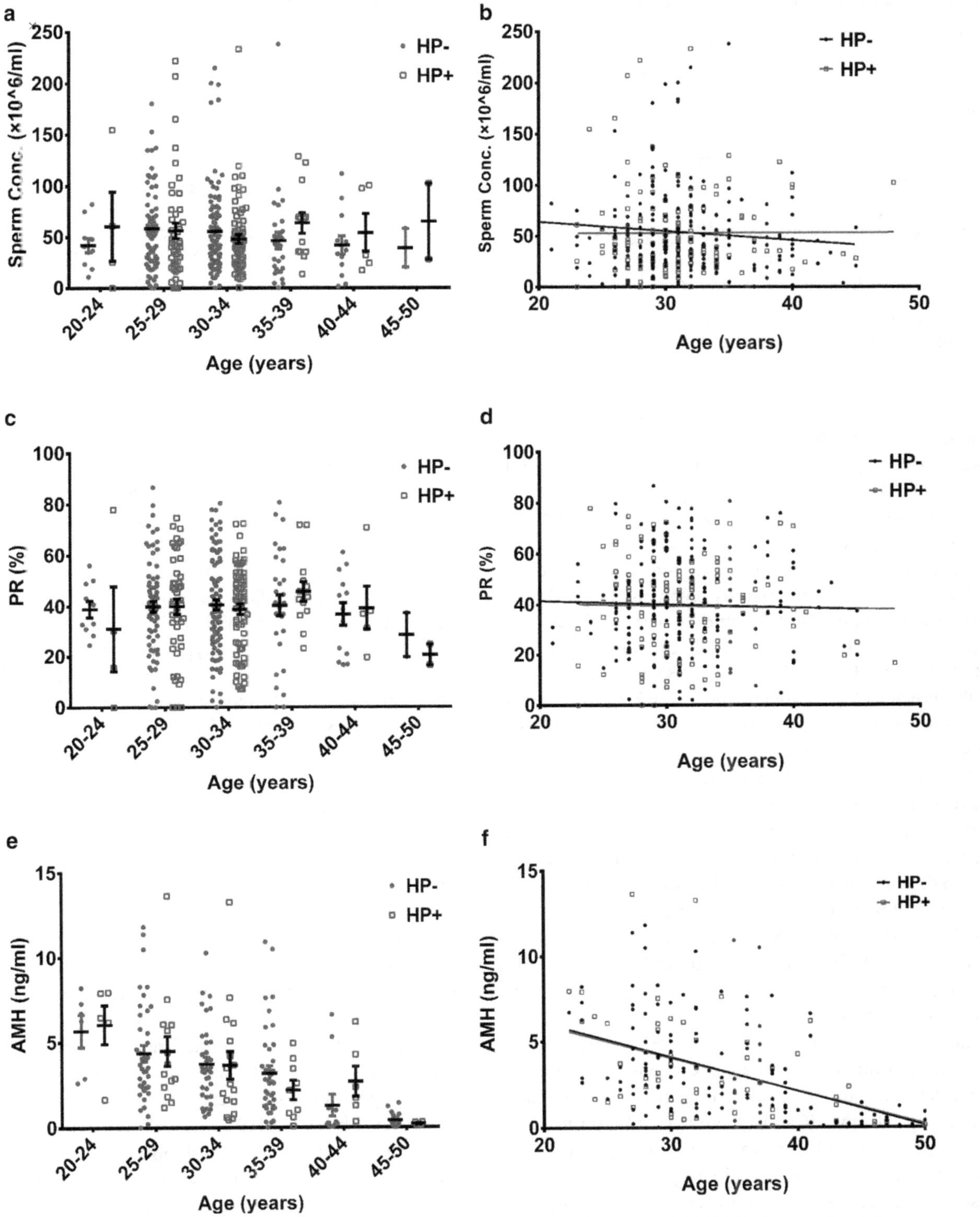

Fig. 2 Correlation between sperm parameters and anti-Müllerian hormone (AMH) and *Helicobacter pylori* (HP) infection. **a**, **b** Correlation between AMH and HP. **c**, **d** Correlation between sperm concentration (Conc.) and HP. **e**, **f** Correlation between progressive motility percentage (PR) and HP

Table 2 Previous studies investigating the impact of HP infection on sperm parameters

Study	Public year	Country	HP (+vs. −)			CagA (+vs. −)			Results
			Population	Conc	PR (%)	Population	Conc	PR (%)	
Moretti [9]	2017	Italy	32 vs. 41	38.0 vs. 55.0*	17 .0 vs. 34.0***	20 vs. 12	33.4 vs. 42.5	10.5 vs. 22.5***	HP+ reduced conc. and PR
Moretti [17]	2015	Italy	28 vs.81	61 vs. 72	32 vs. 32	12 vs. 16	61 vs. 61.5	24 vs. 36.5*	CagA+ reduce PR
El-Garem [18]	2014	Egypt	NA	NA	NA	22 vs. 201	NA	NA	HP treatment improved PR
Moretti [16]	2013	Italy	NA	NA	NA	37 vs. 50	58 vs. 63	18 vs. 32**	CagA+ reduced PR
Moretti [7]	2012	Italy	27 vs. 51	94 vs. 72	32 vs. 30	11 vs. 16	65 vs. 94	24 vs. 38**	CagA+ reduced PR
Collodel [6]	2010	Italy	36 vs.44	24.5 vs. 23.5	22 vs. 28.5	17 vs. 19	25.5 vs. 23	18 vs. 29*	CagA+ reduced PR

NA: not available; Conc.: sperm concentration; PR: progressive motility; CagA: cytotoxin-associated gene A

* $P<0.05$; ** $P<0.01$; *** $P<0.001$

noninvasive method for patients without gastric resection or proton pump inhibitor (PPI) treatment, with both high positive predictive value and negative predictive value [19–21]. A meta-analysis suggested that UBT had high diagnostic accuracy for detecting HP infection in patients with dyspepsia, with a pooled sensitivity of UBT in adult patients of 96% and a pooled specificity of 93% [22, 23]. Another meta-analysis involving 34 studies with serology evaluation and 57 studies with UBT detection reported that the sensitivity of HP diagnosis was 0.94 for ^{13}C-UBT, 0.92 for ^{14}C-UBT, and 0.84 for serology tests. UBT showed a higher diagnostic accuracy than the serology test for HP infection diagnosis [24, 25]. Therefore, in this study, UBT was used, as it provides a more accurate HP diagnosis than serology tests.

Moreover, serology tests cannot distinguish between active and inactive infections [26]. In a letter from Caviglia et al., the authors emphasized that the presence of serological HP antibodies could only indicate previous exposure, not necessarily a current infection, and based on this, they recommended UBT as a direct diagnostic test [27]. Similarly, in the present study, UBT examination represented the status of current HP infection better than serology tests.

CagA is the major virulence factor in HP, encoding the CagA protein in the cag pathogenicity island [28]. HP infection can be divided into two isolates: CagA-producing strains (CagA+) and CagA-nonproducing strains (CagA−). Our meta-analysis of sperm motility and CagA-producing/nonproducing strain infection suggested that PR was 16.18% lower in the CagA+ group than in the CagA− group. The underlying mechanism may be that CagA+ HP infection induces overexpression of miR-543 and downregulation of the p14ARF tumor suppressor to inhibit autophagy and increase cytokine production, which induces inflammatory responses of HP accordingly [29–31]. Anti-CagA antibodies may block spermatozoa acrosomes and disturb fertilization [8].

The prevalence of the CagA genotype in HP infection varies significantly among different regions. In Western countries, CagA+ strains comprise 50–60% of the HP+ population, and in the Chinese population, CagA+ strains occupy nearly 100% of the HP+ population [32, 33]. Studies investigating the CagA status of Chinese HP strains with polymerase chain reaction (PCR) detected CagA genotypes in nearly all strains [34, 35]. Considering the high CagA positivity in the Chinese HP+ population, the sperm concentration and motility should be weakened in HP+ patients, but the present study showed stable parameters. Further study investigating CagA antibody status should be performed to clarify the role of CagA in sperm quality.

The variability of sperm parameters after HP treatment is an interesting question. It was reported that after the treatment of HP, seminal HP IgA level decreased significantly, and meanwhile progressive sperm motility, nonprogressive sperm motility, and sperm normal forms increased significantly ($P=0.001$) [18]. In the present study, sperm analyses were performed before HP test, and most patients with HP+ suspended their plans of pregnancy after HP treatment. Therefore, we did not follow the sperm parameters.

In the present study, there was no difference in serum AMH level between HP+ and HP− groups, which was confirmed with further age-divided subgroup analyses. Published results of the relationship between PCOS and HP infection are inconsistent. Yavasoglu et al. found that HP antibody positivity was significantly more common in the PCOS group than in the age-matched control group [10]. The possible explanation may be that the antigenic mimicry to HP antigens leads to an immune cross-reaction between HP antigens and the ovaries, inducing the onset of PCOS [36]. Nevertheless,

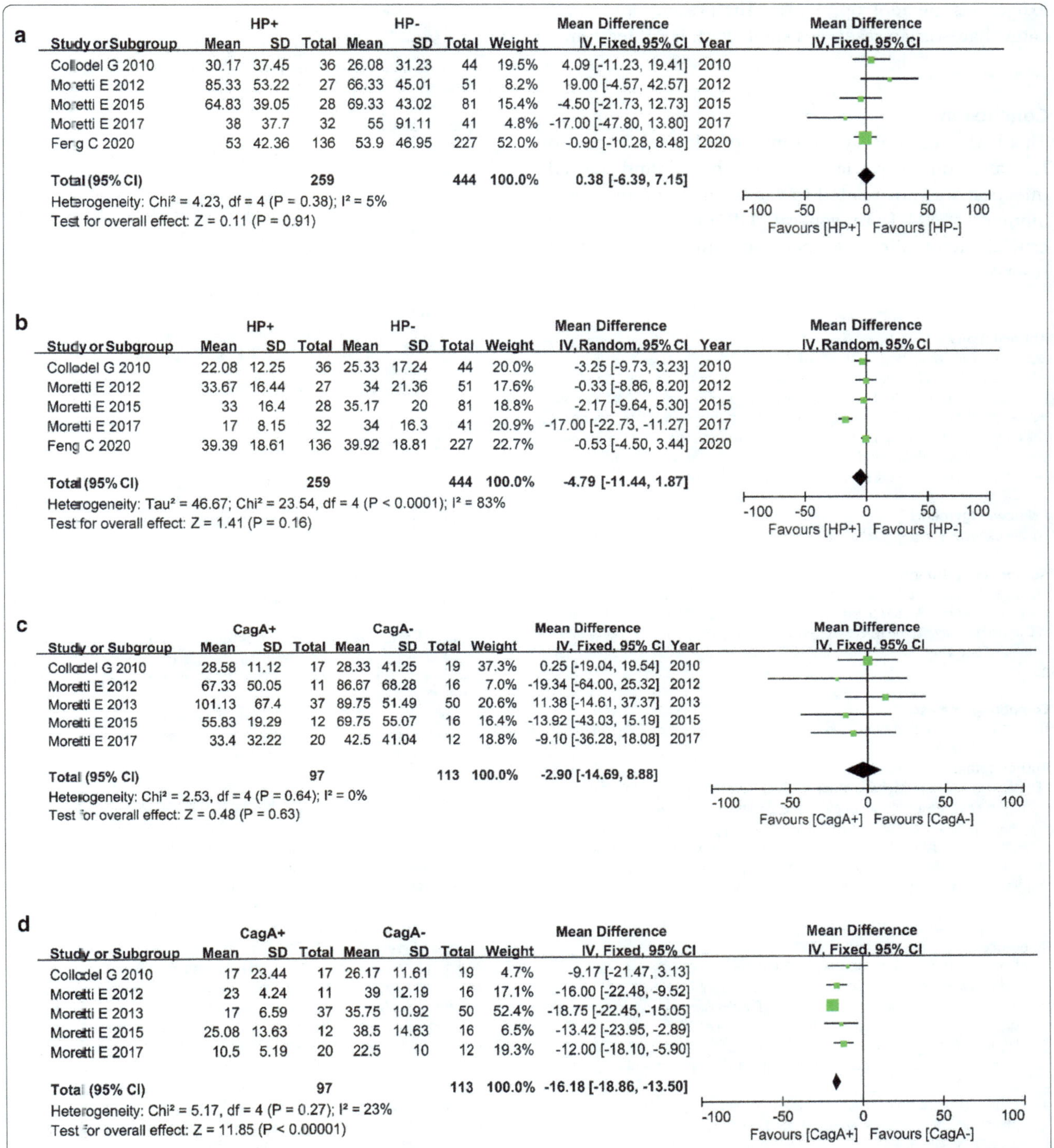

Fig. 3 Forest plot of the association between *Helicobacter pylori* (HP) infection and sperm parameters. **a** Sperm concentration and HP infection. **b** Progressive motility percentage (PR) and HP infection. **c** Sperm concentration and cytotoxin-associated gene A (CagA) strains. **d** PR and CagA strains

Tokmak et al. found no significant difference in HP IgG positivity between PCOS and non-PCOS groups [37]. AMH is a potential future substitute for detecting polycystic ovarian morphology (PCOM) and a useful biomarker for predicting the risk of PCOS [38–40]. Our data indicated no correlation between PCOS and HP infection. Meanwhile, AMH is considered the best serum biomarker of ovarian reserve, reflecting the number of primordial follicles and its response to exogenous gonadotropins [41]. The present study indicates that ovarian reserve is stable with HP infection.

Conclusion

This is the first observation investigating the impact of HP infection on ovarian reserve, which found that HP infection was not related to the serum ovarian reserve biomarker AMH. In general, HP infection is not a crucial factor affecting sperm parameters or ovarian reserve.

Abbreviations

DOB: Delta over baseline; E_2: Estradiol; EPL: Early pregnancy loss; FEM: Fixed-effects model; FSH: Follicle-stimulating hormone; HP: *Helicobacter pylori*; LH: Luteinizing hormone; MD: Mean difference; P: Progesterone; PCOM: Polycystic ovarian morphology; PCOS: Polycystic ovarian syndrome; PCR: Polymerase chain reaction; PPI: Proton pump inhibitor; PR: Progressive motility percentage; PRL: Prolactin; REM: Random-effects model; SD: Standard deviation; T: Testosterone; UBT: Urea breath test; WB: Western blotting.

Acknowledgements

We are especially grateful to Ya-Wen Xing for his kind help in data collection.

Authors' contributions

CF, MJ, and JMS conceived and designed the study; CF, MJ and CCH enrolled the patients and collected the data; CF, PPL, SQY, and QPY analyzed the data; PPL and MJ reviewed the references and extracted the data; CF, MJ, and JMS organized and wrote the manuscript. All authors read and approved the final manuscript.

Competing interests

The authors declare that they have no competing interests.

Author details

[1] Department of Reproductive Medicine, The Second Affiliated Hospital of Zhejiang University School of Medicine, 88 Jiefang Road, Hangzhou 310009, Zhejiang, China. [2] The Women's Hospital of Zhejiang University School of Medicine, Hangzhou 310006, Zhejiang, China. [3] Department of Orthopedics, The First Affiliated Hospital of Zhejiang Chinese Medicine University, 54 Youdian Road, Hangzhou 310006, Zhejiang, China.

References

1. Franceschi F, Covino M, Roubaud BC. Review: *Helicobacter pylori* and extragastric diseases. Helicobacter. 2019;24(Suppl 1):e12636.
2. Ražuka-Ebela D, Giupponi B, Franceschi F. *Helicobacter pylori* and extragastric diseases. Helicobacter. 2018;23(Suppl 1):e12520.
3. Figura N, Piomboni P, Ponzetto A, Gambera L, Lenzi C, Vaira D, et al. *Helicobacter pylori* infection and infertility. Eur J Gastroenterol Hepatol. 2002;14(6):663–9.
4. Kurotsuchi S, Ando H, Iwase A, Ishida Y, Hamajima N, Kikkawa F. The plausibility of *Helicobacter pylori*-related infertility in Japan. Fertil Steril. 2008;90(3):866–8.
5. Hajishafiha M, Ghasemi-Rad M, Memari A, Naji S, Mladkova N, Saeedi V. Effect of *Helicobacter pylori* infection on pregnancy rates and early pregnancy loss after intracytoplasmic sperm injection. Int J Womens Health. 2011;3:329–35.
6. Collodel G, Moretti E, Campagna MS, Capitani S, Lenzi C, Figura N. Infection by CagA-positive *Helicobacter pylori* strains may contribute to alter the sperm quality of men with fertility disorders and increase the systemic levels of TNF-alpha. Dig Dis Sci. 2010;55(1):94–100.
7. Moretti E, Collodel G, Campagna MS, Franci MB, Iacoponi F, Mazzi L, et al. Influence of *Helicobacter pylori* infection on levels of ghrelin and obestatin in human semen. J Androl. 2012;33(5):938–43.
8. Ponzetto A, Holton J. Extragastric diseases correlated with *Helicobacter pylori*. Helicobacter. 2019;24(1):e12549.
9. Moretti E, Figura N, Campagna MS, Iacoponi F, Gonnelli S, Collodel G. Infectious burden and semen parameters. Urology. 2017;100:90–6.
10. Yavasoglu I, Kucuk M, Cildag B, Arslan E, Gok M, Kafkas S. A novel association between polycystic ovary syndrome and *Helicobacter pylori*. Am J Med Sci. 2009;338(3):174–7.
11. WHO laboratory manual for the examination and processing of human semen (Fifth edition). https://www.who.int/reproductivehealth/publications/infertility/9789241547789/en/. 2010.
12. Wan X, Wang W, Liu J, Tong T. Estimating the sample mean and standard deviation from the sample size, median, range and/or interquartile range. BMC Med Res Methodol. 2014;14:135.
13. Luo D, Wan X, Liu J, Tong T. Optimally estimating the sample mean from the sample size, median, mid-range, and/or mid-quartile range. Stat Methods Med Res. 2018;27(6):1785–805.
14. Higgins JPT GS. Cochrane handbook for systematic reviews of interventions version 5.1.0. The Cochrane Collaboration, 2011.
15. Lau J, Ioannidis JP, Schmid CH. Quantitative synthesis in systematic reviews. Ann Intern Med. 1997;127(9):820–6.
16. Moretti E, Collodel G, Mazzi L, Campagna MS, Figura N. CagA-positive *Helicobacter pylori* infection and reduced sperm motility, vitality, and normal morphology. Dis Mark. 2013;35(4):229–34.
17. Moretti E, Figura N, Campagna MS, Gonnelli S, Iacoponi F, Collodel G. Sperm parameters and semen levels of inflammatory cytokines in *Helicobacter pylori*-infected men. Urology. 2015;86(1):41–6.
18. El-Garem Y, El-Sawy M, Mostafa T. Seminal *Helicobacter pylori* treatment improves sperm motility in infertile asthenozoospermic men. Urology. 2014;84(6):1347–50.
19. Tonkic A, Tonkic M, Lehours P, Mégraud F. Epidemiology and diagnosis of *Helicobacter pylori* infection. Helicobacter. 2012;17(Suppl 1):1–8.
20. Kawai S, Arai K, Lin Y, Nishiyama T, Sasakabe T, Wang C, et al. Comparison of the detection of *Helicobacter pylori* infection by commercially available serological testing kits and the ^{13}C-urea breath test. J Infect Chemother. 2019;25(10):769–73.
21. Kusano C, Gotoda T, Ikehara H, Suzuki S, Shibuya H, Horii T, et al. The accuracy of the serum antibody test for *Helicobacter pylori* infection among junior high school students. Digestion. 2019. https://doi.org/10.1159/00050290.
22. Mentis A, Lehours P, Mégraud F. Epidemiology and Diagnosis of *Helicobacter pylori* infection. Helicobacter. 2015;20(Suppl 1):1–7.
23. Ferwana M, Abdulmajeed I, Alhajiahmed A, Madani W, Firwana B, Hasan R, et al. Accuracy of urea breath test in *Helicobacter pylori* infection: meta-analysis. World J Gastroenterol. 2015;21(4):1305–14.
24. Best LM, Takwoingi Y, Siddique S, Selladurai A, Gandhi A, Low B, et al. Non-invasive diagnostic tests for *Helicobacter pylori* infection. Cochrane Database Syst Rev. 2018;3:CD012080.
25. Makristathis A, Hirschl AM, Mégraud F, Bessède E. Review: Diagnosis of *Helicobacter pylori* infection. Helicobacter. 2019;24(Suppl 1):e12641.
26. Miftahussurur M. Noninvasive *Helicobacter pylori* diagnostic methods in Indonesia. Gut Liver. 2019. https://doi.org/10.5009/gnl19264.
27. Caviglia GP, Fagoonee S, Pellicano R. Re: El-Garem et al.: Seminal helicobacter pylori treatment improves sperm motility in infertile asthenozoospermic men (Urology 2014;84:1347–1350). Urology. 2015;85(5):1217.
28. Park JY, Forman D, Waskito LA, Yamaoka Y, Crabtree JE. Epidemiology of *Helicobacter pylori* and CagA-positive infections and global variations in gastric cancer. Toxins (Basel). 2018;10(4):E163.
29. Li N, Tang B, Jia YP, Zhu P, Zhuang Y, Fang Y, et al. *Helicobacter pylori* CagA protein negatively regulates autophagy and promotes inflammatory response via c-Met-PI3K/Akt-mTOR signaling pathway. Front Cell Infect Microbiol. 2017;7:417.
30. Shi Y, Yang Z, Zhang T, Shen L, Li Y, Ding S. SIRT1-targeted miR-543 autophagy inhibition and epithelial-mesenchymal transition promotion in *Helicobacter pylori* CagA-associated gastric cancer. Cell Death Dis. 2019;10(9):625.
31. Horvat A, Noto JM, Ramatchandirin B, Zaika E, Palrasu M, Wei J, et al. *Helicobacter pylori* pathogen regulates p14ARF tumor suppressor and autophagy in gastric epithelial cells. Oncogene. 2018;37(37):5054–65.

32. Yamaoka Y. Mechanisms of disease: *Helicobacter pylori* virulence factors. Nat Rev Gastroenterol Hepatol. 2010;7(11):629–41.
33. Vilaichone RK, Mahachai V, Tumwasorn S, Wu JY, Graham DY, Yamaoka Y. Molecular epidemiology and outcome of *Helicobacter pylori* infection in Thailand: a cultural cross roads. Helicobacter. 2004;9(5):453–9.
34. Zhou J Zhang J, Xu C, He L. cagA genotype and variants in Chinese *Helicobacter pylori* strains and relationship to gastroduodenal diseases. J Med Microbiol. 2004;53(Pt 3):231–5.
35. Yin L, Lu F, Guo C, Wang Q, Pan K, Xu L, et al. Analysis of virulence diversity of 73 *Helicobacter pylori* strains isolated in Guizhou province. China Mol Med Rep. 2018;18(5):4611–20.
36. Yavasoglu I, Kucuk M. Anti-*Helicobacter pylori* antibodies and polycystic ovary syndrome. Eur J Obstet Gynecol Reprod Biol. 2012;163(2):243.
37. Tokmak A, Doğan Z, Sarıkaya E, Timur H, Kekilli M. *Helicobacter pylori* infection and polycystic ovary syndrome in adolescent and young adult patients. J Obstet Gynaecol Res. 2016;42(12):1768–72.
38. Abbara A, Eng PC, Phylactou M, Clarke SA, Hunjan T, Roberts R, et al. Anti-Müllerian hormone (AMH) in the diagnosis of menstrual disturbance due to polycystic ovarian syndrome. Front Endocrinol (Lausanne). 2019;10:656.
39. Calzada M, López N, Noguera JA, Mendiola J, Hernández AI, Corbalán S, et al. AMH in combination with SHBG for the diagnosis of polycystic ovary syndrome. J Obstet Gynaecol. 2019;39(8):1130–6.
40. Teede H, Misso M, Tassone EC, Dewailly D, Ng EH, Azziz R, et al. Anti-Müllerian hormone in PCOS: a review informing international guidelines. Trends Endocrinol Metab. 2019;30(7):467–78.
41. Hansen KR, Hodnett GM, Knowlton N, Craig LB. Correlation of ovarian reserve tests with histologically determined primordial follicle number. Fertil Steril. 2011;95(1):170–5.

26

A performance comparison of the fully automated urine particle analyzer UF-5000 with UF-1000i and Gram staining in predicting bacterial growth patterns in women with uncomplicated urinary tract infections

Stephen Shei-Dei Yang[1,2], Chun-Chun Yang[3], Yi-Sheng Chen[1,2] and Shang-Jen Chang[1,2*]

Abstract

Background: The aim of this study was to compare the performance of the new flow cytometer UF-5000 with the UF-1000i and Gram staining for determining bacterial patterns in urine samples.

Methods: Women who attended our clinic with symptoms suggestive of urinary tract infection were enrolled in the study. Mid-stream urine samples were collected for gram staining, urine analysis and urine cultures. Bacterial patterns were classified using the UF-1000i (none, cocci bacteria or rods/mixed growth), the UF-5000 (none, cocci, rods or mixed growth) and Gram staining.

Results: Among the 102 included samples, there were 10 g-positive cocci, 2 g-positive bacilli, 66 g-negative rods, and 24 mixed growth. The sensitivity/specificity of the UF-1000i was 81.8/91.1% for gram-negative rods and 23.5/96.9% for cocci/mixed. The sensitivity/specificity of the UF-5000 was 80.0/88.2% for gram negative rods and 70.0/86.5% for gram-positive cocci.

Conclusions: The UF-5000 demonstrated good sensitivity and specificity for Gram-negative bacilli and demonstrated an improved sensitivity for detecting Gram-positive cocci compared with the UF-1000i.

Keywords: Urinary tract infection, Diagnosis, Laser flow cytometry, Fully automated urine particle analyzer

Background

Urinary tract infection is a common infectious disease that can cause a significant health care burden, although most cases are uncomplicated infections. It is estimated that 50–60% of women will go through one or more episodes of uncomplicated urinary tract infection (uUTI) in their lifetime [1]. uUTIs usually cause minor symptoms and are rarely life-threatening. However, uUTIs impair quality of life because of their irritative symptoms [2]. uUTIs are diagnosed following the occurrence of positive clinical symptoms and positive urine cultures. The bacterial species that lead to urinary tract infections include *Escherichia coli, Klebsiella* spp., *Enterobacter* spp., *Proteus* spp., *Pseudomonas* spp., *Enterococcus* spp., *Staphylococcus* spp., and *Streptococcus* spp. However, it takes 1–2 days to obtain the results of urine cultures and there is a high contamination rate (0.8–41.6%) during the collection process, which can make interpreting the results difficult or irrelevant [3]. Some experts have suggested that mixed growth in a urine culture may occur among the elderly, the immunocompromised, and those with

*Correspondence: krissygnet@gmail.com
[1] Division of Urology, Department of Surgery, Taipei Tzu Chi Hospital, New Taipei, Taiwan
Full list of author information is available at the end of the article

indwelling catheters, HIV, malignancy, and diabetes [4], but these findings are more commonly regarded as contamination [5]. Manual gram staining of urine specimens has shown a 90% sensitivity when utilized to diagnose bacteriuria, however it is laborious and time consuming [6]. Therefore, a rapid, automatic, reliable and cheaper screening test that can differentiate between gram positive, negative or mixed growth in urine specimens, is required to reduce labor, unnecessary medical costs and waiting time, which would help clinicians improve patient care. Previous studies have examined the efficacy of the UF-1000i (Sysmex UF-1000i; Sysmex Corporation, Kobe, Japan) in differentiating bacilli from cocci/mixed growth [7]. However, the UF-1000i cannot differentiate cocci from mixed growth. Recently, a new model of urine particle analyzer was introduced, the UF-5000 (Sysmex Corporation, Kobe, Japan), where cocci are differentiated from mixed growth bacteria [8, 9]. Therefore, we performed a prospective study to compare the accuracy of gram staining, the UF-1000i and the UF-5000 in differentiating bacterial growth patterns (gram positive, negative or mixed growth) using midstream voided urine specimens from women visiting urological clinics for uUTIs.

Methods

The current study was approved by the Institutional Review Board at our hospital (IRB No: 05-FS02-024) From July 2016 to June 2019, we prospectively enrolled adult women (aged 20–80 years) who visited our clinic presenting with symptoms suggestive of urinary tract infection. Exclusion criteria were a fever (temperature > 38 °C), urolithiasis, pregnancy, congenital urinary tract anomaly, end stage renal disease receiving dialysis, neurogenic bladder with urethral catheterization, a history of bladder cancer, patients who were immunocompromised and recent antibiotics use (within 7 days). After written informed consent was obtained, the patients were asked to complete a questionnaire, including their baseline characteristics (age, medical history including diabetes or hypertension, childbirth, previous abdominal surgery). They were also asked to complete a urinary tract infection symptom assessment (UTISA) [10], which included 7 symptom categories and 7 quality of life categories, with scores for each assessment ranging from 0 to 3. Patients with a total symptom score of ≥ 4 were regarded as positive for symptoms of urinary tract infection.

At the clinic, the patients were asked to collect midstream voided urine in a sterile container for manual gram staining, routine urinalysis and urine culture. A study nurse instructed the patients on proper collection technique to try and reduce the contamination rate. Only specimens with a bacterial growth of $\geq 10^3$ cfu/mL were included in the comparison of bacterial growth pattern differentiation. A 10 ml sample from the sterile collection cup was poured into a urine sediment centrifuge tube (SY, Shih-Yung medical instruments Co., Ltd, Taipei, Taiwan) for automated urine particle analysis (Sysmex UF-1000i; UF-5000, Sysmex Corporation, Kobe, Japan) within half an hour of receiving the specimen. The gram stains of urine specimens were classified as gram positive, negative or mixed by two experienced clinical laboratory scientists with more than 10 years of experience in the field. For each analyzed sample, the bacteria scatter diagram was classified as rods, cocci/mixed growth or none by the UF-1000i. The bacteria scatter gram was also classified as either gram positive, negative, mixed growth or none by the UF-5000 [9, 11].

Gram staining

The centrifuged urine from the urine sediment preparation was used to make slides for Gram staining. These slides were air dried, fixed with heat and then stained according to the Gram stain procedure. The slides were then assessed for the presence of bacteria and the staining characteristics were further described. Slides with bacteria were subsequently evaluated for bacterial morphology to determine whether these bacteria were Gram positive or Gram negative. Slides were classified as positive for bacteriuria if ≥ 1 bacteria/HPF was noted. Then, the specimens were classified as gram positive, negative, mixed growth or none [6].

Microbiological analysis

A 1 μl inoculation loop was applied to the commercial chromogenic agar medium (CPS® ID3, Biomerieux, I'Etoile, France) for the urine culture. The culture plates were then aerobically incubated at 35 °C for 18–24 h. The bacteria were quantified by multiplying the dilution factor by the number of colonies on the agar plate. The growth of more than 2 species of bacteria within the urine culture without a dominant one was regarded as contaminated or mixed growth.

Statistical analysis

The data within the manuscript are expressed as the mean ± standard deviation. We used MedCalc Statistical Software, version 19.1.3 (MedCalc Software bv, Ostend, Belgium; https://www.medcalc.org; 2019) for the statistical analyses. Nominal or categorical data were compared using a X^2 test. Ordinal data were compared using the Mann–Whitney test. Continuous data were compared by an independent t-test. The agreement between two methods was evaluated using kappa statistics. The grading of the agreement complied with Altman's recommendations (<0.2: poor agreement, 0.21–0.40: fair agreement, 0.41–0.60: moderate agreement, 0.61–0.80: good agreement, 0.81–1.00: very good agreement) [12]. Prospective sample size calculations were not performed because the agreement between UF-5000 and urine culture was unavailable at the time the pilot study was designed. A p-value of < 0.05 was considered as statistically significant.

Results

There were 85 patients with no UF-5000 or UF-1000i interpretation and there was 1 specimen with no culture growth, all of which were excluded from the final comparisons. A total of 102 urine specimens from 102 women (mean age $= 58.5 \pm 18.5$ years) with a UTISA score ≥ 4 and bacterial growth $\geq 10^3$ cfu/mL were included for the final analysis. Table 1 summarizes the baseline characteristics of the 102 included patients. The analyzed specimens included 10 g-positive cocci, 2 g-positive bacilli, 66 g-negative rods, and 24 specimens with two or more bacterial species that were regarded as mixed growth (Table 2). Gram-positive bacilli (*Lactobacillus* spp.) were excluded from the agreement analysis. Among the specimens with single bacteria growth, there were Gram positive cocci (2 *Streptococci* spp., 3 *Staphylococci* spp., 1 *Enterococci* spp., 2 *Group B Streptococci, 2 unclassified Gram positive cocci*) and Gram negative rods (53 *Escherichia coli*, 5 *Proteus* spp., 4 *Klebsiella* spp., and 4 *Citrobacter* spp.).

Gram staining

Among the 102 specimens with both UF-1000i and UF-5000 interpretations, there were only 97 specimens with available gram staining results because timely interpretation by the clinical laboratory scientists was not possible. Of the 97 specimens, 29 were classified as negative. Agreement levels between the results of the gram stain and the urine cultures are listed in Table 3 with a kappa value of 0.48 (moderate, 95% CI 0.36 to 0.60). The sensitivity and specificity of the gram stain for gram negative bacteria were 80.6% and 96.7%, respectively, and the sensitivity and specificity of the gram stain for cocci were 60% and 100%, respectively. The sensitivity and specificity of the gram stain for mixed growth were 18.2% and 97.4%, respectively.

UF-1000i

Agreement levels between the results of the Gram-negative bacilli UF-1000i and the urine cultures are listed in Table 4 with a kappa value of 0.49 (moderate, 95% CI: 0.38 to 0.61). The sensitivity and specificity of the UF-1000i for rods were 81.8% and 91.1%, respectively, and the sensitivity and specificity of the UF-1000i for cocci/mixed growth were 23.5% and 96.9%, respectively.

UF-5000

Agreement levels between the results of the UF-5000 laser flow cytometry and urine cultures are listed in Table 5 with a kappa value of 0.46 (moderate, 95% CI: 0.34 to 0.58). The sensitivity and specificity of the UF-5000 for gram negative bacilli (GNB) were 80.0% and 88.2%, respectively, and the sensitivity and specificity for the gram stain for cocci were 70% and 86.5%, respectively. The sensitivity and specificity of the UF-5000 for mixed growth were 4.5% and 94.9%, respectively. For specific gram positive cocci, the UF-1000i identified all *Staphylococci* spp. ($n = 3$), *Enterococci* spp. ($n = 1$) and *Streptococci* spp. (n = 3), except for one Group B Streptococci and two gram positive cocci (10^3 and 2×10^3 cfu/mL, respectively).

For specific GNB, the UF-5000 identified all *Proteus* spp. and *Citrobacter* spp. except for one *Klebsiella* spp. (3×10^3 cfu/mL). However, the UF-5000 only identified 37 of the 49 *E. coli*.

Discussion

To the best of our knowledge, this is the first prospective study that compares the efficacy of automated urine flow cytometry systems (UF-1000i, UF-5000), gram staining and urine cultures for urine specimens from women with uUTIs. The results showed that the UF-5000 had good

Table 1 Baseline characteristics of the included patients

	All n = 102	Menopause(+) n = 56	Menopause(−) n = 44	P value
Age (years, ± SD)	49.56 ± 16.57	62.32 ± 7.55	33.81 ± 9.78	P < 0.001
Diabetes Mellitus, n (%)	12 (11.7)	10 (17.8)	2 (4.5)	P = 0.042
Hypertension, n (%)	21 (20.5)	20 (35.7)	1 (2.2)	P < 0.001
Childbirth, n (%)	65 (63.7)	49 (87.5)	16 (36.6)	P < 0.001
Hysterectomy n(%)	18 (17.6)	17 (30.3)	1 (2.2)	P = 0.001
Abdominal surgery history, n (%)	10 (9.8)	8 (14.2)	2 (4.5)	P = 0.109
Day 0 UTISA score (mean ± SD)	10.71 ± 3.81	10.41 ± 3.73	11.09 ± 4.01	P = 0.383

Table 2 The sensitivity of gram stain, UF1000i and UF5000 for specific bacterial species

Bacterial growth of urine specimens	Number (n)	UF1000i	UF5000	Gram stain
Gram (−)				
Escherichia coli				
≧10^5 cfu/mL	39	Rods = 38/cocci/mixed = 1	G(−) = 31/G(+) = 3/none = 1/mixed = 4	G(−) = 34/None = 5
10^3–10^5 cfu/mL	10	Rods = 3/cocci/mixed = 1/none = 6	G(−) = 6/G(+) = 3/none = 1	G(−) = 4/mixed = 2/None = 4
Klebsiella spp.				
≧10^5 cfu/mL	3	Rods = 3	G(−) = 3	G(−) = 2/G(+) = 1
10^3–10^5 cfu/mL	1	None = 1	None = 1	None = 1
Proteus mirabilis				
≧10^5 cfu/mL	2	Rods = 2	G(−) = 2	G(−) = 1/None = 1
10^3–10^5 cfu/mL	2	Rods = 1/none = 1	G(−) = 2	G(−) = 1/None = 1
Citrobacter spp.				
≧10^5 cfu/mL	3	Rods = 2/none = 1	G(−) = 3	G(−) = 2/None = 1
10^3–10^5 cfu/mL	1	None = 1	G(−) = 1	None = 1
Gram (+)				
Streptococci spp.	1	cocci/mixed = 1	G(+) = 2	G(+) = 1
Staphylococci spp.	3	Rods = 1/cocci/mixed = 1/none = 1	G(+) = 3	G(+) = 2/None = 1
Enterococci spp.	1	Rods = 1	G(+) = 1	G(+) = 1
Group B Streptococci	2	None = 2	G(+) = 1/none = 1	G(+) = 1/None = 1
G(+)cocci	2	None = 2	None = 2	None = 2
Lactobacillus species	2	cocci/mixed = 1/none = 1	G(+) = 1/none = 1	None = 2
Mixed growth				
≧10^5 cfu/mL	3	Rods = 1/cocci/mixed = 1	G(+) = 1/G(−) = 1/mixed = 1	Mixed = 2/None = 1
10^3–10^5 cfu/mL	19	cocci/mixed = 3/None = 16	G(+) = 5/G(−) = 3/None = 11	G(−) = 1/G(+) = 1/mixed = 2/None = 15

Table 3 Agreement levels between the results of gram stain and urine cultures

Urine culture	Gram stain			
	GNB	GPC	Mixed	None
GNB	50	0	2	10
GPC	0	6	0	4
Mixed	1	0	4	16

GNB gram negative bacilli, *GPC* gram positive cocci, *Mixed* mixed growth

Table 4 Agreement levels between the results of UF1000i and urine cultures

Urine culture	UF 1000i		
	Rods	Cocci/Mixed	None
Rods	54	2	10
Cocci/Mixed	3	8	23

Table 5 Agreement levels between the results of UF5000 and urine cultures

Urine culture	UF 5000			
	GNB	GPC	Mixed	None
GNB	52	6	5	2
GPC	0	7	0	3
Mixed	4	6	1	13

GNB gram negative bacilli, *GPC* gram positive cocci, *Mixed* mixed growth

sensitivity (80.0%) for identifying gram negative bacteria with an acceptable specificity (88.2%). With regard to gram positive bacteria, the UF-5000 outperformed the UF-1000i in detecting gram positive cocci (UF-5000 sensitivity: 70% and specificity: 86.5%) with good specificity, which was comparable to gram staining (sensitivity: 60% and specificity: 100%). However, the sensitivity of the UF-5000 for identifying mixed growth bacteria was poor.

The UF-5000 is an automated urine analyzer produced by Sysmex Corporation, which performs flow cytometry analysis with a higher level of accuracy and more precise data [13]. Several previous studies have investigated legacy models of automated urine particle analyzers (including the UF500i and the UF-1000i) for screening urine cultures, while few studies have evaluated the ability of the newer UF-5000 model in the differentiation of bacterial growth patterns. Compared with the legacy systems, the current study showed that the UF-5000 had comparable sensitivity and specificity for GNB (80.0% and 88.2%, respectively). For specific bacteria (Table 2), the current results revealed that the UF-5000 could identify *Klebsiella* spp. *Proteus* spp., and *Citrobacter* spp. but it only identified 37 out of the 49 *E coli.* cases.

However, a retrospective study by Kim et al. [11] reported that the UF-5000 had good performance in identifying *E coli.* Further studies are required to check the performance of the UF-5000 in identifying *E coli.* As for Gram-positive bacteria, the UF-5000 showed high sensitivity and specificity for *Enterococcus* spp., however, the sensitivity for *Streptococci* spp. was much lower. In the current study, the UF-5000 identified all *Staphylococci* spp. (n = 3), *Enterococci* spp. ($n = 1$) and *Streptococci* spp. (n = 3), except for one *Group B Streptococci* (2*104 cfu/mL) and two gram positive cocci (103 and 2 × 103 cfu/mL, respectively). With regard to gram positive bacteria, the UF-5000 outperformed the UF-1000i in detecting gram positive cocci, which was comparable to gram staining.

Gram staining is associated with a sensitivity rate of 88%, a specificity rate of 95%, a negative predictive value of 96%, and a positive predictive value of 84% for identifying bacteriuria [6, 14]. When differentiating bacterial growth patterns, gram staining has good sensitivity and specificity for gram negative (80.6% and 96.7%, respectively) and gram positive bacteria (60% and 100%, respectively). Although real-time reporting of gram staining could reduce the blind initiation of antibiotics, and thus prevent unnecessary expenditure and drug treatment, gram staining is time consuming and labor-intensive. The UF-5000 offers comparable efficacy and a much faster and far easier way of providing the same information, compared with the classic method of Gram staining.

Detecting Gram positive bacteria has significant clinical implications. First, the most commonly isolated Gram-positive uropathogens are *Staphylococcus saprophyticus*, *Enterococcus faecalis*, and *Streptococcus agalactiae*. A previously published review suggested that urologic diseases involving Gram-positive bacteria may be easily overlooked due to the limited culture-based assays that are typically utilized for urine analysis in hospital microbiology laboratories [4]. Hooton et al. [12] found that only *Staphylococcus saprophyticus* correlated well with catheterized urine whereas, enterococci and streptococci were poorly correlated with catheterized urine cultures. Therefore, patients with gram positive bacteria shown on the UF-5000 may not have uUTI by classical GNB and may not need empirical antibiotics. Second, in patients with Gram positive cocci as determined by the UF-5000, a urine culture is recommended as well as the administration of antibiotics targeting Gram positive bacteria, as opposed to empirical antibiotics for gram negative bacteria. In this way, patients can avoid unnecessary waiting times, the overuse of antibiotics and increased medical costs. Third, immediately identifying Gram positive bacteria in ascites [13], cerebral spinal fluids [14] and pleural fluids may help clinicians make appropriate and timely antibiotic choices for these life threatening infections. More clinical studies to explore the use of the UF-5000 in these situations is encouraged.

About 21.6% of urine cultures revealed mixed growth (n = 22, 21.6%) and lactobacillus (n = 2, 1.9%), which were regarded as contamination due to improper collection, transportation, preservation or storage. The study only included female participants, which may explain the relatively high contamination rate. Because females have a short on 102 specimens with both UF1000i and UF5000 interpretation, there were only 97 specimens with gram stain results available. There were only 5 specimens that were not examined with gram staining because of unavailability of laborators. Therefore, we did not compare the background differences between the three specimen. urethral length and their urethra meatus is proximal to the vagina and anus, urine specimens from women are more easily contaminated than men. Our study showed that the sensitivity and specificity of the UF-5000 for mixed growth were 4.5% and 94.9%, respectively. Further improvements in laser flowcytometry for the identification of mixed growth could help health care workers and save time, labor and money.

The current study did have some limitations. Although the study was prospective and compared the efficacy of the three methods (gram stain, the UF-1000i and the UF 5000), the major limitation was the limited number of included samples. To prove the efficacy of UF-5000, a sample size of 684 specimens is indicated based on the kappa value (0.46) of the current study (acceptable kappa: 0.6, alpha: 0.05, power: 80%), but the current study only included 102 [15]. In addition, a significant proportion of patient specimens yielded gram negative bacteria and mixed growth culture, so evidence supporting the promising efficacy of the UF-5000 in detecting gram positive bacteria is limited due to the low number of specimens with gram positive bacteria. The menopause can lead to vaginal atrophy and an inability for the vagina to maintain its acidity, which could impact the bacterial strains [16]. Due to the limited number of participants, we did not analyze the effect of menopause on the agreement. A strength of the current study was its prospective nature and the fact that it compares two automated urine particle analyzers. Further studies are still warranted to evaluate the generalizability of the UF-5000 in a larger subset of patients, institutions and populations. In addition, the role of the UF-5000 in detecting bacterial patterns in other type of specimens, *i.e.,* ascites, cerebral spinal fluids and pleural effusion, should be investigated further.

Conclusions

The UF-5000 demonstrated that is has potential utility as a rapid screening method for bacterial morphology, which correlated well with the legacy analyzer UF-1000i for GNB bacteria, while showing improved sensitivity for detecting Gram-positive cocci.

Abbreviations

GNB: Gram negative bacilli; UTISA: Urinary tract infection symptoms assessment score; uUTI: Uncomplicated urinary tract infection.

Author contributions

SSY and SJC were involved in project development, data collection and the writing of the manuscript. YSC and CCY conducted the data collection. All authors have read and approved the final version of the manuscript.

Competing interests

The authors declare that they have no competing interests.

Author details

[1] Division of Urology, Department of Surgery, Taipei Tzu Chi Hospital, New Taipei, Taiwan [2] School of Medicine, Tzu Chi University, Hualien, Taiwan. [3] Division of General Laboratory, Taipei Tzu Chi Hospital, New Taipei, Taiwan.

References

1. Medina M, Castillo-Pino E. An introduction to the epidemiology and burden of urinary tract infections. Ther Adv Urol. 2019;11:1756287219832172.
2. Foxman B, et al. Risk factors for second urinary tract infection among college women. Am J Epidemiol. 2000;151(12):1194–205.
3. Jolkkonen S, et al. Screening of urine samples by flow cytometry reduces the need for culture. J Clin Microbiol. 2010;48(9):3117–21.
4. Kline KA, Lewis AL. Gram-positive uropathogens, polymicrobial urinary tract infection, and the emerging microbiota of the urinary tract. Microbiol Spectr. 2016;4(2):1–31.
5. Bekeris LG, et al. Urine culture contamination: a College of American Pathologists Q-Probes study of 127 laboratories. Arch Pathol Lab Med. 2008;132(6):913–7.
6. Wiwanitkit V, Udomsantisuk N, Boonchalermvichian C. Diagnostic value and cost utility analysis for urine Gram stain and urine microscopic examination as screening tests for urinary tract infection. Urol Res. 2005;33(3):220–2.
7. Yang CC, et al. Rapid differentiation of cocci/mixed bacteria from rods in voided urine culture of women with uncomplicated urinary tract infections. J Clin Lab Anal. 2017;31(5):e22071.
8. Seghezzi M, et al. Preliminary evaluation of UF-5000 Body Fluid Mode for automated cerebrospinal fluid cell counting. Clin Chim Acta. 2017;473:133–8.
9. De Rosa R, et al. Evaluation of the new Sysmex UF-5000 fluorescence flow cytometry analyser for ruling out bacterial urinary tract infection and for prediction of Gram negative bacteria in urine cultures. Clin Chim Acta. 2018;484:171–8.
10. Chang SJ, et al. Reliability and validity of a Chinese version of urinary tract infection symptom assessment questionnaire. Int Braz J Urol. 2015;41(4):729–38.
11. Kim SY, et al. Rapid screening of urinary tract infection and discrimination of gram-positive and gram-negative bacteria by automated flow cytometric analysis using Sysmex UF-5000. J Clin Microbiol. 2018;56(8):e0200417.
12. Bland JM, Altman DG. Statistical methods for assessing agreement between two methods of clinical measurement. Lancet. 1986;1(8476):307–10.
13. Previtali G, et al. Performance evaluation of the new fully automated urine particle analyser UF-5000 compared to the reference method of the Fuchs-Rosenthal chamber. Clin Chim Acta. 2017;472:123–30.
14. Olson ML, et al. The slide centrifuge gram stain as a urine screening method. Am J Clin Pathol. 1991;96(4):454–8.
15. Donner A, Eliasziw M. A goodness-of-fit approach to inference procedures for the kappa statistic: confidence interval construction, significance-testing and sample size estimation. Stat Med. 1992;11(11):1511–9.
16. Amabebe E, Anumba DOC. The vaginal microenvironment: the physiologic role of lactobacilli. Front Med (Lausanne). 2018;5:181.

27

Primary pure angiosarcoma of the testis: A vanishingly rare malignancy

J. Walravens-Evans[1*†], M. Yao[2†], S. Grannò[3], D. Arul[4] and S. Chitale[5]

Abstract

Background: Primary pure angiosarcoma of the testis is an exceptionally rare testicular malignancy, which is poorly understood. We present the fifth and youngest case in the current medical literature. Additionally, all cases of angiosarcoma of the testicle, both occurring with associated germ cell tumour and without, were compared in an extended tabular format.

Case presentation: A 56-year old man presented with unilateral scrotal pain, swelling and erythema. Ultrasonography revealed two testicular lesions with a high suspicion of malignancy but serum tumour markers were negative. A radical orchidectomy was performed with clear surgical margins. Diagnosis of primary pure angiosarcoma of the testis was confirmed on subsequent histopathology.

Conclusions: Primary pure angiosarcoma is a rare testicular neoplasm. We present the fifth case in the literature. Clinical and radiological features are non-specific. The diagnosis is purely histological, with the pathologist choosing immunohistochemistry based on abnormal morphology. Local invasiveness is variable but metastatic sites are typical for extra-gonadal angiosarcomas. Primary pure testicular angiosarcoma diagnosis confers a relatively better prognosis compared to angiosarcoma arising in the context of a testicular germ cell tumour. While extra-gonadal angiosarcomas are associated with high rates of local recurrence following resection, in all cases of testicular angiosarcoma there were no local recurrences following radical orchidectomy. Surgical resection remains the most effective treatment for both subtypes of testicular angiosarcoma.

Keyword: Angiosarcoma, Testicular malignancy, Immunohistochemistry, Cisplatin, Radiotherapy, Embryonal carcinoma

Background

Angiosarcomas are an uncommon group of malignancies that arise from vascular endothelial cells and generally carry a poor prognosis. Reported five-year survival rate is 35% in non-metastatic disease [1]. Incidence is highest in the sixth and seventh decades of life, although angiosarcoma can develop at any age [2]. Aetiological factors known to give rise to angiosarcoma include radio- or chemotherapy, vinyl chloride, arsenic and thorium dioxide [2, 3]. These malignancies behave aggressively, with extensive local invasion, early and widespread metastases and high rates of local recurrence following resection [2, 3]. Metastasis is thought to occur via haematogenous spread [4]. The most frequent sites of metastasis are the lungs, liver, bones and lymph nodes [4]. In most cases of angiosarcoma, extensive metastatic disease is present at the time of diagnosis [4]. Surgical resection, where possible, comprises the mainstay of treatment. Angiosarcomas are relatively unresponsive to chemotherapy and

*Correspondence: j.walravens-evans@nhs.net
†J. Walravens-Evans and M. Yao equally contributed to this work
[1] Kingston Hospital NHS Foundation Trust, Galsworthy Road, Surrey KT2 7QB, UK
Full list of author information is available at the end of the article

radiotherapy [5–7]. Angiosarcoma arising as a primary malignancy in the testis (PPAS) is extremely rare.

Germ cell tumours (GCT) are the most common testicular neoplasm, which most frequently comprises teratoma or seminoma [8, 9]. GCTs affect young men, the majority of cases occur between the ages of 20–39 years [10, 11]. Two to four percent of teratomatous elements within GCTs undergo malignant transformation [6, 12, 13], and sarcomatous transformation predominates over carcinoma [7, 14]. Transformation of testicular GCT to angiosarcoma is extremely rare, with eight cases reported in the literature to date. Once angiosarcoma arises, it can metastasise with, or independently, of other tumour cell types and its behaviour is usually aggressive [15].

For the purposes of this paper, the following subtypes of angiosarcoma are henceforth referred to as: extra-testicular soft tissue angiosarcomas (extra-gonadal), and two gonadal subtypes: primary pure angiosarcoma of the testis (PPAS), and angiosarcoma as a component of a testicular germ cell tumour (AS-GCT). In the latter, the angiosarcoma component might arise either within the testicular primary or within a germ cell tumour metastasis.

PPAS and AS-GCT are extremely rare, thus little is known about these conditions and further work is required. Here, we describe the fifth and youngest case of PPAS. Following, we summarise all previous cases of PPAS [16–19] and AS-GCT [7, 13, 15, 20–23] via an extended tabular approach.

Case presentation

We report our case of a 56-year-old man of Bulgarian origin working in the UK, who initially presented to primary care with a four-day history of right scrotal swelling, redness and pain, with a palpable abnormal testicular mass on examination. The patient had no past medical or family history of note. He was a 30-pack year smoker, with no occupational exposure, nor any history of previous chemo- or radio-therapy. He was treated with oral antibiotics for presumptive clinical diagnosis of epididymo-orchitis and an urgent ultrasound scan was arranged in secondary care. All blood tests were normal, including a full blood count and differential, urea and electrolytes, β-HCG, lactate dehydrogenase (LDH), and alpha-fetoprotein (AFP).

Ultrasonography demonstrated two discrete, heterogenous, hypoechoic lesions within the parenchyma of the right testis, with some cystic changes. The larger lesion measured 2 cm in diameter. There was no evidence of extension beyond the testicular tunica albuginea. Angiosarcomas typically appear highly vascular on ultrasonography, however in this case was there was no evidence of internal vascularity (Fig. 1a). Bilateral simple epididymal cysts were noted, as well as a small volume hydrocele of the left testis.

In the context of partially treated epididymo-orchitis, our differential diagnoses at that time included intra-testicular abscess and primary testicular neoplasm, potentially a teratoma. The case was discussed at local multi-disciplinary team (MDT) meeting and a right radical orchidectomy as a definitive therapeutic procedure was performed.

Pathological examination revealed the right testis to measure 50 × 40 × 40 mm (average male 50 × 20 × 30 mm), and the spermatic cord measured 45 × 20 × 25 mm. This gives an estimated testicular volume of 41.6 ml, where a normal range is 12–30 ml [24]. On gross inspection, two discrete, adjacent lesions distorted the testicular parenchyma. The first lesion was a cream-coloured tumour that measured 17 × 19 × 17 mm. The second lesion comprised an irregular haemorrhagic area with an ill-defined edge that measured 20 × 20 × 20 mm. The surrounding parenchyma appeared macroscopically normal. Neither lesion appeared to infiltrate the tunica or hilum.

Microscopically, both lesions displayed similar appearances (Fig. 1b–e). Each comprised sheets of cells, mainly with a lace-like pattern of infiltration, although in places solid sheets of cells were visualised. The cells exhibited markedly pleomorphic nuclei with prominent nucleoli. The cytoplasm contained eosinophilic granules of variable sizes. Large areas of haemorrhage and focal necrosis were noted. Separate to these nodules, tumour was noted to infiltrate between seminiferous tubules (Fig. 1c) and into the stroma of the rete testis, but not into the hilum. Resected surgical margins were negative.

Immunohistochemical analysis was performed. The lesions were diffusely and strongly positive for vascular markers, CD31 and CD34. The markers looking for potential background germ cell tumour (AFP, Oct3/4, Glypican 3, Beta-HCG, CD30 and CD117) were negative. The following antibodies were also negative: EMA, S100, CAM5.2, MNF116, BerEp4 and calretinin.

In light of these findings, the final histopathological diagnosis was given as high-grade angiosarcoma ie PPAS. The patient had a re-staging CT scan three months post operatively due to lower back pain, which demonstrated no evidence of recurrence or metastatic disease. Subsequent follow up continued with active surveillance at a tertiary centre. The patient remained well at review six months after initial presentation.

Discussion and conclusions

We have reported the fifth case of primary pure angiosarcoma (PPAS) of the testis. The four existing cases of PPAS, plus the index case, are summarised in Tables 1

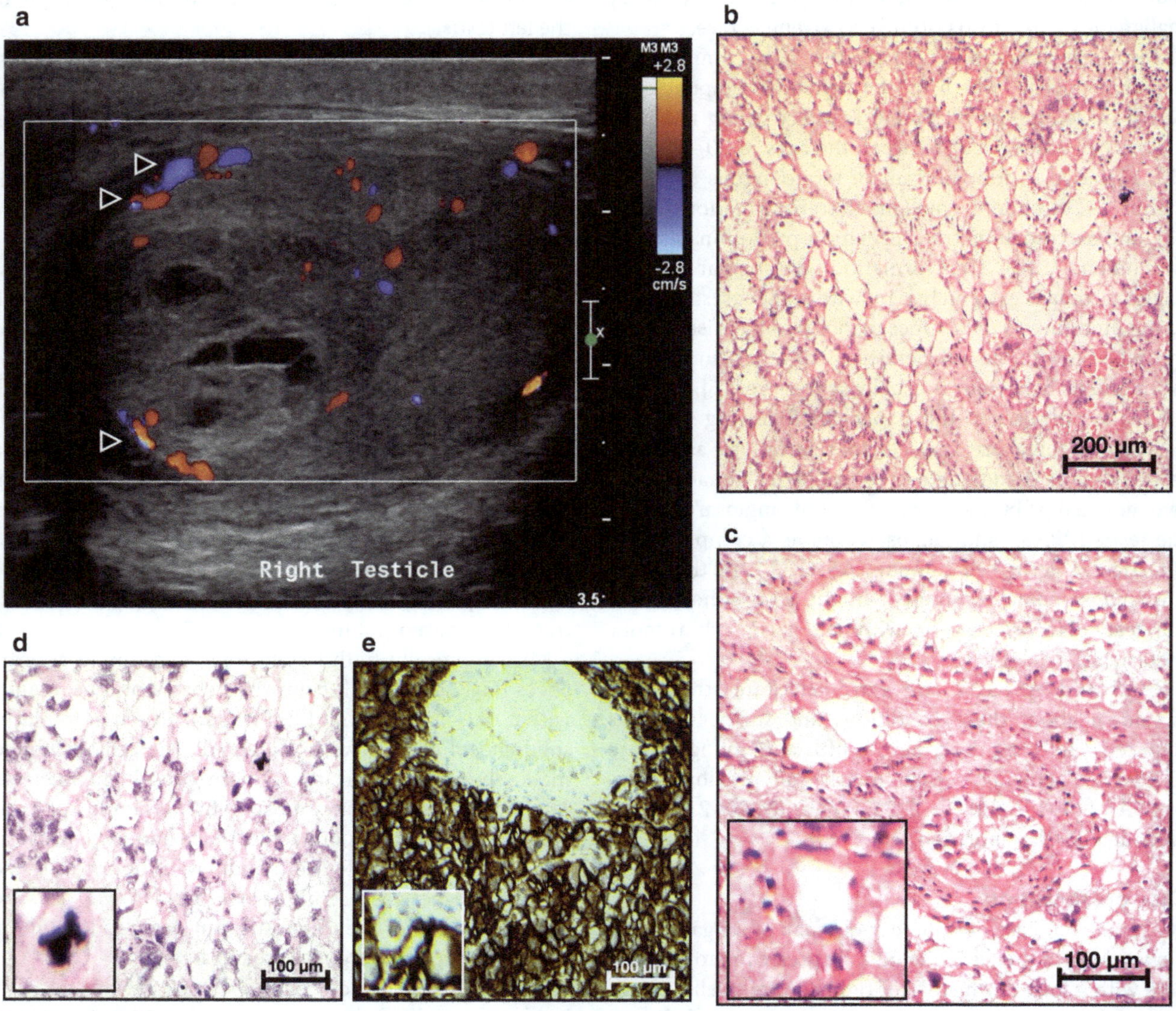

Fig. 1 Micro- and Macroscopic appearance of this case of PPAS. **a** Doppler ultrasound scan of the patient's right testicle, demonstrating one of the suspicious lesions (white square), with areas of vascularity that surrounds the lesion but not evident within it (black arrowheads with white border). **b** Hematoxylin and eosin stain of primary testicular AS at 10 × magnification. **c** Hematoxylin and eosin stain of PPAS at 20 × magnification, demonstrating a seminiferous tubule and several malignant cells infiltrating in and around the tubules. **d** Hematoxylin and eosin stain of PPAS at 20 × magnification, demonstrating markedly atypical, plump endothelial cells with atypical mitoses. **e** CD31 staining at 20 × magnification, demonstrating strong and diffuse CD31 immunopositivity

and 2 [16–19]. The eight previous cases of AS-GCT are summarised in Tables 3 and 4 [7, 13, 15, 20–23].

PPAS tends to occur in elderly patients (median 63 years, 56–80, $n=5$), whereas AS-GCT affects younger men (median 27 years, 16–38, $n=8$). The aetiology of all four previous cases of PPAS, plus the index case presented, remains unknown. Previous radiation therapy and chemotherapy are known causative factors in the pathogenesis of extra-gonadal angiosarcomas [2, 3]. Indeed, angiosarcoma first developed in three of the eight cases of AS-GCT following the use of platinum-based chemotherapy regimens and/or radiotherapy to treat primary testicular germ cell tumours. It has been hypothesised that these systemic therapies might have triggered clonal progression to angiosarcoma as well as hastening metastasic disease due to selective eradication of less aggressive germ cell tumour cell types [5, 7, 13, 21]. However, while some of the testicular primaries were extensively sampled, it is possible that components of angiosarcoma had already been present within the primary germ cell tumours prior to systemic treatment, but were missed. In contrast, the remaining five cases of

Table 1 Clinical and pathological features of all known cases of PPAS

Case	Age (years)	Diagnosis	Presentation		Investigations		Macroscopic features of testicular lesion		
			Symptoms (duration)	Patient noticed lump? (duration)	Bloods	Testicular ultrasound	Site	Appearance	Size (mm)
Current case	56	PPAS	Testicular pain, swelling, redness (4 days)	No	Normal	Two lesions Heterogenous, hypo-echoic, some cysts, no vascularity	Parenchyma, rete testis, tunica	*A:* cream-coloured, Solid *B:* Haemorrhagic, infiltrative	*A:* 17 × 17 × 19 *B:* 20 × 20 × 20
Piotrowski et al. [19]	58	PPAS	Hip pain, back pain (3 months)	No	Normal	Two lesions	*A:* Parenchyma, epididymis *B:* Spermatic cord	*N/A*	*A:* 120 × 68 × 68 *B:* 35 × 24 × 20
Jain et al. [18]	63	PPAS	Testicular enlargement (8 months), preceding testicular firmness (10 years)	Yes (10 years)	Normal	Solid lesion	Parenchyma replaced by tumour	Haemorrhagic, necrotic, focal solid white	110 × 80 × 70
Armah et al. [17]	80	PPAS	Painless lump (2 months), hydrocoele (7 years)	Yes (2 months)	*N/A*	*N/A*	Parenchyma, epididymis	Haemorrhagic, solid	30
Mašera et al. [16]	74	PPAS, epithelioid	Fever unknown cause (3 weeks)	No	CRP↑ ESR↑	Transonic, vascularity	Parenchyma	Haemorrhagic, brown-white, infiltrative	17

Table 2 Therapeutic strategies and outcomes for all known cases of PPAS

Case	Testicular lesion		Metastases	Outcome
	Treatment (margins)	Local recurrence		
Current case	Orchidectomy (clear)	No	No	Alive and well after 6 months
Piotrowski et al. [19]			*At presentation:* Bones, lungs, right retroperitoneum, right pelvic LN's	Died after 6 months
Jain et al. [18]			*3 months after presentation:* Widespread bones	Died after 3 months
Armah et a . [17]			No	Alive and well after 20 months
Mašera et al. [16],			No	Died after 1 month from stroke

AS-GCT did not occur in association with any known risk factor for extra-gonadal angiosarcoma [15, 20, 22, 23]. Angiosarcoma was identified as a component of teratomatous germ cell tumours prior to the administration of systemic therapies. In these cases, the angiosarcoma components were postulated to occur as a consequence of malignant transformation within teratomatous foci [15, 20, 22, 23].

In comparison, none of the four previous cases of PPAS, nor the index case, were exposed to any identifiable risk factor for angiosarcoma. Malignant transformation of a teratoma is unlikely to explain the pathogenesis of PPAS, because no teratomatous components were identified on microscopic or

Table 3 Clinical and pathological features of all known cases of AS-GCT

Case	Age (years)	Diagnosis	Presentation		Testicular lesion				
			Symptoms (duration)	Bloods	Diagnosis	Site	Size (mm)	Definitive treatment (margins)	Local recurrence
Primary angiosarcoma in germ cell tumour									
Malagón et al. [15]	25	AS-GCT	*N/A*	*N/A*	Teratoma, yolk sac tumour, angiosarcoma	*N/A*	*N/A*	Orchidectomy (*N/A*)	*N/A*
Malagón et al. [15],	35	AS-GCT	*N/A*	*N/A*	Teratoma, yolk sac tumour	*N/A*	*N/A*	Orchidectomy (*N/A*)	*N/A*
Sahoo et al., [23]	23	AS-GCT, epithelioid	Right flank pain, back pain	Normal	Teratoma	Parenchyma	65 × 60 × 55	Orchidectomy (clear)	No
Steele et al. [22]	24	AS-GCT, epithelioid	Left testis mass (6 months)	Normal	Teratoma, epithelioid angiosarcoma	Parenchyma, rete testis, epididymis, spermatic cord	80 × 70	Orchidectomy (clear)	No
Hughes et al. [20]	16	AS-GCT	Right testis mass (1 months)	Normal	Teratoma, angiosarcoma	Parenchyma	90 × 70 × 65	Orchidectomy (clear) post-op RT	No
Therapy-related angiosarcoma in germ cell tumour									
Idrees et al. [7]	38	AS-GCT	Abdominal pain	AFP 8320	Teratoma, yolk sac tumour, seminoma	Parenchyma, epididymis, para-testicular soft tissue	*N/A*	Orchidectomy (clear)	No
Lee et al. [21]	35	AS-GCT, epithelioid	*N/A*	*N/A*	Seminoma	*N/A*	80	Orchidectomy (clear)	No
Ulbright et al. [6]	17	AS-GCT	Testis mass, back pain (1 years)	*N/A*	Teratoma	*N/A*	*N/A*	Orchidectomy (*N/A*)	No

immunohistochemical evaluation of any case. Furthermore, malignant teratomas seldom occur in the elderly [25]. Therefore, the etiology of PPAS remains unclear.

Clinical and radiological features prior to definitive surgery (radical orchidectomy) are *not* diagnostic of PPAS [20, 22, 23]. On ultrasonography, the index case did not display the internal vascularity that is regarded as a characteristic feature of extra-gonadal angiosarcomas (Fig. 1a). This is in contrast to a previous case of PPAS which demonstrated prominent internal vascularity on ultrasound [16]. Diagnosis is made following radical orchidectomy, by microscopic identification of characteristic morphologic features and confirmation employing immunohistochemistry. Nevertheless, this approach should be undertaken cautiously, since AS-GCT and PPAS are similar in both morphology and immunophenotype [4]. AS-GCT, however, demonstrates background germ cell tumour, whereas PPAS appears to arise de novo. Histologically, angiosarcoma comprises two main subtypes: classic (spindled cells) and epithelioid (plump epithelial-like cells). These malignancies also display variable architecture (solid or vasoformative) [4]. Epithelioid angiosarcomas are often macro- and microscopically similar to embryonal carcinomas [20, 22, 23]. They are distinguishable by subtle differences on microscopy and stain differently upon immunohistochemistry, however [20, 22, 23].

Initial misdiagnosis as embryonal carcinoma with teratoma occurred upon macroscopic and microscopic evaluation of two surgical AS-GCT specimens [22, 23]. Since embryonal carcinoma and epithelioid angiosarcoma often exhibit similar morphological characteristics, [22, 23] we highlight the importance of considering the diagnosis of angiosarcoma when examining unusual testicular malignancies, with use of appropriate immunohistochemistry if necessary. Accurate diagnosis of testicular angiosarcoma is of extreme clinical relevance. Missing this diagnosis indeed has a significant detrimental effect on patient management and prognosis [22, 23].

Local invasiveness was variable between cases of PPAS (Table 1). In the index case there was no evidence of local invasion, with two discrete lesions confined within the

Table 4 Disease progression, treatment and misdiagnosis of all known cases of AS-GCT

Case	Diagnosis				Treatment after angiosarcoma developed		Outcome at follow-up (time interval)
	Primary testicular diagnosis	Metastatic sites (tumour diagnosis)	Risk factors for angiosarcoma	Misdiagnosis	Chemotherapy	Surgery	
Primary angiosarcoma in germ cell tumour							
Malagón et al. [15]	Mature teratoma, yolk sac tumour, angiosarcoma	Retroperitoneum (N/A)	No	No	Cisplatin, Cyclophosphamide and Adriamycin	*N/A*	Alive with mets (8 months)
Malagón et al. [15]	Mature teratoma, angiosarcoma	Lungs, LNs (MT, AS)	No	No	Cisplatin, Cyclophosphamide and Adriamycin	*N/A*	Alive with mets (72 months)
Sahoo et al. [23]	Mature teratoma	Retroperitoneum (MT, AS), liver (AS), lungs, pleura (AS), retroperitoneal LNs (AS)	No	Yes, met: MT with epithelioid AS diagnosed as MT with embryonal carcinoma	Thalidomide Cisplatin and Gemcitabine	Resection, LND	Alive with mets (22 months)
Steele et al. [22]	Mature teratoma, epithelioid angiosarcoma	Lungs (AS), renal hilum (AS), pre-aortic, interaortocaval and renal hilar LNs (AS)	No	Yes, primary: MT with epithelioid AS diagnosed as MT with embryonal carcinoma	Cisplatin, Etoposide and Bleomycin Ifosfamide and Doxorubicin	Resection, RPLND	Alive with recurrent mets
Hughes et al. [20]	Mature teratoma, angiosarcoma	No	No	No	No	No	Alive with no mets (9 months)
Therapy-related angiosarcoma in germ cell tumour							
Idrees et al. [7]	Mature teratoma, seminoma, yolk sac tumour	Lungs (MT), retroperitoneum (MT), para-iliac, para-caval and retrocrural LNs (MT), LNs near thoracic duct (MT), posterior mediastinum (AS)	Cisplatin, Etoposide and Bleomycin (40 months) Vinblastine, Ifosfamide and Cisplatin (40 months)	No	No	6 Resections over 4 years	Alive with no mets (58 months)
Lee et al. [21]	Seminoma	Paravertebral (AS), lungs (AS), thorax (AS), liver (AS)	RT (10 years) Cisplatin, Vinblastine and Bleomycin (13 months)	No	MTX and leucovorin	Resections	Died (13 months after mets)
Ulbright et al. [6]	Mature teratoma	Retroperitoneum (MT), lungs, liver (AS), kidneys (AS), adrenals (AS), spleen (AS)	RT (5 years) Cisplatin, Vinblastine and Bleomycin (5 years)	No	No	No	Died (5 years)

rete testis and tunica albuginea. In the case of Piotrowski et al. [19] one tumour minimally extended into ipsilateral proximal spermatic cord and another into the epididymis. In the cases of Jain et al. [18] and Masera et al. [16] there was no local invasion. In the former case the entire testicular parenchyma was replaced by tumour and the patient complained of testicular firmness dating back ten years. In Armah et al. [17], there was invasion into the epididymis. We found no apparent explanation for the discrepancy in extent of local invasion between cases of PPAS.

The contralateral testis was not affected by metastatic disease in any of the cases of PPAS or AS-GCT. Metastatic sites of the PPAS and AS-GCT cases were similar to those of extra-gonadal angiosarcoma (Tables 2 and 4) [4].

Although extra-gonadal soft tissue angiosarcomas are associated with high rates of local recurrence [4], none of the thirteen testicular cases (index case included) experienced local recurrence following radical orchidectomy. This could be a consequence of negative surgical margins due to resection high up at the level of the spermatic cord, which enabled total oncological clearance via radical orchidectomy.

All cases of PPAS were treated using radical orchidectomy only (Table 2). In contrast, five of the eight cases of AS-GCT were treated using surgery with adjuvant chemotherapy after the angiosarcomatous component arose (Table 4). However, none of the chemotherapy regimens that were employed to treat AS-GCT eradicated disease [7, 13, 15, 21–23]. Surgery thus remains the most effective treatment for PPAS and AS-GCT. This is in keeping with extra-gonadal angiosarcomas, which also appear to be resistant to chemotherapies and radiotherapy [5, 15, 23]. Radical orchidectomy is also the mainstay surgical treatment for GCTs [8, 9, 26]. Platinum-based chemotherapy is the standard treatment for testicular germ cell tumours with heightened potential for metastasis or proven pre-existing metastasis [9, 27]. Teratomas are highly sensitive to cisplatin-based chemotherapy [9, 27]. Seminomatous metastases are particularly responsive to radiotherapy [28–30]. In general, testicular germ cell tumours are associated with excellent prognoses, even in the presence of metastatic disease [8–10].

Overall, two (40%) of the five PPAS cases suffered metastatic disease and died shortly thereafter, whereas three (60%) were alive without metastasis at follow-up, including the index case (Table 2). In contrast, only two (25%) of the eight cases of AS-GCT were alive without metastasis at follow-up and two (25%) had died (Table 4).

While follow-up was limited for most cases, survival for gonadal PPAS appeared superior to primary angiosarcoma that arises in extra-gonadal sites [1, 4, 15]. This is in keeping with a previous study that noted differential outcomes between testicular (gonadal) and mediastinal germ cell tumours (extra-gonadal) with sarcomatous transformation [15]. This might be because testicular angiosarcomas present earlier due to their location, ie easy access to self-examination, frequently prior to metastasis, and are amenable to complete resection using radical orchidectomy, compared to extra-gonadal angiosarcomas [4, 15].

In conclusion, PPAS is a rare testicular neoplasm. We present the fifth case in the literature. Clinical and radiological features are non-specific. The diagnosis is purely histological, with the pathologist choosing immunohistochemistry based on abnormal tumour morphology. Local invasiveness is variable but metastatic sites are typical for extra-gonadal angiosarcomas. PPAS confers a relatively better prognosis as compared to AS-GCT. While extra-gonadal angiosarcomas are associated with high rates of local recurrence following resection, in all cases of PPAS and AS-GCT there were no local recurrences following radical orchidectomy. Chemotherapy is associated with poor outcomes, thus surgical resection remains the most effective treatment for both subtypes of testicular angiosarcoma.

Abbreviations

AFP: Alpha-fetoprotein; AS: Angiosarcoma; AS-GCT: Angiosarcoma associated with germ cell tumour; CRP: C-reactive protein; CT: Chemotherapy; ESR: Erythrocyte sedimentation rate; LDH: Lactate dehydrogenase; LNs: Lymph nodes; MDT: Multi-disciplinary team; Met: Metastasis; MT: Mature teratoma; MTX: Methotrexate; N/A: Not communicated in original case report; PPAS: Primary pure angiosarcoma; RPLND: Retroperitoneal lymph node dissection; RT: Radiotherapy; β-HCG: Beta-human chorionic gonadotrophin.

Acknowledgements

The authors thank James Arrich for his contribution to the tabulated summaries, and Brendan Berry for the acquisition of the ultrasound images.

Authors' contributions

JWE wrote the first draft of the paper and edited at later stages. MY coordinated all author efforts, wrote and edited the paper and managed patient communication. JWE and MY contributed equally to the paper. SG wrote and edited the paper and assembled all graphics. DA generated and analysed histopathological data, wrote and edited the paper. SC made first contact with the patient, held final responsibility pertaining all clinical activities concerned, conceived the study and edited the paper. All authors read and approved the final manuscript.

Competing interests

The authors declare that they have no competing interests.

Author details

[1] Kingston Hospital NHS Foundation Trust, Galsworthy Road, Surrey KT2 7QB, UK. [2] Department of Urology, Kent and Canterbury Hospital, Ethelbert Road, Canterbury CT1 3NG, UK. [3] UCL School of Life and Medical Sciences, Gower St, London WC1E 6BT, UK. [4] Department of Pathology, Whittington Hospital, Magdala Avenue, London N19 5NF, UK. [5] Department of Urology, Whittington Hospital, Magdala Avenue, London N19 5NF, UK.

References

1. Fury MG, et al. A 14-year retrospective review of angiosarcoma: clinical characteristics, prognostic factors, and treatment outcomes with surgery and chemotherapy. Cancer J. 2005;11(3):241–7.

2. Mark RJ, et al. Angiosarcoma. A report of 67 patients and a review of the literature. Cancer. 1996;77(11):2400–6.
3. Meis-Kindblom JM, Kindblom LG. Angiosarcoma of soft tissue: a study of 80 cases. Am J Surg Pathol. 1998;22(6):683–97.
4. Gaballah AH, et al. Angiosarcoma: clinical and imaging features from head to toe. Br J Radiol. 2017;90(1075):20170039.
5. Motzer RJ, et al. Teratoma with malignant transformation: diverse malignant histologies arising in men with germ cell tumors. J Urol. 1998;159(1):133–8.
6. Ulbright TM. Testis risk and prognostic factors. The pathologist's perspective. Urol Clin North Am. 1999;26(3):611–26.
7. Idrees MT, et al. Clonal evidence for the progression of a testicular germ cell tumor to angiosarcoma. Hum Pathol. 2010;41(1):139–44.
8. Bahrami A, Ro JY, Ayala AG. An overview of testicular germ cell tumors. Arch Pathol Lab Med. 2007;131(8):1267–80.
9. Winter C, Albers P. Testicular germ cell tumors: pathogenesis, diagnosis and treatment. Nat Rev Endocrinol. 2011;7(1):43–53.
10. Hayes-Lattin B, Nichols CR. Testicular cancer: a prototypic tumor of young adults. Semin Oncol. 2009;36(5):432–8.
11. Ruf CG, et al. Changes in epidemiologic features of testicular germ cell cancer: age at diagnosis and relative frequency of seminoma are constantly and significantly increasing. Urol Oncol. 2014;32(1):33.e1–6.
12. Ahmed T, Bosl GJ, Hajdu SI. Teratoma with malignant transformation in germ cell tumors in men. Cancer. 1985;56(4):860–3.
13. Ulbright TM, Clark SA, Einhorn LH. Angiosarcoma associated with germ cell tumors. Hum Pathol. 1985;16(3):268–72.
14. Fizazi K, et al. Germ cell tumors in patients infected by the human immunodeficiency virus. Cancer. 2001;92(6):1460–7.
15. Malagon HD, et al. Germ cell tumors with sarcomatous components: a clinicopathologic and immunohistochemical study of 46 cases. Am J Surg Pathol. 2007;31(9):1356–62.
16. Masera A, Ovcak Z, Mikuz G. Angiosarcoma of the testis. Virchows Arch. 1999;434(4):351–3.
17. Armah HB, Rao UN, Parwani AV. Primary angiosarcoma of the testis: report of a rare entity and review of the literature. Diagn Pathol. 2007;2:23.
18. Jain S, Cantley R, Philip J. Primary pure angiosarcoma of the testis: a case report. Transl Univ Toledo J Med Sci. 2014;1:C1-3.
19. Piotrowski JT, et al. Primary angiosarcoma of the testis with retroperitoneal metastasis. Urol Case Rep. 2018;21:116–8.
20. Hughes DF, Allen DC, O'Neill JJ. Angiosarcoma arising in a testicular teratoma. Histopathology. 1991;18(1):81–3.
21. Lee KC, et al. Angiosarcoma following treatment of testicular seminoma: case report and literature review. J Urol. 1995;153(3 Pt 2):1055–6.
22. Steele GS, et al. Angiosarcoma arising in a testicular teratoma. J Urol. 2000;163(6):1872–3.
23. Sahoo S, et al. Angiosarcoma masquerading as embryonal carcinoma in the metastasis from a mature testicular teratoma. Arch Pathol Lab Med. 2003;127(3):360–3.
24. Behre HM. Andrology: male reproductive health and dysfunction. Berlin: Springer; 1997.
25. Berney DM, et al. Malignant germ cell tumours in the elderly: a histopathological review of 50 cases in men aged 60 years or over. Mod Pathol. 2008;21(1):54–9.
26. Heidenreich A, et al. Organ sparing surgery for malignant germ cell tumor of the testis. J Urol. 2001;166(6):2161–5.
27. Dearnaley DP, et al. Combination chemotherapy with bleomycin, etoposide and cisplatin (BEP) for metastatic testicular teratoma: long-term follow-up. Eur J Cancer. 1991;27(6):684–91.
28. Hamilton C, et al. Radiotherapy for stage I seminoma testis: results of treatment and complications. Radiother Oncol. 1986;6(2):115–20.
29. Classen J, et al. Radiotherapy for stages IIA/B testicular seminoma: final report of a prospective multicenter clinical trial. J Clin Oncol. 2003;21(6):1101–6.
30. Patel HD, et al. Radiotherapy for stage I and II testicular seminomas: Secondary malignancies and survival. Urol Oncol. 2017;35(10):606.e1-606.e7.

Risk factors for incident delirium among urological patients: A systematic review and meta-analysis with GRADE summary of findings

L. Sanyaolu[1*], A. F. M. Scholz[1], I. Mayo[1], J. Coode-Bate[2], C. Oldroyd[3], B. Carter[4,5], T. Quinn[3] and J. Hewitt[1]

Abstract

Background: Post-operative delirium is an important, yet under-researched complication of surgery. Patients undergoing urological surgery may be at especially high risk of POD, as they are often older, and interventions can be associated with conditions that trigger delirium. The main aim of this systematic review was to evaluate the available evidence for risk factors in this patient group.

Methods: Five databases were searched (MEDLINE, Web of Science, EMBASE, CINAHL and PsychInfo) between January 1987 and June 2019. The Newcastle–Ottawa Scale was used to assess for risk of bias. Pooled odds ratio or mean difference (MD) for individual risk factors were estimated using the Mantel–Haenzel and inverse variance methods.

Results: Seven articles met the inclusion criteria, giving a total population of 1937. The incidence of POD ranged from 5 to 29%. Three studies were deemed low risk of bias and four at a high risk of bias. Nine risk factors were suitable for meta-analysis, with age (MD 4.314 95% CI 1.597, 7.032 $p=0.002$) and the clock drawing test (MD − 2.443 95% CI − 3.029, − 1.857 $p<0.001$) having a statistically significant association with POD in pooled analyses.

Conclusion: Delirium is common in urological patients. This review has identified a lack of studies in this surgical population, with wide heterogeneity and high risk of bias. It also highlights a number of potential risk factors for post-operative delirium, of which some are modifiable. However, the strength of evidence is weak at present and so future research should focus on assessing comparable risk factors in this patient group in order to inform future clinical practice.

Keywords: Delirium, Elderly, Urology, Epidemiology

Background

Delirium, derived from the Latin *deliriare* "go off the furrow", describes a disturbance, or clouding, of consciousness and is diagnosed by fulfilling diagnostic criteria such as those proposed in the Diagnostic and Statistical Manual of Mental Disorders (DSM) [1, 2]. Additional features include agitation, hallucinations and disturbance in the sleep–wake cycle. Delirium is a multifactorial syndrome, associated with significant morbidity and mortality. A previous meta-analysis of hospitalised patients reported that a single episode of delirium was associated with a doubling of mortality rate [3, 4]. Although traditionally

*Correspondence: SanyaoluLN@cardiff.ac.uk
[1] Division of Population Medicine, Cardiff University, Cardiff, UK
Full list of author information is available at the end of the article

considered a transient phenomenon, increasing research shows that delirium can become persistent and is a risk factor for incident dementia [5].

Delirium can be described as prevalent, i.e. found on admission, or incident, when it develops during the hospital admission. Incident delirium is a serious concern in surgical disciplines; delirium rates of over 50% have been reported in older adults undergoing major non-cardiac surgery [4]. Previous research into post-operative delirium (POD) has focused on major orthopaedic or cardiac surgery, with urological patients under-represented [6, 7].

There are reasons to believe that delirium may be a particular issue in Urology. Common urological diseases, including cancers and benign prostatic hyperplasia (BPH), are strongly associated with increasing age which is a generally accepted risk factor for delirium [8, 9]. Urological interventions can be associated with infection, electrolyte disturbance or prescription of anticholinergic drugs—all of which can be triggers to a delirium episode. With changing population demographics and changing expectations of surgery, the urological surgeon is increasingly managing older adults living with frailty and comorbidity, which may further increase the risk of delirium.

A better understanding of urological POD epidemiology and risk factors could inform decisions about treatment. Multicomponent interventions may prevent delirium and if high risk patients could be identified these resources could be applied appropriately [10].

The aim of this study was to identify risk factors for delirium in patients undergoing urological surgery. Systematic reviews of POD in other surgical areas reported small sample sizes and uncertainty in conclusions [6, 11–16]. In this context a comprehensive evidence synthesis can offer the clarity needed to inform practice, research and policy.

Methods

The preferred reporting items for systematic reviews and meta-analyses (PRISMA) statement guidelines were followed for reporting and the review protocol was prospectively registered with the PROSPERO database (reference CRD42017054613). The study design used in this review was based on previous reviews related to POD in older general and vascular surgical patients [11, 12].

Search strategy and study eligibility

A comprehensive search strategy was developed using search syntax based on medical subject heading (MeSH) terms and other controlled vocabulary relating to urological surgery, delirium and potential risk factors. The full search strategy is presented in Additional file 1: Fig. 1 (S1) (supporting information). Gastrointestinal and vascular terms were included in the search criteria in case of mixed surgical population studies. It was predicted that such studies would include larger numbers. To ensure these studies were relevant to this review they needed to include at least 50% of patients undergoing urological surgery.

Literature searches were undertaken between January 1987 and June 2019 inclusive. January 1987 was chosen as this coincided with the introduction of the first validated delirium assessment tools [17–19]. Literature searches were conducted across multiple cross-disciplinary electronic databases including: CINAHL® (EBSCO), Embase (Ovid), MEDLINE (Ovid), PSYCinfo® (Ovid) and Web of Science (Thompson Reuters). Citation lists of included studies and relevant reviews were also searched and repeated until no new relevant papers were identified. The grey literature was not assessed. Study selection was performed by two independent authors (AS and IS) and any disagreements were mediated by a third author (JH).

Inclusion criteria were studies of humans published in English, using a validated delirium diagnostic/assessment tool and evaluating risk factors for incident POD. Only full papers published in a peer-reviewed scientific journal were considered. Eligible study designs were primary research evaluating risk factors for incident delirium only, cohort, case–control and cross-sectional studies. The population of interest was patients undergoing elective or emergency urological surgery. The primary outcome of interest was the development of POD (Table 1). The outcome of POD was defined as the proportion of patients experiencing POD following surgery. Exposure(s) for this systematic review were variables or risk factors associated with POD. To develop a provisional set of risk factors to analyze, the NICE delirium guidelines and previous review articles were used [7, 11, 17, 20, 21]. The list was then expanded as additional risk factors were identified. For the full set of risk factors assessed and how they were measured see Additional file 1: Table 1. POD can occur either early or late after surgery, so the duration of follow-up was not defined in the inclusion criteria, but was noted in the analysis, and used to assess risk of bias. Exclusion criteria were studies relating exclusively to delirium tremens and studies based solely in intensive care.

Quality assessment

An assessment of methodological quality and risk of bias of included studies was conducted by two independent authors using the Newcastle–Ottawa Scale (NOS) [22]. The NOS assesses the design quality of non-randomized studies including case–control and cohort studies. Scores were assigned for selection criteria, comparability and outcome (cohort) or exposure (case–control) with an overall score out of 9. Overall study risk of bias was deemed as high, some concerns or low according to the NOS score (Fig. 2). Studies were deemed to be at high risk of bias overall if any domain (selection criteria, comparability or outcome) received a high risk of bias rating.

Data analysis

To analyse associations with POD, each risk factor reported in the included studies was recorded with the size of association and statistical significance. Meta-analysis was used to estimate the pooled odds ratio (OR) for dichotomous data, or mean difference (MD) for continuous data, between patients developing POD and those not developing POD. The quality of evidence for each risk factor was assessed using the GRADE criteria and presented in a summary of findings table.

Studies were pooled into a meta-analysis if study designs were considered sufficiently homogeneous and where two or more studies examined the same risk factor in a comparable manner (numerical data available and comparable units of measurement) [23, 24]. Meta-analyses and forest plots were undertaken using Comprehensive meta-analysis (version 3) [25]. A random-effects model was used to pool data. A p value of <0.05 was considered statistically significant. Statistical heterogeneity was assessed by visual inspection of data and using the Higgins I^2 statistic, caution was highlighted where I^2 was greater than 60%.

Sensitivity analyses were conducted based on risk of bias (pre-specified), excluding studies at high risk of bias based on NOS score and overall assessment of bias. Sensitivity analyses were also performed based on heterogeneity of studies in terms of urological operations included.

Results

Study selection and incidence

After removal of duplicates, the initial literature search identified 2331 articles. After title and abstract screening, 44 articles were fully reviewed and 5 met the inclusion criteria [26–30]; see PRISMA flow chart (Fig. 1). A total of 1937 subjects were studied, with 336 (17%) cases of POD. Incidence of POD varied between studies, ranging from 5 to 29%, with the largest study of 640 patients (Gani et al.) having a POD incidence of 26%. Through peer review and further citation searching, we found two new eligible studies [31, 32]. We updated our narrative and quantitative data synthesis to include this new evidence.

Study characteristics

The main characteristics of the seven included studies are summarised in Table 1. Published between 2005 and 2016, all were prospective cohort studies and studied in patients undergoing urological surgery. Most patients were male (n = 1831, 95%). Studies generally included older adults, one study had an age range 60 years or older [27], four included those 65 years or older [26, 28, 29, 31], another 66 years or older [30]. Finally one study did not restrict inclusion based on age [32]. The overall age for the study population was reported in four studies with a median of 67 years in Sato et al. [32] and the mean age ranging from 71.3 to 74.3 years [27, 29, 30].

A range of urological procedures were included, and Table 1 includes a summary of those included in each paper. Three of the included studies were from Europe [26, 27, 30], two based in China [29, 31], one from Japan [32] another from the USA [28]. Six of the included studies used the Confusion Assessment Method (CAM) [33] to screen for delirium, one [32] used DSM-V and one used DSM-IV[30]. Five studies employed CAM once per day for seven days postoperatively [27–30] and one assessed for delirium once or twice daily till discharge from hospital [32]. The seventh study [26], did not specify how frequently or for how long post-operatively they assessed for delirium. Two studies [27, 29] used the World Health Organization's International Classification of Diseases (ICD-10) criteria [34].

Study quality

The seven studies scored between 4 to 9 on the NOS, the majority scoring 7 [27, 29, 30]. Apart from three papers [28, 31, 32], all papers lost two points due to lack of control for age or other factors. Three studies were deemed to be at a low risk of bias overall [28, 31, 32] and four were at high risk of bias overall [26, 27, 29, 30]. The studies at high risk of bias had an overall NOS ranging from 4 to 7 (Fig. 2) [26, 27, 29, 30].

Risk factors

A total of 26 separate risk factors were studied, with 14 studied in two or more analyses (Table 2). However, only nine risk factors had data suitable for meta-analysis. Six risk factors had pooled results based on data from greater than two studies. The pooled odds ratio (OR, for categorical outcomes) or mean difference (MD, for continuous outcomes) were estimated (Table 3). See Additional file 1: figure (S2) for forest plots.

Sensitivity and subgroup analyses

Sensitivity analyses were conducted based on study overall risk of bias where possible and studies at a high risk of bias were excluded. This significantly affected the results in the pooled results of two risk factors (Age and ADL) but did not affect the overall result in the other analyses undertaken. Study heterogeneity existed in terms of the operations included within some

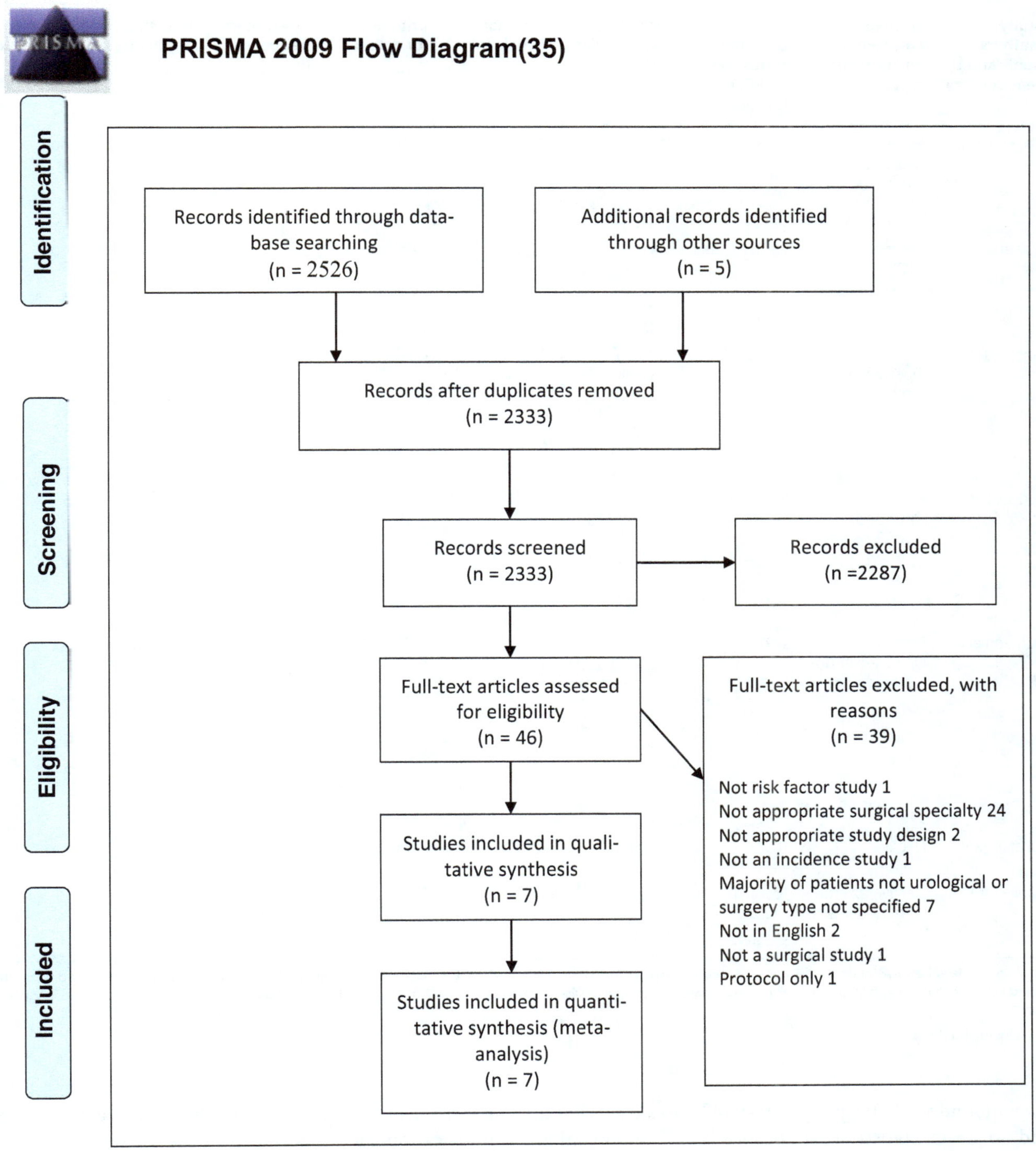

Fig. 1 PRISMA flow diagram of results of database literature searching [35]

studies. To assess their impact, sensitivity analyses were performed but the overall result was unchanged in all analyses. A Meta-regression analysis was also considered but due to lack of data and heterogeneity this was not feasible.

Demographics

Age

Age as a risk factor was studied in all the included papers. Five of the studies found older age was a statistically significant risk factor for developing POD [28–32]. One

Table 1 Study characteristics

Study (authors, publication year, country)	Elective/ emergency and operation type	Study outcome status: POD/ no POD (incidence)	Age: mean (SD)/median (IQR)	Sex: male/ female (n)	Criteria for delirium	Assessment frequency (h)	Assessment length (days)	Study overall risk of bias
Large et al. [28]	Elective Radical cystectomy	14/35 (29%)	*Median* With POD 77.8 (73.5–83.5) No POD 73.1 (70.1–76.5)	40/9	CAM	24	3 then days 5, 7	Good
Xue et al. [31]	Elective TURP	28/330 (7.8%)	*Mean* With POD 78.1 (5.33) No POD 74.8 (6.39)	358/0	CAM	24	7	Good
Sato et al. [32]	NS Open and endoscopic surgery	10/205 (4.7%)	*Median* Overall 67 (63–75) With POD 79 (77–80) No POD 67 (62–74)	175/40	DSM-V	12–24	3, then daily during hospital LOS	Good
Tognoni et al. [30]	NS Open and TURP > 60mins length	8/82 (8.8%)	*Mean* Overall 74.3 (0.40) With POD 77 (1.7) No POD 74 (0.4)	81/9	CAM, DSM-IV	24	7	Poor
Hamann et al. [27]	Elective Open and endoscopic surgery	7/93 (7.0%)	Overall mean age 71.9 (SD not stated) *Median* With POD 75.1 (IQR not stated) No POD 71.5 (IQR not stated)	77/23	CAM, ICD-10	24	7 or discharge	Poor
Tai et al. [29]	Elective TURP	103/382 (21.2%)	*Mean* 71.3 (2.35)	485/0	CAM, DSM-IV	24	7	Poor
Gani et al. [26]	Elective, all urology patients	166/474 (26.0%)	Median age range 71–75	615/25	CAM	NS	NS	Poor
Totals		336/1601		1831/106		Mean: 24[a]		

SD standard deviation, *IQR* interquartile range, *CAM* confusion assessment method, *DSM IV/V* the diagnostic and statistical manual of mental disorders 4th edition/ 5th edition, *ICD 10* World Health Organization's International Classification of Diseases version 10, *TURP* transurethral resection of the prostate, *NS* not stated, *LOS* length of stay

[a] Excluding Gani et al.

paper found the POD group had an older mean age, but it did not reach statistical significance [27]. The remaining paper examined POD based on age groups, with no significant difference [26]. Pooling of data from three studies [30–32] demonstrated older age was significantly associated with an increased risk of developing POD (Table 3) (MD 4.314; 95% confidence intervals (95% CI) 1.597, 7.032; $p=0.002$). A sensitivity analysis based on study risk of bias resulted in a larger mean difference and larger p-value (MD 6.961 95% CI − 1.144, 15.066; $p=0.092$). A further sensitivity analysis removing Sato et al. (based on urological operations included in the study) led to narrower CI and a smaller p-value (MD 3.010 95% CI 2.571, 3.448; $p<0.001$).

Sex

The effect of male sex was examined in all but two papers [29, 31], as these studies only included male participants. Sex was not found to be associated with an increased risk of POD in any study and did not reach statistical

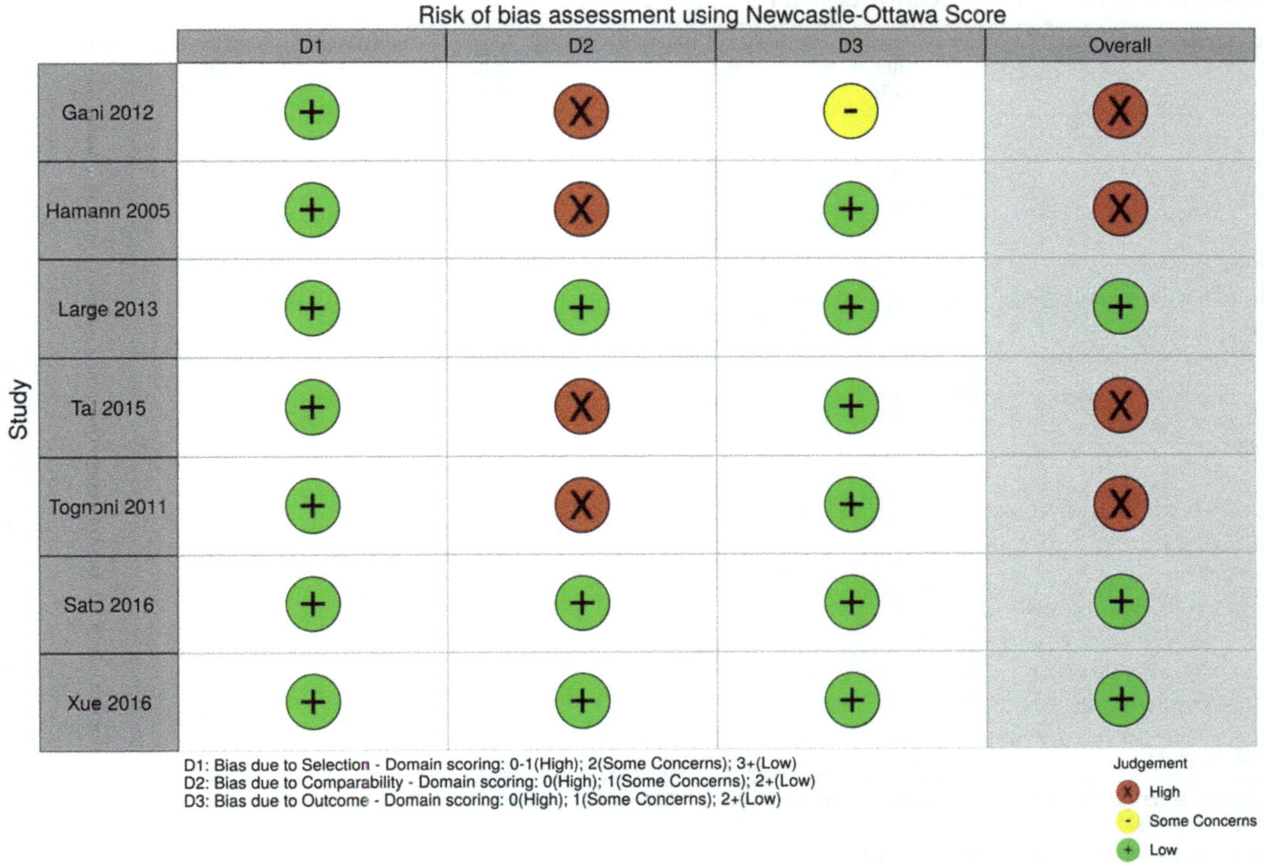
Risk of bias assessment using Newcastle-Ottawa Score
D1
D2
D3
Overall
Study
Gani 2012
Hamann 2005
Large 2013
Tai 2015
Tognoni 2011
Sato 2016
Xue 2016
D1: Bias due to Selection - Domain scoring: 0-1(High); 2(Some Concerns); 3+(Low)
D2: Bias due to Comparability - Domain scoring: 0(High); 1(Some Concerns); 2+(Low)
D3: Bias due to Outcome - Domain scoring: 0(High); 1(Some Concerns); 2+(Low)
Judgement
High
Some Concerns
Low

Fig. 2 Risk of bias assessment using Newcastle–Ottawa score[22]. Risk of bias assessment for each study according to NOS. Plots created using risk-of-bias visualization (robvis) tool [43]

significance in the meta-analysis (OR 1.284 95% CI 0.421, 3.910, p = 0.660). The result remained not statistically significant after sensitivity analyses removing studies at high risk of bias (OR 1.147 95% CI 0.358, 3.675; p = 0.817) and removal of three studies [26, 28, 32] based on the urological operations included in these studies (OR 0.649 95% CI 0.103, 4.098; p = 0.645).

Marriage

Marriage was recorded in three papers [28, 29, 31], with differing results. One study found an association which was statistically significant [29] whereas the other two found no association.

Physical status

Five studies recorded co-morbidities, but only two were comparable as the others used different measurements. The Charlson Co-morbidities Index (CCI) was used in two papers [27, 28] but analysed according to a score ≥ 3 or the mean. Another collectively looked at hyperlipidaemia, hypertension and diabetes as potential risk factors, but no significant difference was found [29]. Two studies used ≥ 2 diseases as a definition of co-morbidity [30, 31]. One of these studies demonstrated a significant association between co morbidities and POD [31], whereas the other did not but did show higher rates of co-morbidity in the POD population [27, 28, 30]. Pooling of results suggests a possible association between having ≥ 2 co-morbidities and an increased risk of POD (OR 1.959 95% CI 0.984, 3.903; p = 0.056).

Meta-analysis of activities of daily living (ADL) scores from three studies found no statistically significant association (MD 0.061 95% CI − 0.776, 0.898; p = 0.886) [28, 29]. Heterogeneity was high in this analysis with an I^2 of 98%. Sensitivity analysis based on type of surgery did not reach statistical significance (MD 0.227 95% CI − 0.792, 1.246; p = 0.662). Excluding studies at high risk of bias in a further sensitivity analysis resulted in a significantly smaller p-value (MD-0.300 95% CI − 0.514, − 0.086; p = 0.006) and reduced statistical heterogeneity (I^2 0%). A poor Instrumental Activities of Daily Living (IADL) score was found to be statistically significant risk factor for

Table 2 Risk factors for post-operative delirium

Risk factor	Hamann 2005 [27]	Large 2012 [28]	Tai 2015 [29]	Tognoni 2010 [30]	Gani 2012 [26]	Sato 2016 [32]	Xue 2016 [31]
Demographic factors							
Older age*	=	+	+	+	=	+	+
Male sex±	=	=		=	=	=	
Married±		=	=				=
Education length in years				=			=
Mental status (mean MMSE/mean CDT)	=	+	+	=/+			=
History of delirium±				+			
Depression (DSI > 40 or GDS)	=		+	=			
Comorbidity (based on mean age-adjusted CCI, CCI > 3 or ≥ 2 co-morbidities)	=	=		=			+
Mean BMI		=	=			=	=
ADL (mean score or functions lost)		=	=	=			=
IADL (mean score or functions lost)			+	+			
Surgical							
Operation time (mean or median)	+	=				=	
Blood loss (mean or median)		=				=	
Intraoperative hypotension±				+	?		=
GA versus regional Anaesthesia	=			=		=	=
Alcohol intake (active consumption or excess/abuse)	=	=	=	=			=

* Age was described by a variety of methods in the included studies such as mean, median or age range. The results presented represent if increasing age was associated with POD

±Proportion of patients with the exposure/risk factor

+ increased risk of POD, = no increased risk of POD, ? not clear due to absence of data. See Additional file 1: Table 1 (S1) for full details

MMSE mini mental state examination, *CDT* clock drawing test, *DSI* Depression Status Inventory, *GDS* geriatric depression scale, *CCI* Charlson Comorbidity Index, *BMI* body mass index, *ADL* activities of daily living, *IADL* Instrumental Activities of Daily Living, *GA* general anaesthetic, *CAGE* CAGE questionnaire relates to drinking habits [24]

Table 3 Meta-analyses of risk factors for post-operative delirium

Risk factor	Studies/total sample (n/n)	Statistical method	Pooled OR/MD** [95% CI]	Heterogeneity I^2 (%)
1. Age*	3/663	IV, Random	4.314 [1.597, 7.032]**	73
2. Male Sex	5/1094	M–H, Random	1.284 [0.421, 3.910]	40
3. BMI	4/1107	IV, Random	0.372 [− 0.121, 0.865]**	0
4. ADL score	3/892	IV, Random	0.061 [− 0.776, 0.898]**	98
5. Pre-op MMSE Score	4/982	IV, Random	− 0.476 [− 1.570, 0.618]**	96
6. Education	2/448	IV, Random	− 0.878 [− 1.758, 0.002]**	80
7. CDT mean*	2/575	IV, Random	− 2.443 [− 3.029, − 1.857]**	90
8. Regional anaesthesia	4/763	M–H, Random	0.826, [0.445, 1.533]	0
9. ≥ 2 Co morbidities	2/448	M–H, Random	1.959 [0.984, 3.903]	0

M–H Mantel–Haenszel, *IV* inverse variance, *OR* odds ratio, *MD* mean difference, *BMI* body mass index, *ADL* activities of daily living, *MMSE* mini mental state examination, *CDT* clock drawing test

*p-value< 0.05. See Additional file 1: figure 1 for corresponding forest plots.

POD in two studies [29, 30]. The results were not suitable for meta-analysis as they were not comparable with one study presenting the mean for IADL whereas the other study presented the median score.

The mean BMI of the POD and non-POD groups were comparable in four studies [28, 29, 31, 32] but no association was demonstrated (MD 0.372 95% CI – 0.121 to 0.865; p = 0.139). Sensitivity analyses of pooled data based on operations included in the studies or study risk of bias also did not demonstrate an association.

Only one study [32] assessed risk factors associated with frailty (handgrip strength, get-up and Go test and falls risk assessment score). The authors found an association with all three risk factors.

Depression and cognition

Depression was included in three studies, and was found to be associated with POD in one study [29]. Use of antidepressant medication [27] or psychotropic medication [31] was assessed in two papers but not suitable for pooling and neither found an association with POD. Two of the papers measured depression using the Geriatric Depression Score (GDS) and compared the mean score between the groups [29, 30]. The GDS mean in both POD groups was higher than the non-POD groups, with one study [29] finding an association with a p-value of 0.038 whereas in the other study [30] the p-value was > 0.05 (exact p-value not stated). Results were not pooled due to very high statistical heterogeneity (I^2 100%).

Five of the seven studies recorded pre-operative MMSE, but only one found a low score to be associated with an increased risk of POD [28]. Pooled analysis of four study results demonstrated no association (MD – 0.476, 95% CI – 1.570 to 0.618; p = 0.394). Heterogeneity was also high in this analysis with an I^2 of 96%. Excluding studies at high risk of bias in a sensitivity analysis did not significantly affect the result (MD – 1.104 95% CI – 2.573, 0.365; p = 0.141) but did reduce statistical heterogeneity (I^2 67%). A sensitivity analysis based on operations included in the studies also did not demonstrate an association (MD – 0.143 95% CI – 1.315, 1.030; p = 0.811). The majority of the studies excluded patients with a pre-existing history of Alzheimer's disease. A history of previous delirium was reported statistically significant risk factor for developing POD in one study (Delirium 37.5% vs no Delirium 6%; p = 0.003) [30].

Two studies [29, 30] analysed the association between pre-operative clock drawing test (CDT) and POD. The CDT is an established neuropsychological test of free-hand clock drawing used to screen dementia [36]. Both studies found a significant difference when looking at CDT score as a risk factor for delirium. Tognoni et al. [30] and Tai et al. [29] had similar results; those patients who developed POD had a mean CDT score 2.12 (p = 0.040) and 2.72 (p = 0.038) respectively, less than those who did not develop POD. Pooling of the study results demonstrated a statistically significant association between low CDT score and risk of POD (MD – 2.443 95% CI – 3.029, – 1.857; p < 0.001).

Education, in years, was assessed pre-operatively in two studies [30, 31]. Pooling of the data from the two studies suggests a possible association between shorter education length and an increased risk of POD (MD – 0.878 95% CI – 1.758, 0.002; p = 0.051).

Intraoperative factors

No statistically significant impact on risk of developing POD was seen between general and regional anaesthesia. This was the case in individual studies, in the meta-analysis [27, 30–32] (OR 0.826, 95% CI 0.445 to 1.533 p = 0.544) and following sensitivity analyses based on operations included in the study (OR 0.842 95% CI 0.441, 1.607; p = 0.602). Operation time was recorded in three papers, two studies found no association whereas Hamann et al. found longer operation times were associated with POD. [27, 28, 32]. It was not possible to pool the data from these studies. Intra-operative hypotension of less than 90 mmHg systolic, was examined in only one paper and was found to be statistically significant [30]. Xue et al. also assessed hypotension during surgery but it was not possible to pool this data as they did not state how they defined hypotension. They found no association between intra-operative hypotension and POD [31]. Another study mentioned haemodynamic complications appearing to contribute to POD in their 65–70 year old age group, but did not provide data [26].

Risk of bias across studies

Based on the asymmetry of the funnel plot (Fig. 3) there is a suggestion of publication bias.

GRADE evaluation of certainty of findings

A 'Summary of findings table' for the nine pooled risk factors analysed within the meta-analysis was created (see Table 4 and Additional file 1: Table 2). The quality of evidence for each outcome was assessed using the five GRADE criteria: risk of bias, consistency of effect, imprecision, indirectness, and other factors including size of effect as well as risk of publication bias (GRADEpro GDT) [37, 38]. Decisions and justifications to down—or upgrade the quality of studies are documented within footnotes.

Based on the GRADE certainty of evidence assessment, all nine risk factors had a very low certainty of evidence.

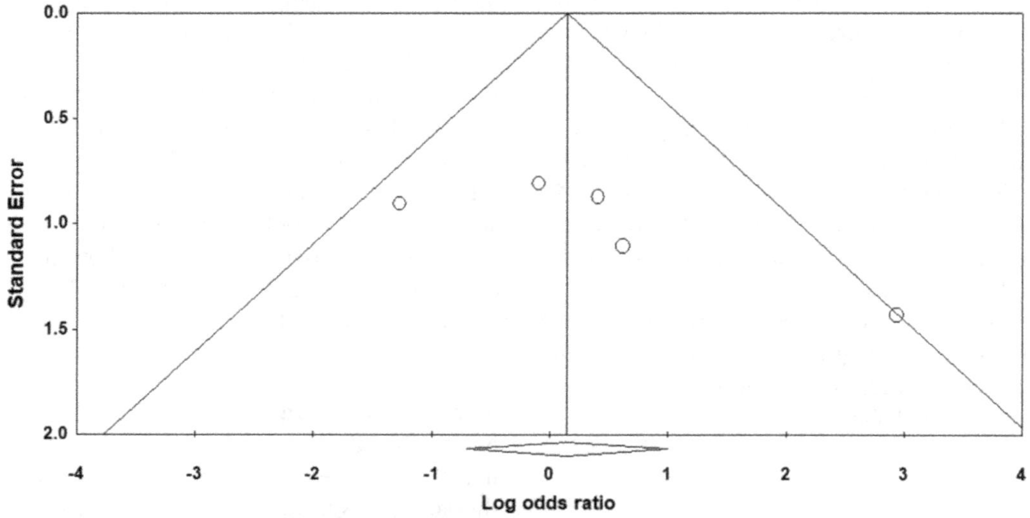

Fig. 3 Funnel plot to assess for publication bias. Funnel plot to assess for publication bias[25]

Discussion

Seven studies [26–30] were identified for inclusion in this systematic review assessing risk factors associated with POD in urological surgical patients. The included studies had a predominantly elderly male patient population and analysed a variety of risk factors for their association with delirium post operatively. The 16 broad risk factors were reported using 26 different methods and studies included patients undergoing very different operations, allowing only nine risk factors to undergo meta-analysis; the majority only containing data from 2 studies. Of the risk factors included in meta-analysis, the clock drawing test and age were the only two that reached statistical significance.

Although the other risk factors were not found to be significantly associated with delirium, it is important to interpret these with caution as four of the included studies were deemed to be at a high risk of bias. In addition, the majority of risk factors assessed within the meta-analysis contained data from two studies. Meta-analysis was limited by the heterogeneity of the data and the types of operations included, with a number of risk factors unable to be pooled or limited studies for the meta-analysis. These included co-morbidities and IADLs, both found within the individual studies to be associated with the development of post-operative delirium.

With regard to co-morbidity, this was higher within the delirium group in four of the studies [27, 28, 30, 31] with one study finding a significant association [31]. Pooling was only possible for two studies (two or more co-morbidities). The result suggests that having two or co-morbidities is associated with POD, although it did not achieve our cut off for statistical significance ($p=0.056$) and included one study at high risk of bias. This could be either to true lack of association or due to lack of statistical power. Therefore, research with a larger cohort of patients, using the same assessment method and possibly looking at specific co-morbidities such as dementia, depression and visual/hearing impairment would be of use. A shorter duration of education also appears to be associated with an increased risk of POD despite again not achieving significance within the meta-analysis ($p=0.051$) possibly for the same reasons as co-morbidity.

The two significant results in the meta-analysis were a lower mean CDT score and higher mean age in those who developed POD. These results should be interpreted with caution as both analyses included studies at high risk of bias. The sensitivity analysis conducted, based on study risk of bias, also suggests the result for the association between older age and POD is not very robust and limits its interpretation. Despite this, advancing age is a well-recognised risk factor for delirium and similar associations have been demonstrated within the literature [12–15, 39]. CDT is a screening tool for cognitive impairment and dementia [36], and the association with delirium may justify its use to establish underlying cognitive impairment preoperatively and delirium risk postoperatively [20]. Finally, ADL was not initially found to be associated with POD, but after excluding studies at high risk of bias, there appeared to be an association. However, its interpretation is limited due to small study sample sizes.

Numerous systematic reviews have been undertaken in both surgical and non-surgical patient populations. Reviews in post-operative surgical patients have mainly focused on Vascular [12], Gastrointestinal [11], Cardiac

Table 4 GRADE summary of findings table

Certainty assessment							№ of patients		Effect		Certainty	Importance
No. of studies	**Study design**	**Risk of bias**	**Inconsistency**	**Indirectness**	**Imprecision**	**Other considerations**	**Delirium**	**Non-delirium**	**Relative (95% CI)**	**Absolute (95% CI)**		
Clock drawing test												
2	Observational studies	Very serious [a]	Not serious	Not serious	Not serious	None	111	464	–	MD 2.443 lower (3.029 lower to 1.857 lower)	⨁◯◯◯ VERY LOW	IMPORTANT
Age												
3	Observational studies	Very serious [c]	Not serious	Not serious	Serious [b]	None	46	617	–	MD 4.314 higher (1.597 higher to 7.032 higher)	⨁◯◯◯ VERY LOW	IMPORTANT

Bibliography: Tai et al. [29], Tognoni et al. [30], Sato et al. [32], Xue et al. [31]

CI confidence interval, *MD* mean difference, *OR* odds ratio

*p-value < 0.05. See Additional file 1: Fig. 1 for corresponding forest plots

Explanations

a. Downgraded as both studies did not control for age or other factors associated with delirium

b. Wide confidence intervals

c. Downgraded as all 3 studies did not control for age or other factors associated with delirium

[13, 14] and Orthopaedic [6, 15, 16] specialties, with incidence ranges (4%-55%) aligning with the results from this systematic review. Incidence ranges are also similar in the medical inpatient setting [17, 40], but significantly higher within intensive care [39, 41]. A multitude of risk factors have been analysed via meta-analyses or multivariable analyses for an association with incident delirium. Most commonly, increasing age [12–15, 39], cognitive impairment [6, 13, 14, 16] and alcohol excess [11, 39] have been identified to increase the risk of developing delirium. Other factors were more mixed, similar to results observed within this review, such as BMI and sex [12, 15–17, 39].

These previous systematic reviews on incident delirium have also highlighted the heterogeneity in the risk factors analysed within the included studies and difficulties pooling results in a similar manner to this review. As discussed above, a low mean CDT score was identified within this review to be associated with POD, a result not replicated within the current body of systematic reviews. Although not technically a risk factor, it does present a potential screening tool to identify those at risk of delirium who could then be targeted for interventions to reduce the risk of POD occurring. Although promising, these results do have limitations and therefore the CDT would need extensive further evaluation before use as a screening tool within clinical practice. A recently published prospective study of over 1000 patients identified a different cognitive screening tool for dementia was associated with development of POD [42]. The authors found that a Hasegawa Dementia Scale-Revised (HDS-R) score of less than 20 was an independent risk factors for POD in elderly urological patients [42]. However, they also identified that its use for all urological patients would be limited as only 3% of patients with this as their only risk factor developed POD [42]. These considerations would need to be taken into account for CDT also.

This review does have a number of limitations. The main one being that there are relatively few studies on this subject within the literature and the numbers of patients within those studies are relatively small. Therefore, the lack of association found may be a result of a lack of statistical power rather than there being no true association. The largest study was not well detailed [26] and the majority of studies are at a high risk of bias. The heterogeneity of the risk factors studied and inconsistency between the studies in how the data were recorded makes it difficult to fully assess the various risk factors. In terms of limitations of the studies themselves, the major issue was with assessment of delirium. This occurred once per day in the majority of the studies which, in view of the fact delirium has a fluctuating course, may mean some cases were missed and thus the true incidence of post-operative delirium is likely to have been under reported. A final limitation is that two of the studies excluded patients with Alzheimer's and dementia without adequate explanation. This is especially important, as dementia is known to be a risk factor for the development of delirium [14].

This review has highlighted that there is a lack of research in post-operative delirium in urological patients and within the relevant studies there is heterogeneity between the risk factors assessed, often with small numbers of patients. Importantly, this review has identified a number of potential areas for future research. A number of statistically significant risk factors in individual studies, including MMSE, CDT, depression, IADL functions, previous delirium, severity of urological disease, duration of surgery and intra-operative hypotension, were reported as being associated with the development of post-operative delirium. To improve our understanding of delirium in this group of patients, future studies should focus on comparable risk factors and methods of data collection as well as possible collaborative work.

Conclusion

In summary, research into post-operative delirium within the urological surgical population is limited. Of those studies included in this systematic review, there is high risk of bias and the heterogeneity of risk factors assessed was restrictive to pooling of data and meta-analysis. It has, however, raised a number of risk factors worthy of further research, and highlighted the importance of future collaborative and comparative work to increase our understanding of risk factors associated with post-operative delirium within the urological patient population.

Abbreviations

POD: Post-operative delirium; NOS: Newcastle–Ottawa scale; OR: Odds ratio; MD: Mean difference; CI: Confidence interval; CDT: Clock drawing test; DSM: The diagnostic and statistical manual of mental disorders; BPH: Benign prostatic hyperplasia; PRISMA: Preferred reporting items for systematic reviews and meta-analyses; NICE: National Institute for Health and Care Excellence; MeSH: Medial subject heading; CAM: Confusion assessment method; ICD: World Health Organisation's International Classification of Diseases; MMSE: Mini mental state examination; CCI: Charlson Co-morbidities Index; ADL: Activities of daily living; IADL: Instrumental Activities of Daily Living; BMI: Body mass index; GDS: Geriatric Depression Score; DSI: Depression Status Inventory; GA: General anaesthetic; SD: Standard deviation; IQR: Interquartile range; TURP: Trans-urethral resection of the prostate; M-H: Mantel Haenszel; IV: Inverse variance.

Authors' contributions

Conception and Design—JH, AS; Data acquisition—AS, IM, LS (re-running search); Data analysis and interpretation—AS, IM, LS, JCB, CO, TQ, BC, JH; Drafting of manuscript—AS, IM, LS, JCB, CO, TQ, JH; Critical revision of manuscript—AS, IM, LS, JCB, CO, TQ, BC, JH; Statistical analysis—AS, IM, LS, BC, JH. All authors have read and approved the manuscript.

Competing interests

The authors declare that they have no competing interests.

Author details
[1] Division of Population Medicine, Cardiff University, Cardiff, UK. [2] Addenbrooke's Hospital, Cambridge, UK. [3] Institute of Cardiovascular and Medical Sciences, University of Glasgow, Glasgow, UK. [4] Department of Biostatistics and Health Informatics, Institute of Psychiatry, Psychology and Neuroscience, King's College London, London, UK. [5] Cochrane Skin Group, School of Medicine, The University of Nottingham, Nottingham, UK.

References

1. Smith J, Seirafi J. Delirium and dementia. In: Marx JA III, Hockberger RS, Walls RM, editors. Rosen's emergency medicine concepts and clinical practices. 7th ed. Philadelphia, PA: Elsevier; 2010.
2. American Psychiatric Association. Diagnostic and statistical manual of mental disorders. 5th ed. Arlington: American Psychiatric Association; 2013.
3. McDaniel M, Brudney C. Postoperative delirium: etiology and management. Curr Opin Crit Care. 2012;18(4):372–6.
4. Mangnall LT, Gallagher R, Stein-Parbury J. Postoperative delirium after colorectal surgery in older patients. Am J Crit Care. 2011;20(1):45–55.
5. Saczynski JS, Marcantonio ER, Quach L, Fong TG, Gross A, Inouye SK, et al. Cognitive trajectories after postoperative delirium. N Engl J Med. 2012;367(1):30–9.
6. Dasgupta M, Dumbrell AC. Preoperative risk assessment for delirium after noncardiac surgery: a systematic review. J Am Geriatr Soc. 2006;54(10):1578–89.
7. Dyer CB, Ashton CM, Teasdale TA. Postoperative delirium. A review of 80 primary data-collection studies. Arch Intern Med. 1995;155(5):461–5.
8. Barry MJ, Fowler FJ, Jr., Bin L, Oesterling JE. A nationwide survey of practicing urologists: current management of benign prostatic hyperplasia and clinically localized prostate cancer. J Urol. 1997;158(2):488–91; discussion 92.
9. Cancer research UK website. https://www.cancerresearchuk.org/about-cancer/prostate-cancer. Last accessed 20th November 2017.
10. Siddiqi N, Harrison JK, Clegg A, Teale EA, Young J, Taylor J et al. Interventions for preventing delirium in hospitalised non-ICU patients. Cochrane Database Syst Rev. https://doi.org/10.1002/14651858.CD005563.pub3.
11. Scholz AF, Oldroyd C, McCarthy K, Quinn TJ, Hewitt J. Systematic review and meta-analysis of risk factors for postoperative delirium among older patients undergoing gastrointestinal surgery. Br J Surg. 2016;103(2):e21–8.
12. Oldroyd C, Scholz AFM, Hinchliffe RJ, McCarthy K, Hewitt J, Quinn TJ. A systematic review and meta-analysis of factors for delirium in vascular surgical patients. J Vasc Surg. 2017;66(4):1269-79.e9.
13. Koster S, Hensens AG, Schuurmans MJ, van der Palen J. Risk factors of delirium after cardiac surgery: a systematic review. Eur J Cardiovasc Nurs. 2011;10(4):197–204.
14. Gosselt AN, Slooter AJ, Boere PR, Zaal IJ. Risk factors for delirium after on-pump cardiac surgery: a systematic review. Crit Care. 2015;19:346.
15. Smith TO, Cooper A, Peryer G, Griffiths R, Fox C, Cross J. Factors predicting incidence of post-operative delirium in older people following hip fracture surgery: a systematic review and meta-analysis. Int J Geriatr Psychiatry. 2017;32(4):386–96.
16. Oh ES, Li M, Fafowora TM, Inouye SK, Chen CH, Rosman LM, et al. Preoperative risk factors for postoperative delirium following hip fracture repair: a systematic review. Int J Geriatr Psychiatry. 2015;30(9):900–10.
17. Ahmed S, Leurent B, Sampson EL. Risk factors for incident delirium among older people in acute hospital medical units: a systematic review and meta-analysis. Age Ageing. 2014;43(3):326–33.
18. Grover S, Kate N. Assessment scales for delirium: a review. World J Psychiatry. 2012;2(4):58–70.
19. American-Psychiatric-Association. Diagnostic and statistical manual of mental disorders. 3rd ed, revised (dsm-iii-r); 1987.
20. Young J, Murthy L, Westby M, Akunne A, O'Mahony R. Diagnosis, prevention, and management of delirium: summary of NICE guidance. BMJ. 2010;341:c3704.
21. Elie M, Cole MG, Primeau FJ, Bellavance F. Delirium risk factors in elderly hospitalized patients. J Gen Intern Med. 1998;13(3):204–12.
22. Wells GA, Shea B, O'Connell D, Peterson J, Welch V, Losos M et al. The Newcastle–Ottawa Scale (NOS) for assessing the quality of non randomised studies in meta-analyses; 2011. https://www.ohri.ca/programs/clinical_epidemiology/oxford.asp. Last accessed 20 Nov 2017.
23. Reeves BC, Deeks JJ, Higgins JPT, Shea B, Tugwell P, Wells GA. Chapter 24: in-cluding non-randomized studies on intervention effects. In: Higgins JPT, Thomas J, Chandler J, Cumpston M, Li T, Page MJ, Welch VA, editors. Cochrane Handbook for systematic reviews of interventions version 6.0 (updated July 2019). Cochrane, 2019. www.training.cochrane.org/handbook. Last accessed 10 Sept 2020.
24. Deeks JJ, Higgins JPT, Altman DG, editors. Chapter 10: analysing data and under-taking meta-analyses. In: Higgins JPT, Thomas J, Chandler J, Cumpston M, Li T, Page MJ, Welch VA, editors. Cochrane handbook for systematic reviews of interventions version 6.0 (updated July 2019). Cochrane, 2019. www.training.cochrane.org/handbook. Last accessed 10 Sept 2020.
25. Borenstein M, Hedges L, Higgins J, Rothstein H. Comprehensive meta-analysis version 3 biostat. NJ: Englewood; 2013.
26. Gani H, Prifti P, Naco M, Domi R, Beqiri V, Torba D, et al. The incidence of postoperative delirium in elderly patients undergoing urologic surgery. Anaesth Pain Intensive Care. 2012;16(3):262–5.
27. Hamann J, Bickel H, Schwaibold H, Hartung R, Forstl H. Postoperative acute confusional state in typical urologic population: incidence, risk factors, and strategies for prevention. Urology. 2005;65(3):449–53.
28. Large MC, Reichard C, Williams JT, Chang C, Prasad S, Leung Y, et al. Incidence, risk factors, and complications of postoperative delirium in elderly patients undergoing radical cystectomy. Urology. 2013;81(1):123–8.
29. Tai S, Xu L, Zhang L, Fan S, Liang C. Preoperative risk factors of postoperative delirium after transurethral prostatectomy for benign prostatic hyperplasia. Int J Clin Exp Med. 2015;8(3):4569–74.
30. Tognoni P, Simonato A, Robutti N, Pisani M, Cataldi A, Monacelli F, et al. Preoperative risk factors for postoperative delirium (POD) after urological surgery in the elderly. Arch Gerontol Geriatr. 2011;52(3):e166–9.
31. Xue P, Wu Z, Wang K, Tu C, Wang X. Incidence and risk factors of postoperative delirium in elderly patients undergoing transurethral resection of prostate: a prospective cohort study. Neuropsychiatr Dis Treat. 122016. p. 137–42.
32. Sato T, Hatakeyama S, Okamoto T, Yamamoto H, Hosogoe S, Tobisawa Y et al. Slow gait speed and rapid renal function decline are risk factors for postoperative delirium after urological surgery. PloS one. 2016;11(5).
33. Inouye SK, van Dyck CH, Alessi CA, Balkin S, Siegal AP, Horwitz RI. Clarifying confusion: the confusion assessment method. A new method for detection of delirium. Ann Intern Med. 1990;113(12):941–8.
34. World Health Organization. (2004). ICD-10 : international statistical classification of diseases and related health problems: tenth revision. 2nd ed. World Health Organization.
35. Moher D, Liberati A, Tetzlaff J, Altman DG. Preferred reporting items for systematic reviews and meta-analyses: the PRISMA statement. BMJ. 2009;339:b2535.
36. Mendez MF, Ala T, Underwood KL. Development of scoring criteria for the clock drawing task in Alzheimer's disease. J Am Geriatr Soc. 1992;40(11):1095–9.
37. GRADEpro GDT: GRADEpro Guideline Development Tool [Software]. McMaster University, 2015 (developed by Evidence Prime, Inc.).
38. Schünemann H, Brożek J, Guyatt G, Oxman A, editors. GRADE handbook for grading quality of evidence and strength of recommendations. Updated October 2013. The GRADE Working Group, 2013. Available fromguidelinedevelopment.org/handbook.
39. Zaal IJ, Devlin JW, Peelen LM, Slooter AJ. A systematic review of risk factors for delirium in the ICU. Crit Care Med. 2015;43(1):40–7.
40. Siddiqi N, House AO, Holmes JD. Occurrence and outcome of delirium in medical in-patients: a systematic literature review. Age Ageing. 2006;35(4):350–64.
41. Van Rompaey B, Schuurmans MJ, Shortridge-Baggett LM, Truijen S, Bossaert L. Risk factors for intensive care delirium: a systematic review. Intensive Crit Care Nurs. 2008;24(2):98–107.
42. Matsuki M, Tanaka T, Takahashi A, Inoue R, Hotta H, Itoh N, et al. Incidence and risk factors of postoperative delirium in elderly patients undergoing urological surgery: A multi-institutional prospective study. Int J Urol. 2020;27(3).
43. McGuinness L, Higgins J. Risk-of-bias VISualization (robvis): an R package and Shiny web app for visualizing risk-of-bias assessments. Res Syn Meth. 2020; 1-7. https://doi.org/10.1002/jrsm.1411.

Permissions

All chapters in this book were first published by BioMed Central; hereby published with permission under the Creative Commons Attribution License or equivalent. Every chapter published in this book has been scrutinized by our experts. Their significance has been extensively debated. The topics covered herein carry significant findings which will fuel the growth of the discipline. They may even be implemented as practical applications or may be referred to as a beginning point for another development.

The contributors of this book come from diverse backgrounds, making this book a truly international effort. This book will bring forth new frontiers with its revolutionizing research information and detailed analysis of the nascent developments around the world.

We would like to thank all the contributing authors for lending their expertise to make the book truly unique. They have played a crucial role in the development of this book. Without their invaluable contributions this book wouldn't have been possible. They have made vital efforts to compile up to date information on the varied aspects of this subject to make this book a valuable addition to the collection of many professionals and students.

This book was conceptualized with the vision of imparting up-to-date information and advanced data in this field. To ensure the same, a matchless editorial board was set up. Every individual on the board went through rigorous rounds of assessment to prove their worth. After which they invested a large part of their time researching and compiling the most relevant data for our readers.

The editorial board has been involved in producing this book since its inception. They have spent rigorous hours researching and exploring the diverse topics which have resulted in the successful publishing of this book. They have passed on their knowledge of decades through this book. To expedite this challenging task, the publisher supported the team at every step. A small team of assistant editors was also appointed to further simplify the editing procedure and attain best results for the readers.

Apart from the editorial board, the designing team has also invested a significant amount of their time in understanding the subject and creating the most relevant covers. They scrutinized every image to scout for the most suitable representation of the subject and create an appropriate cover for the book.

The publishing team has been an ardent support to the editorial, designing and production team. Their endless efforts to recruit the best for this project, has resulted in the accomplishment of this book. They are a veteran in the field of academics and their pool of knowledge is as vast as their experience in printing. Their expertise and guidance has proved useful at every step. Their uncompromising quality standards have made this book an exceptional effort. Their encouragement from time to time has been an inspiration for everyone.

The publisher and the editorial board hope that this book will prove to be a valuable piece of knowledge for researchers, students, practitioners and scholars across the globe.

List of Contributors

Salah E. Shebl
Urology Department, Faculty of Medicine for Girls, Al-Azhar University, Cairo, Egypt

Eugen Widmeier
Department of Medicine IV, Medical Center – University of Freiburg, Faculty of Medicine, University of Freiburg, Freiburg, Germany

Hannah Füllgraf
Institute of Surgical Pathology, Faculty of Medicine, University of Freiburg, Freiburg, Germany

Cornelius F. Waller
Department of Medicine I, Medical Center – University of Freiburg, Faculty of Medicine, University of Freiburg, Hugstetter Strasse 55, 79106 Freiburg, Germany

Fang Zhou
School of Nursing, Xuzhou Medical University, Xuzhou, China

Kaikai Xue
School of Nursing, Xuzhou Medical University, Xuzhou, China
School of Nursing and Midwifery, Jiangsu College of Nursing, Huai'an, China

Mary H. Palmer
School of Nursing, University of North Carolina at Chapel Hill, CB 7460, Chapel Hill, USA

Asma Babar
CHU de Québec-Laval University Research Center, Québec City, Canada
Department of Social and Preventive Medicine, Faculty of Medicine, Laval University, Québec City, Canada

Lynne Moore
Department of Social and Preventive Medicine, Faculty of Medicine, Laval University, Québec City, Canada

Vicky Leblanc, Stéphanie Dudonné, Yves Desjardins and Simone Lemieux
Institute of Nutrition and Functional Foods, Laval University, Québec City, Canada

Valérie Bochard
Diana Food, Rennes, France

Denis Guyonnet
Diana Nova, Paris, France

Sylvie Dodin
CHU de Québec-Laval University Research Center, Québec City, Canada
Department of Social and Preventive Medicine, Faculty of Medicine, Laval University, Québec City, Canada
Department of Obstetrics and Gynecology, Saint-Francois D'Assise Hospital, Laval University, 10 Espinay Road, Québec City G1V 0A6, Canada

Behzad Mesbahzadeh
Department of Physiology, School of Allied Medical Sciences, Birjand University of Medical Sciences, Birjand, Iran

Mohammadmehdi Hassanzadeh-Taheri and Mehran Hosseini
Cellular and Molecular Research Center, Birjand University of Medical Sciences, Birjand, Iran
Department of Anatomical Sciences, Faculty of Medicine, Birjand University of Medical Sciences, Birjand, Iran

Mohadese-sadat Aliparast and Pardis Baniasadi
Student Research Committee, Birjand University of Medical Sciences, Birjand, Iran

Yuefan Shen, Anping Xiang and Sihai Shao
Department of Urology, The First People's Hospital of Huzhou, No.158 Guangchanghou Road, Huzhou, Zhejiang Province, China

Matthew A. Anderson
Department of Renal Medicine and Renal Transplant, Royal Prince Alfred Hospital, Missenden Rd, Camperdown, NSW, Australia

Tracey Ying, Kate Wyburn, Steve Chadban and David M. Gracey
Department of Renal Medicine and Renal Transplant, Royal Prince Alfred Hospital, Missenden Rd, Camperdown, NSW, Australia
Kidney Node, Charles Perkins Centre, University of Sydney, Camperdown, NSW, Australia
Central Clinical School, Faculty of Medicine, University of Sydney, Camperdown, NSW, Australia

Peter M. Ferguson
Central Clinical School, Faculty of Medicine, University of Sydney, Camperdown, NSW, Australia
Department of Tissue Pathology, Royal Prince Alfred Hospital, Missenden Rd, Camperdown, NSW, Australia

Madeleine C. Strach
Department of Medical Oncology, Chris O'Brien Lifehouse, Camperdown, NSW, Australia

Peter Grimison
Central Clinical School, Faculty of Medicine, University of Sydney, Camperdown, NSW, Australia
Department of Medical Oncology, Chris O'Brien Lifehouse, Camperdown, NSW, Australia

Jan Hrbacek and Roman Zachoval
Department of Urology, 3rd Faculty of Medicine, Charles University and Thomayer University Hospital, Videnska 800, 140 59 Prague, Czech Republic

Pavel Cermak
Department of Clinical Microbiology, Thomayer University Hospital, Videnska 800, Prague 14059, Czech Republic

Abdikarim Hussein Mohamed, Hussein Ali Mohamud and Adem Yasar
Mogadishu Somalia Turkish Training and Research Hospital, Mogadishu, Somalia

Sat Prasad Nepal, Takehiko Nakasato, Takashi Fukagai, Takeshi Shichijo, Jun Morita, Yoshiko Maeda, Kazuhiko Oshinomi, Yoshihiro Nakagami, Tsutomu Unoki, Tetsuo Noguchi, Tatsuki Inoue, Ryosuke Kato, Satoshi Amano, Moyuru Mizunuma, Masahiro Kurokawa, Yoshiki Tsunokawa, Sou Yasuda and Yoshio Ogawa
Department of Urology, Showa University School of Medicine, 1-5-8 Hatanodai, Shinagawa-Ku, Tokyo 142-8555, Japan

Qais T. Ahmad, Jaffar H. Saffarini, Ahmad M. Samara, Dima S. Jabri, Zaina H. Safarini and Yousra M. Banijaber
Department of Medicine, College of Medicine and Health Sciences, An- Najah National University, Nablus 44839, Palestine

Ahmad Jaradat and Faris Abushamma
Department of Medicine, College of Medicine and Health Sciences, An- Najah National University, Nablus 44839, Palestine
Department of Urology, An-Najah National University Hospital, Nablus 44839, Palestine

Sa'ed H. Zyoud
Department of Clinical and Community Pharmacy, Department of Pharmacy, College of Medicine and Health Sciences, An-Najah National University, Nablus 44839, Palestine
Poison Control and Drug Information Center (PCDIC), College of Medicine and Health Sciences, An-Najah National University, Nablus 44839, Palestine
Clinical Research Center, An-Najah National University Hospital, Nablus 44839, Palestine

Pagano Carmine
Clinica Nostra Signora di Lourdes, Somma, Italy

Faenza Mario, Guastafierro Antonio, Manfellotto Vincenzo, Grella Elisa, Pieretti Gorizio and Izzo Sara
Multidisciplinary Department of Medical Surgical and Dental Sciences - Plastic Surgery Unit, Università degli Studi della Campania "Luigi Vanvitelli", Caserta, Italy

Cosenza Angelo
Department of Advanced Medical and Surgical Sciences - General Surgery Unit, Università degli Studi della Campania "Luigi Vanvitelli", Caserta, Italy

Hui-Yin Yow and Sze-Han Lok
School of Pharmacy, Faculty of Health and Medical Sciences, Taylor's University (Lakeside Campus), Subang Jaya, Malaysia

John Jeh Lung Tiong
Ferring Pharmaceuticals Malaysia & Singapore, Kuala Lumpur, Malaysia

Chun-Wai Mai
School of Pharmacy, International Medical University, Kuala Lumpur, Malaysia

Esther van der Werf
Louis Bolk Institute, Bunnik, The Netherlands

Zulkifli Md Zainuddin
Urology Unit, Department of Surgery, Universiti Kebangsaan Malaysia, Kuala Lumpur, Malaysia

Charng-Chee Toh
Department of Urology, Hospital Selayang, Selangor, Malaysia

Kay-Seong Ngoo
Department of Surgery, Hospital Angkatan Tentera Tuanku Mizan, Kuala Lumpur, Malaysia

Eng-Hong Goh
Urology, Nephrology & Men's Health Clinic, Prince Court Medical Centre, Kuala Lumpur, Malaysia

Ahmad Nazran Fadzli and Teng-Aik Ong
Department of Surgery, Faculty of Medicine, University of Malaya, 50603 Kuala Lumpur, Malaysia

M. Korn, L. Reitnauer, F. B. Maurer, J. Hennenlotter, T. Todenhofer, J. Bedke and A. Stenzl
Department of Urology, University of Tuebingen Hospital, Hoppe-Seyler-Str. 3, 72076 Tübingen, Germany

P. C. Black
Vancouver Prostate Centre, University of British Columbia, Level 6, 2775 Laurel St, Vancouver, BC V5Z 1M9, Canada

Wilhelm K. Aicher
Department of Urology, University of Tuebingen Hospital, Hoppe-Seyler-Str. 3, 72076 Tübingen, Germany
Department of Urology, Center for Medical Research, University of Tuebingen Hospital, Waldhoernlestrasse 22, 72072 Tübingen, Germany

Celina M. T. Martelli
Instituto de Pesquisa Aggeu Magalhães - Fiocruz, Recife, Pernambuco, Brazil

Elizabeth B. Brickley
London School of Hygiene and Tropical Medicine, London, UK

Rômulo A. L. de Vasconcelos, Adriano A. Calado, Maria A. W. Rocha and Demócrito de B. Miranda-Filho
Universidade de Pernambuco, Rua Arnóbio Marques, 310 - Santo Amaro, Recife, PE 50100-130, Brazil

Ricardo A. A. Ximenes and Andreia V. Gonçalves
Universidade de Pernambuco, Rua Arnóbio Marques, 310 - Santo Amaro, Recife, PE 50100-130, Brazil
Universidade Federal de Pernambuco, Recife, Brazil

Thalia V. B. de Araújo
Universidade Federal de Pernambuco, Recife, Brazil

Si Hyun Kim, Hee Jo Yang, Doo Sang Kim, Chang Ho Lee, Youn Soo Jeon and Ki Hong Kim
Department of Urology, Soonchunhyang University Cheonan Hospital, Soonchunhyang University College of Medicine, 31 Suncheonhyang 6-gil, Dongnam-gu, Cheonan 31151, Korea

Dong In Jo, Song Hyun Han and Soon Heum Kim
Department of Plastic and Reconstructive Surgery, Konkuk University School of Medicine, Chungju, Republic of Korea

Hye Young Kim
Department of Anesthesiology and Pain Medicine, Konkuk University School of Medicine, Chungju, Republic of Korea

Hong Chung and Hong Sup Kim
Department of Urology, Konkuk University School of Medicine, Gukwon-daero 82, 27376 Chungju, Chungbuk, Republic of Korea

Andrea Necchi
Department of Medical Oncology, Fondazione IRCCS Istituto Nazionale Dei Tumori, 20133 Milan, Italy

Hiroyuki Nishiyama
University of Tsukuba, Tsukuba, Japan

Nobuaki Matsubara
National Cancer Center Hospital East, Chiba, Japan

Jae-Lyun Lee
Asan Medical Center, University of Ulsan College of Medicine, Seoul, Republic of Korea

Daniel P. Petrylak
Yale University, New Haven, CT, USA

Ronald de Wit
Erasmus MC Cancer Institute, Rotterdam, Netherlands

Alexandra Drakaki
University of California Los Angeles, Los Angeles, CA, USA

Astra M. Liepa, Huzhang Mao and Katherine Bell-McGuinn
Eli Lilly and Company, Indianapolis, IN, USA

Thomas Powles
Barts Cancer Institute, London, UK

Wei-Kang Chen, Dong-Dong Yu, Zhi-Xia Chen, Peng-Fei Li and Jian Cai
Department of Andrology, The First Affiliated Hospital of Wenzhou Medical University, Wenzhou 325000, Zhejiang, China

Yu-Peng Liu
School of Public Administration and Health, Wenzhou Medical University, Wenzhou 325000, Zhejiang, China

Zhi-Gang Wu
Department of Andrology, The First Affiliated Hospital of Wenzhou Medical University, Wenzhou 325000, Zhejiang, China
Reproductive Health Research Center, Health Assessment Center of Wenzhou Medical University, Wenzhou 325000, Zhejiang, China

Clinton T. Yeaman, Kimberly Maciolek, Mei Tuong, Perri Nelson, Chandler Morris and Tracey L. Krupski
Department of Urology, UVA Medical Center, Fontaine Research Park, 500 Ray C. Hunt Drive, Charlottesville, VA 22908, USA

Andrew Winkelman
University of Virginia School of Medicine, Charlottesville, VA, USA

Stephen Culp and Sumit Isharwal
Department of Urology, UVA Medical Center, Fontaine Research Park, 500 Ray C. Hunt Drive, Charlottesville, VA 22908, USA
University of Virginia School of Medicine, Charlottesville, VA, USA

Chien-Sheng Wang, Ching-Chia Li and Wen-Jeng Wu
Department of Urology, School of Medicine, College of Medicine, Kaohsiung Medical University Hospital, No.100, Shiquan 1st Rd., Sanmin Dist., Kaohsiung City 807, Taiwan

Wen-Chin Liou
Department of Surgery, St. Joseph Hospital, Kaohsiung City, Taiwan

Wei-Chuan Chen
Department of Urology, School of Medicine, College of Medicine, Kaohsiung Medical University Hospital, No.100, Shiquan 1st Rd., Sanmin Dist., Kaohsiung City 807, Taiwan
Department of Surgery, St. Joseph Hospital, Kaohsiung City, Taiwan

Yusen Eason Lin
Graduate Institute of Human Resource and Knowledge Management, National Kaohsiung Normal University, Kaohsiung City, Taiwan
CleanWave Medical Co., LTD, Kaohsiung City, Taiwan

Yoshitaka Sekine, Daisuke Oka, Hiroshi Nakayama, Yoshiyuki Miyazawa, Takahiro Syuto, Seiji Arai, Masashi Nomura, Hidekazu Koike, Hiroshi Matsui, Yasuhiro Shibata and Kazuhiro Suzuki
Department of Urology, Gunma University Graduate School of Medicine, 3-39-22 Showa-Machi, Maebashi 371-8511, Japan

Kazuhiko Kotani
Division of Community and Family Medicine, Department of Clinical Laboratory Medicine, Jichi Medical University, Shimotsuke, Japan

Masami Murakami
Department of Clinical Laboratory Medicine, Gunma University Graduate School of Medicine, Maebashi, Japan

Ming Liu, Xiao-Feng Zhao, Lan-Ting Hu, Zheng-Xin Wang, Wei-Guo Ma, Xiao Chen, Jing-Yi Lu and Bin-Jie Su
Department of Urology, Karamay Central Hospital, Karamay 834000, Xinjiang, China

Ting-Shuai Zhai, Jian Zhang and Xu-Dong Yao
Department of Urology, Shanghai Tenth People's Hospital, Tongji University School of Medicine, No.301, Middle Yan-Chang Rd., Jing-An District, Shanghai 200072, China

Lin Ye
Department of Urology, Karamay Central Hospital, Karamay 834000, Xinjiang, China
Department of Urology, Shanghai Tenth People's Hospital, Tongji University School of Medicine, No.301, Middle Yan-Chang Rd., Jing-An District, Shanghai 200072, China

Li-Jin Feng
Department of Pathology, Shanghai Tenth People's Hospital, Tongji University School of Medicine, Shanghai 200072, China

Xin-Sheng Lyu
Department of Radiology, Karamay Central Hospital, Karamay 834000, Xinjiang, China

Daniel McClelland, Luke P. O'Connor, John Barnard, Ali Hajiran, Chad Crigger, Tyler Trump, Emma Bacharach, Amr Elbakry, Zach Werner, Chad Morley and Adam Luchey
Department of Urology, West Virginia University, 1 Medical Center Drive, Morgantown, WV 26506-9251, USA

Daniel Grabo
Department of Surgery, West Virginia University, Morgantown, WV, USA

Chun Feng, Chang-Chang Huang, Song-Qing Yang, Qiu-Ping Yao and Min Jin
Department of Reproductive Medicine, The Second Affiliated Hospital of Zhejiang University School of Medicine, 88 Jiefang Road, Hangzhou 310009, Zhejiang, China

Ping-Ping Lv
The Women's Hospital of Zhejiang University School of Medicine, Hangzhou 310006, Zhejiang, China

Jin-Ming Shen
Department of Orthopedics, The First Affiliated Hospital of Zhejiang Chinese Medicine University, 54 Youdian Road, Hangzhou 310006, Zhejiang, China

Stephen Shei-Dei Yang, Yi-Sheng Chen and Shang-Jen Chang
Division of Urology, Department of Surgery, Taipei Tzu Chi Hospital, New Taipei, Taiwan
School of Medicine, Tzu Chi University, Hualien, Taiwan

Chun-Chun Yang
Division of General Laboratory, Taipei Tzu Chi Hospital, New Taipei, Taiwan

J. Walravens-Evans
Kingston Hospital NHS Foundation Trust, Galsworthy Road, Surrey KT2 7QB, UK

M. Yao
Department of Urology, Kent and Canterbury Hospital, Ethelbert Road, Canterbury CT1 3NG, UK

S. Granno
UCL School of Life and Medical Sciences, Gower St, London WC1E 6BT, UK

D. Arul
Department of Pathology, Whittington Hospital, Magdala Avenue, London N19 5NF, UK

S. Chitale
Department of Urology, Whittington Hospital, Magdala Avenue, London N19 5NF, UK

L. Sanyaolu, A. F. M. Scholz, I. Mayo and J. Hewitt
Division of Population Medicine, Cardiff University, Cardiff, UK

J. Coode-Bate
Addenbrooke's Hospital, Cambridge, UK

T. Quinn and C. Oldroyd
Institute of Cardiovascular and Medical Sciences, University of Glasgow, Glasgow, UK

B. Carter
Department of Biostatistics and Health Informatics, Institute of Psychiatry, Psychology and Neuroscience, King's College London, London, UK
Cochrane Skin Group, School of Medicine, The University of Nottingham, Nottingham, UK

Index